T0366822

What people are s[

The Ultimate Book on Vocal
Sound Healing

A very important contribution, indeed a gift, for people who want to exercise their innate power to experience wholeness. (Book I)
Richard Moss, physician, author and spiritual teacher (USA)

I have read Githa's fantastic book and my copy is full of red and blue underlines! The book has started so many exciting thoughts in my head. You have done in practice what I intuitively got close to and believed in when I made the film *As It Is in Heaven* (Oscar nominated in 2005). (Book II)
Kay Pollak, writer and director of the Academy Award nominated film *As It Is in Heaven* (Sweden)

Githa is, as far as I know, the most advanced and most brilliant vocal sound healer in the world. The depth of her knowledge is extraordinary. I can attest that her sound healing really does work as she has practiced it on me with immediate and astonishing results. (Books I, II, III)
Michael Mann, Former Founder and Chairman of Element Books

Githa Ben-David is one of the pioneers in Vocal Sound Therapy. The methods she has developed are based on her wealth of experience. This book will contribute to even more people discovering the undreamt of possibilities lying within our natural voice. (Books I, II)
Audun Myskja, Professor in musical therapy, Doctor Med. (Norway)

What a wonderful eye- and heart-opening book! *The Note from Heaven* is for anyone who is wounded in body and soul. The miracles lie right in front of us, we just need to bend down and pick them up. (Book III)

Hella Joof, award-winning actress, television star and director (Denmark)

The Ultimate Book on Vocal Sound Healing is nothing less than a treasure trove of knowledge. It is a masterpiece and a pedagogic work of art. (Books I, II, III)

Helle Hewau, psychologist, spiritual mentor and sound healer (Denmark)

The Ultimate Book on Vocal Sound Healing

The Ultimate Book on Vocal Sound Healing

Githa Ben-David

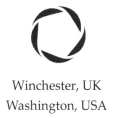

Winchester, UK
Washington, USA

JOHN HUNT PUBLISHING

First published by O-Books, 2022
O-Books is an imprint of John Hunt Publishing Ltd., 3 East St., Alresford,
Hampshire SO24 9EE, UK
office@jhpbooks.com
www.johnhuntpublishing.com
www.o-books.com

For distributor details and how to order please visit the 'Ordering' section on our website.

ISBN: 978 1 78904 862 9
978 1 78904 863 6 (ebook)
Library of Congress Control Number: 2021932915

A CIP catalogue record for this book is available from the British Library.

Design: Matthew Greenfield
Illustrations: Githa Ben-David

UK: Printed and bound by CPI Group (UK) Ltd, Croydon, CR0 4YY
Printed in North America by CPI GPS partners

We operate a distinctive and ethical publishing philosophy in
all areas of our business, from our global network of authors to
production and worldwide distribution.

Contents

Book I: The Note from Heaven: How To
Sing Your Self To Higher Consciousness   **1**

Introduction   **3**
What is the "Note from Heaven"?   5
How much time will I need to spend?   6

Part 1: Establishing Contact with The Note
From Heaven   **7**

Discipline, Hearing and Fear of Failure   **9**
Discipline   9
The importance of listening   10
Fear of failure/performance anxiety   11

Energy Centers   **14**
Root chakra (*muladhara*)   17
Sacral chakra (*hara*)   18
Solar plexus chakra (*manipura*)   18
Heart chakra (*anahata*)   20
Throat chakra (*vishuddha*)   22
The third eye (*ajna*)   24
Crown chakra (*sahasrara*)   26

Before You Start   **28**
Environment   28
Warming up the body   29
Singing posture   31

Breathing   **32**
Physical effect of an extended exhalation   33

Key images   35

Awareness of Tone   **38**
  The root note   39
  "Aaar"   42
  The soft palate   45
  Strengthening a slack soft palate   48

The Note from Heaven   **49**
  The primal sound behind the Note from Heaven   51
  The strength behind the weakness   52

Part 2: Singing with The Note From Heaven   **57**

Note Names   **59**
  The location of specific vowels in the body   59

Deepening the Voice   **61**
  How low can you go? • Using the Note from Heaven
  to build up your voice • Example of a work method

Indian Note Names   **65**
  Sa • Re • Gha • Ma • Pa • Dha • Ni
  Writing the note names   71
  Benefits of the note names   72

Scale   **73**
  The vibration of a scale   74
  Learning the feeling of a scale   76
  The raga, a state   77
  Common Western ragas   77
  Other scales   79
  Scale exercises   79

Part 3: Creative Music-Making   81

Improvisation   83
   Addiction to notes   83
   Composition   86
   Tone deafness   87

Children, Adults and Voices   87
   Calming a noisy child   90
   Understanding through imitation   91

Creative Writing   92
   An approach to creative writing   93

Performance   94

Epilogue   97
   Tree   97

Appendix   98
   Physical Exercises   98

The Practice CD   111
   Track-by-track comments   112
   Contents of each track   114

Applying the Tanpura Accompaniment to the Piano   118
Chakra Overview   119

Book II: Sing Yourself Free: Regressive Cell-singing   121

Introduction   123

Part 1: Collective Traumatization **125**
The path 128
The pain body 129
Plus power 132
How to truly listen to your self 133

Preparing for Regressive Cell-singing **134**
The Note from Heaven – a gateway to Oneness 137
Grounding 138
The experience of being sung by a higher power 139
Contact with the Note from Heaven 140

Breathing and the Note from Heaven **140**
How a listener can support the opening of
   a traumatized breath 143
How a singer can work alone with a
   traumatized breath 144

Images and the Note from Heaven **144**

We Are Tone-Deaf **146**

Part 2: Regressive Cell-Singing **149**

Principles and Practice **151**
Listener and singer 152
Overview of a one-day course in regressive
   cell-singing 152
Providing a comfortable environment 154
The listener's role 155
Ethical considerations 158
The Oneness level 161
Trust and faith 162
The placebo effect 164

Wishes and Primary Feelings   **165**
The four primary feelings   166
Formulation of wish and primary feeling   171
Examples of formulating wishes   172
Code words   174
Navigation signs   177

Riding on Feelings   **178**
How to lead a singer up to the light   180
Expression   180
Cry-toning   184

Storytelling   **187**
Story examples • 1 Back to Nature • 2 Strengthening Faith • 3 Dissolving a Social Phobia

Situations the Listener Must Be Prepared For   **195**
When a choice needs to be made   195
When other feelings obscure the primary feeling   197
When a singer wants to tell their life story   197
Issues of confidentiality   198

A Few Common Symbols   **200**

Animals   **200**
Birds • Riding animals • Embracing animals

Crosses   **202**
Union of ego and soul •
Freedom from an austere upbringing

Revealing the Light in a Singer's Voice   **204**
"Hamster in the Wheel"   205
Care and physical contact   208

Encouraging openness about sexuality 210
Shared themes 211
Getting locked into tonal patterns 212
When a question is practical 212
Manifestation of Jesus 213

The Wall 214
Example 1: Nooo, I don't want to sing! 214
Example 2: Wishing for more than you can handle 217

General Problems 220
When a singer does not hear the story 220
When a singer does not recognize a miracle 220

Trauma Due To Being Ignored 223
Experiment with rice 223
Examples of being ignored 225
Treating people who have been ignored 227
Physical touch 228

Paula Technique 229
Pulse and rhythm 231

Release Through Changing the Story 231
Readiness for release 231
Considerations 233
Changing the first layer of a multilayered trauma 234
Changing the story 235
Forgiveness 237
Personal tools 239

When the Singer Sees Images 241
Example 1: A successful distraction maneuver 242
Example 2: Images without a main thread 243

Regression 244
  My personal experience with regression 244
  Regression to heaven 247
  Women in orgasmic ceremonies 248
  A special regression 249

Boundaries 250
  People who lack boundaries 250
  People who have overly controlled boundaries 252
  When a person's foundation collapses 253

Release of Guilt 255
  Release through contact with wise light beings 257
  Gratitude ritual 258

Physical Reactions 259
  During regressive cell-singing 259
  After regressive cell-singing 260
  Yawning 262
  Giving birth supported by the Note from Heaven 263

Gender and Sexuality 264
  The gateway between Oneness and duality 264
  The power of the feminine 266

Part 3: Resonance with Domino Effect 271

What is Resonance with Domino Effect (RDE)? 273
  Principles of RDE singing 275
  Practical organization 280
  Example from a course of RDE singing 281

Book III: Sound Healing: With the Note from Heaven 283

Introduction 285

Part 1: My Path Into the Universe of Sound Healing 289
Meeting with The Note from Heaven 291
Dr. Karl 292
Spiritual knockout 294
How can I serve the whole? 295
"Is it so that the type of sound I have described is
dependent on being open to you, the spirits?" 296
"Should I sing jazz...?" 297
"What about healing? Is that something
I should do?" 298
"When you heal others, is there a risk of taking on
their problems?" 298
Transformation 299
Dr. Karl's words hold water 300
Working with the other side 301
Opening 302
A physical initiation 304
A change of identity 306
An attempt to cure tinnitus 309
Measuring brain waves during singing and
Sound Healing 310

Part 2: The Effects of Sound Healing 313
Lectures and Sound Healing Demonstrations 315
The concert pianist's curse (tinnitus/deafness) 315
The Psychologists' Association (tinnitus) 317
Measurements with an audiometer 318
Sacré Cœur 319
The Primary Cilium 321
Conducive conditions for Sound Healing 321

Non-conducive conditions for Sound Healing 322
Sound Healing of tinnitus 323
Sound Healing of hearing problems 323
Sound Healing of cancer 324
Cancer cells sound different than healthy cells 326
Sound Healing of stress 327
Pain Relief with Sound Healing 327
The body's chemistry during singing and
    Sound Healing 328

Part 3: Spiritual Science and Traditional Science 331
Einstein, H.C. Ørsted, and Dr. Karl 331
Sound and Science 333
Meeting with Spiritual Scientists 336
Excerpts from the Sound and Science Session
    with Graham Bishop and Dr. Karl 337
General notes 337
Introductory lecture 338
A voice's flair for healing specific illnesses 339
"Does each human represent a specific tone?" 342
"Is it possible to know your own tone?" 343
"Is it the cells that resonate during Sound Healing?" 343
"How many treatments are necessary?" 344
Time between treatments 345
Sound Healing and side effects 345
"Does gender polarity have any significance in
Sound Healing?" 347
Vocal, mechanical or electronic sound? 348
Difference in quality between live and
    recorded sound 349
A reprimand for healers 351
Sound, Light, Magnetism 352
Crystals 354
Chromaticism 355

Part 4: Being a Sound Healer   **357**

On saying "Yes" to being a Sound Healer   359
On the necessity of cleaning your flute   362
Fear of intuition   364
The Ego and the Soul in fruitful cooperation   366
The Nature of the Soul   367
The Nature of the Ego   367
Robert Johnson's seesaw   368

Vocal Prayer   **370**

Inflation of the ego   **370**

How to create a healthy relationship with the ego   372
When the ego takes on the role of the Soul   373
Distinguishing between ego and intuition   374
Pitfalls   376
Eliminating the influence of the ego in
     Sound Healing   377

Part 5: Vocal Sound Healing   **381**

The signature sound of the voice   383
The vocal light   384
Vowels   384
Exercise I: Vertical and Horizontal Movements
     with Vowels   387
Exercise II: The Gate of Life   387
Exercise III: The Great Breath   388
Exercise IV: The Vowel Circle   389
Exercise V: Sound Scanning   390
a) The Primary Vowel   390
b) Scanning the Energy Body   391
c) Scanning the Stomach   392
If the Recipient Doesn't Feel Anything   393
Exercise VI: Glissando Exercises   394

Exercise VII: The foundation for Sound Healing
   with the Note from Heaven　　　　　　　　396
Sound Scanning exercises 1-5　　　　　　　　396
Undertones　　　　　　　　398
1) The outward sounding undertone　　　　　　　　399
2) The inward sounding undertone　　　　　　　　399
3) Uninvited undertones　　　　　　　　400
4) Trauma sound　　　　　　　　401
Instructions for outward sounding undertones　　　　　　　　401
Sound scanning with outward
   sounding undertones　　　　　　　　403
Personal Boundaries Regarding Undertones　　　　　　　　406
Sound Healing exercise with sounding undertones　　　407
Undertones and tumors　　　　　　　　409
Undertones and tinnitus　　　　　　　　409
Undertones and broken bones　　　　　　　　411
Undertones and trauma sound　　　　　　　　412
Undertones and colic　　　　　　　　412
Undertones and hernias　　　　　　　　413
Undertones and leukemia　　　　　　　　414
The Feeling of Sound Healing　　　　　　　　415
An inexplicable phenomenon　　　　　　　　415
Physical reactions of clients during Sound Healing　　　416
Three Personal Experiences as a Recipient of
   Healing/Sound Healing　　　　　　　　417
Sensitivity to sound　　　　　　　　419
Men who are sensitive to sound　　　　　　　　420
Duration of Sound Healing　　　　　　　　421
Preparations for Sound Healing　　　　　　　　422
Protection　　　　　　　　423

The Structure of a Sound Healing Session　　　**425**
Opening Ritual　　　　　　　　425
Sound Scanning the Energy Field　　　　　　　　428

Open the Antenna/Silver thread   428
Sound Scanning the Body   428
Rounding off and concluding a Sound
    Healing Session   440
Gratitude Ritual   441
The Structure of a Sound Healing   443

Examples of Special Sound Healing Sounds   443
Dolphin sounds • Silver thread notes •
Asinine sounds/Trauma sound • Vibrato sounds •
Your own sounds
The Use of Organ During Sound Healing   446
Alternative Sound Healing Positions   447
About Offering Sound Healing   448
Too few clients   450
Too many clients   451
Sound Healing Combinations   452
Sound Healing Two Recipients   452
Sound Healing of Groups   453
Sound Healers on the Same Wavelength   454
Sound Healing as a Duo   455
The Fifth   456
Choral Sound Scanning   457
Sound Healing based on the Sound of the Heart   458
Communal Sound Healing   459
Remote Sound Healing   462
Grail Meditation   464
Sound Healing as a Profession   466

Part 6: Selected Case Stories   469
Written Feedback from Recipients   471
Edema on the retina   471
Asthma   471
Whiplash   472

Terminal Cancer   472
Shoulder pain   473
Enlarged Knuckle   473
Sound Healing of hearing loss/deafness   474
Examples of pain relief   477
Examples of Sound Healing on cancer   478
Sound Healing of stress   482
Sound Healing for lack of sex drive   483
Sound Healing ADHD   484
Sound Healing struma/goiter   485
Sound Healing a limb/leg
Other Sound Healers' cases   486

Part 7: Research In Sound   **489**
Chromatic Toning of Cancer Cells   491
The Importance of the Vagus Nerve   493
Nerve Impulses are Sound Waves   496
Research on the Cat's Purr   498
Bioacoustics   499
Research into the Relationship between
    the Immune System and Cancer Cells   502
Structured Water   503

Postscript   **505**
Endnotes   **507**
Inspirational Film Links   **515**
Bibliography   **516**
About the Author   **518**
Biography • Education • Musical Career •
    Current Work • Internet Resources •
    Book Publications • CD Releases •
    Practical Information

Other books by Githa Ben-David:

Tonen fra himlen
Borgen 2002, Gilalai 2009-2020 (ISBN 9788799235650)

Syng dig Fri
Universal Gratefulness 2008 (ISBN 9788799235612)

Lyd er Liv
Gilalai 2011 (ISBN 9788799235681)

Terapeuternes Mysterieskole (with Lars Muhl)
Gilalai 2012 (ISBN 9788799235698)

Liluja
Gilalai 2015 (ISBN 9788799736645)

The Songs of Lars Muhl & Githa Ben-David
2015 (ISBN 9788799736621)

The Note from Heaven
Watkins 2016 (ISBN 9781780289359)

Hjaelp – En personlig historie...
Gilalai 2018 (ISBN 9788797052808)

Heal the Pineal – Detox with Hung Song
Gilalai 2020 (ISBN 9788797052860)

My Heartfelt Thanks To

First and foremost, Mangala Tiwari, my teacher of classical Indian singing, who led me to my path.

Lars Muhl, my friend and partner in Gilalai for support.

My two singing sons for their wonderful voices, open minds, purity and support.

Special thanks to Michael Mann for his genuine and professional attitude to my work. Jane Helbo, Susan Andersen, Julie Rosendal and Janne Wind for translation, dedication and commitment. Elizabeth Radley for the editing and Matthew Greenfield for graphical design.

Course participants, students, clients and colleagues for their trust in the Note from Heaven.

Richard Moss for his recommendation.

Graham Bishop, Doctor Karl and the White Brotherhood for their invaluable support.

All of you who are open to surrender to the inspiration of the other side.

Pioneering Researchers, quantum physicists, neurobiologists, for being passionate about their specialist fields.

The Medical doctors, scientists and holistic therapists that truly serve mankind.

Overture

A bush and a tree. They stand there in the middle of the field, marking my turning point.

The walk has taken me through snow-covered fields in December's hazy darkness. It's about five pm. Imagine this never-ending white landscape, which seems to merge into the sky, is merely a small section of an endless Mongolian steppe...

In the distance the hum of traffic can be heard. It doesn't help to cover my ears. The sound vibrates imperceptibly through my body. The silence of nature is indescribably healing, and right now, my whole being yearns for it.

So, here we are, the bush, the tree, and I – tranquilly drawing breath. The trees humbly spread out their arms to receive whatever comes from above. It strikes me that the serene silence expressed in this humility makes up for the absence of a Mongolian steppe. The trees seem unaffected by the cars passing by on the distant horizon. Even if threatened by a chainsaw, they would firmly stand their ground, unshakable in their faith. The branches unfold the best they can. If there is too much western wind, they bend. If a neighboring branch gets in the way, they twine around it.

Obstacles make us bend and look for another way. No matter how complicated, the way forward is towards the light.

The snow drifts gently down onto my head. I welcome these magic crystals with reverence and feel blessed. There are many different types of vegetation in the patchwork of fields. On closer inspection it is clear that each one has its own distinctive character – trees, bushes, all equally beautiful in their existence.

I too raise my arms to the heavens and, for a moment, experience eternity within myself.

Why do we have to make ourselves so all important?

In times of hardship, life will block your path. At some point, you bend, find the way forward – or perhaps break down. It all depends on what you are up against, and who you are. Fate, combined with the fact that you did what you could.

So simple and beautiful. The thought appears naked in this greyish, opaque darkness.

Notes:

The Note from Heaven: Description of a sound-based being state, written in capitals.

The Note from Heaven: The title of Book I in this trilogy.

Certain words and expressions have been created specifically for this book:

"Vocal light": The vocal sound that the Sound Healer uses to find resonance.

"Recipient" and *"Sound Healer"*: Capitalized when used as nouns.

"Primary vowel": The vowel that is easiest for a Sound Healer to scan with.

"Sing Yourself Free": The title of Book II in the trilogy.

In one particular chapter, and throughout *The Ultimate Book on Vocal Sound Healing*, there is a reference to an audio recording from 2007 of a sitting with the British medium, Graham Bishop. The German spirit, Dr. Karl, speaking through Graham Bishop, answers general questions regarding Sound Healing with the Note from Heaven.

Disclaimer

1. No advice

1.1 This book contains general medical information.

1.2 The medical information is not advice and should not be treated as such.

2. Medical assistance

2.1 You must not rely on the information in this book as an alternative to medical advice from your doctor or other professional healthcare provider.

2.2 If you have any specific questions about any medical matter, you should consult your doctor or other professional healthcare provider.

2.3 If you think you may be suffering from any medical condition, you should seek immediate medical attention.

2.4 You should never delay seeking medical advice, disregard medical advice or discontinue medical treatment because of information on our website.

Book I

The Note from Heaven: How To Sing Your Self To Higher Consciousness

In memory of Mangala Tiwari (1955-2010)

Introduction

My first encounter with India and Indian singing, in December 1986, led me into something that I am only now beginning to understand. This inexplicable something made my career as a classical/rhythmic saxophone player seem pale and uninteresting by comparison. I felt drawn to singing, to creativity for its own sake, and my efforts to achieve public success worked against that.

In 1999, I started writing a book about this "something", because I felt that writing would enable me to reach out wholeheartedly to my surroundings with my music. At first, the process felt more like a duty than something I really wanted to do, so I tried to get it over with as quickly as possible. However, that was not to be. It took no fewer than three rewritings and a substantial editing down before *The Note from Heaven* was born.

Writing the book caused remarkable changes in my spiritual life. There was a pleasant tingling in my scalp, and with every page I wrote I learned more and more from all the information and ideas that simply fell into my lap.

The Note from Heaven is based mainly on my own personal experience. It was only after completing the book that I compared its contents to material from other relevant books. (See the Bibliography at the end of the book.)

In 1986 my singing teacher in India, Mangala Tiwari, said to me: "Go home, and sing 'Aaar' on your root note[1] for one hour every day." In fact, this single instruction is really everything you need to know. Anyone who perceives the value of this instruction and follows it will be whirled into a process of spiritual development. However, I have shared my experiences and developed them further, so this book is longer than the above mentioned sentence.

Working with the Note from Heaven has set me on fire and put a wind behind me. I am never alone, as long as I listen to that wind and spread out my wings, doing whatever I possibly can to stay on track. The Note from Heaven is pure inspiration and love. My heart quivers daily with gratitude. Gratitude for gratitude. Love, love, love.

The Note from Heaven gives the singer a vibrating experience of oneness, a sound to which each of us brings our own qualities – a healing sea, full of light.

The sound of the Note from Heaven has a healing effect. The first time I healed someone through my voice was when a woman with a headache regained hearing in her totally deaf left ear. I didn't even know she was deaf in that ear. I have healed people several times since then.[2] The first time I tried to heal tinnitus, it went down. I got very excited, thinking that now I could heal anyone with tinnitus. But that's not how energy works. This kind of thinking is the voice of the ego popping up and will cause the healing power of the Note from Heaven to vanish.

The "I" is a flute. It is nothing in itself, but the wind can make it sound like heaven. Our duty as flutes is to keep our Selves open and humble.

Go and sweep the chamber of your heart.
Prepare it for dwelling in the abode of the Beloved one.
As you go, He will come.
In you, emptied of yourself, He will unfold His beauty.
Mahmud Shabistari: Rose Garden of Mystery (13th century)

The tangible effects that have come from working with the Note from Heaven include the ability to see color and images in my mind's eye, a tingling, mainly in the hands and on the top of my head when healing or doing other work in an inspired state.

If you experience these kinds of effects, don't attribute more significance to them than they deserve. They are the manifestation of an opening of the contact to higher energies, a natural spiritual development. It is important to let this growth process happen gradually, without letting the ego get carried away by thinking, "Oh, now I see colors, so I'm spiritual." All human beings are spiritual. Just treat these kinds of extra ordinary experiences as positive signs on your path.

What is the "Note from Heaven"?

The Note from Heaven is not in itself the goal. Its function is to free the voice, and through that to expand consciousness. It balances the body's energy system, in preparation for conscious work with meditation and healing and for expressing yourself directly from the heart through song. It develops your intuition, your ability to sense and trust that what feels good deep inside is truly valid.

The Note from Heaven is the tonal expression of a divine state that we all have within us and we can all contact.

When you experience the Note from Heaven, the note seems to sing you, rather than you singing it. Therefore my method is addressed for all readers who have an interest in spirituality.

Since song is an expression of how we breathe, and breathing is influenced by our state of mind and body, it is hard to provide a self-help method that everyone can use. Traditional singing teachers might even claim that it is impossible.

But I am going to try anyway, because the listening process required to find the Note from Heaven is such an invaluable aid to self-discovery.

The experience of being able to find the way to a divine state *by yourself* is the overriding goal.

In this way the degree of healing that occurs when the voice opens up is dependent upon the degree to which the performer has been capable of inwardly listening to him or herself. A student who follows my instructions in a teacher/student situation, for example, will most likely experience the Note from Heaven, but at the same time will not quite be convinced that it belongs to him or her. Our fear of perceiving our own divine nature will give rise to all kinds of excuses to justify not doing this or that thing ourselves. This fear makes us dependent on our surroundings and gives us a false sense of security, since we cannot completely control them. Therefore, the purpose of *The Note from Heaven* Book I and the accompanying practice CD is to inspire you to sing yourself. It is this self that is the source of true learning. **The practice session for this book can be downloaded for free at www.gilalai.com on the English page under** *free downloads.*

I recommend that you read the first part of Book I and, for approximately one month, practice opening up to the Note from Heaven by singing a single note, the root note. This is really important, because such intense absorption in the sound is the only way to really understand and experience the point of this book.

How much time will I need to spend?

If you are a beginner, you will need to practice for about an hour each day for a month to establish good contact with your support (the laughter muscles in the stomach area) and to learn to find your way into the state of the Note from Heaven by singing the root note. Remember, the idea is to concentrate on one note only. Find a place where you will not be disturbed, so that you can listen intently to yourself. Once you have established the experience of finding the Note from Heaven in your body, you will be able to return to it at any time. This also works for people who believe that they are tone-deaf.

Then it will take approximately one year of daily practice to extend your connection to the Note from Heaven to the rest of the notes in the register, as well as to learn to sing the note language at a slow speed.

Part 1:

Establishing Contact with The Note From Heaven

Discipline, Hearing and Fear of Failure

Discipline

Devoting one hour a day to singing requires a great deal of discipline. Following through with regular practice, regardless of your mood or unexpected events in daily life, is a beneficial process in itself that gives great joy and self-respect. For it is through this persistence that you curb your ego and become uncompromisingly faithful to your innermost desires. When you give up on something you had seriously decided to do, you, on some deep level, disregard your higher self and let yourself be controlled by your ego.

The result is that you end up with a flat feeling, and that kind of experience drains self-confidence.

Most of us have ingrained ways of viewing ourselves that tell us what we are good at and what we are not good at. They are part of our self-image. Strict discipline is necessary to break such patterns. Years of repeating thoughts and statements like, for example, "I can't sing," leave their mark in the brain and form a habitual thinking. It is the ego that is responsible for these habits – it pops up full of angst and seduces us into arresting all personal growth. Only when becoming aware of our thought patterns, can we change them, and the road ahead is free: Our potential is infinite.

Your ego is the doubtful inner voice saying, "No, that can't be true for me."

Discipline is your weapon. Follow through with your decision at all costs, despite negative feelings such as boredom, fear, doubt, frustration and low self-worth which you may be stronger at facing, the more you open up to the light within.

The importance of listening

Most of us are born like tiny, fully developed angels. Our hearing has functioned since we were four-month-old embryos. As babies we rely on our surroundings to stimulate our senses. The fact that some people's hearing has not been correctly stimulated does not mean that the original sense, for example, the ability to listen to oneself, has been lost. Like Sleeping Beauty, it is merely hidden behind the thorn bushes in a deep sleep. In order to take the decision to penetrate the thorn bushes and liberate this Sleeping Beauty, we first need to recognize that she exists.

Once we fully understand that we are divine in our essence and therefore have the potential to sing from a divine place in ourselves, the ego's fears quickly dissolve. It is impossible to gain such an insight by reading even the wisest of theories in a book. It has to be experienced as a physical state, as a part of oneself.

When you first access the Note from Heaven, it is like a spiritual appetizer; the body is granted a spiritual experience through the ears.

The fact that the sound of your own voice might disturb you at first, because it doesn't sound as you expect it to, is a positive sign, a confirmation that your listening function is active.

Since the voice can express only what the ears can hear, it is important not to focus on your singing performance, but instead attach greater importance to sensing what kind of sound your ears would like to hear.

When the soul has its way, the ears want to hear something that feels good in the body. However, if the ego pops up it can make us aspire to sound like a singing idol instead of our ultimate self. In that case, push the ego aside. We are looking for the authentic nightingale, not the artificial one.

When you start listening to what feels good for you, your whole sensory system develops. Everything that we can sense, but not express in words, is made up of vibrations of differing frequencies, just as sound is. Science has long pointed out that all matter is actually composed of vibrations with differing degrees of density. We, too, are vibrating masses. Therefore, people develop intuition when they begin listening closely to themselves. We improve our sensitivity to vibrations as we develop the ability to listen.

Fear of failure/performance anxiety

When fear of failure arises during a practice session, all you can do is face it and fight it. It is not necessarily an easy battle, but recognizing the fear is already a big step. As mentioned before, an ego on the loose will naturally want to prevent us from experiencing ourselves as divine.

By looking the fear straight in the eye and continuing to sing, you will eventually succeed. Concentrating on the knowledge that you are essentially divine will cause the fear to evaporate. The following exercise is another, more tangible approach to curing the fear of failure.

Physically, fear manifests itself as a tightening of the throat and/or solar plexus. It is possible to restore free breathing by concentrating your thoughts on the solar plexus, for example, and then imagining that you are moving the tension from that area up to the middle of your forehead (the "third eye"). The blocked emotional energies, expressed as tension, can most easily be moved with the help of one's breathing.

Remedy for tightness in the solar plexus or the throat

- Close your eyes and breathe through your nose. Make a nasal sound like someone deeply asleep, but not snoring, as you breathe in and out.
- On the in breath, draw the energy in your body upwards along the spine.
- By surfing on the flow of energy created by the in breath,

you can move the tensions from the solar plexus or throat up to the forehead.

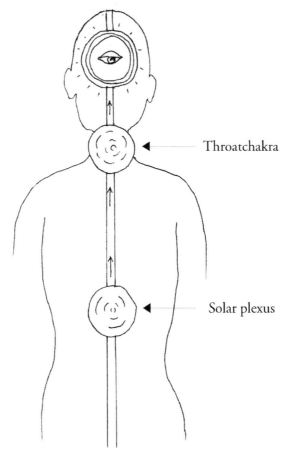

Throatchakra

Solar plexus

Use your in breath to unblock energy in the throat or solar plexus by moving it up through the spine to the forehead (the third eye).

- On the out breath, pull the energy downwards along the spine. Surf on this flow of energy in order to move it back down to the solar plexus or throat.
- Imagine the field of tension as a transparent, round, white disc that you can move up the front of your body using the flow of your breath.

12

- Move the disc up to your forehead (the third eye) by using a couple of breaths.
- Following this, meditate by concentrating on the middle of the forehead until you are breathing freely through the solar plexus. Carry on doing this for 5-8 minutes.

If this exercise brings on a headache, try moving the disc to the top of the head (the crown chakra) instead.

Fear of failure is natural and can be regarded as a gift that we humans would have difficulty living without. We are able to become conscious of our divinity only when we acknowledge its opposite – namely, our fear of failure. Those who seem to have been given everything in life tend to be lost on a deeper level: they take their paradise for granted because they do not have anything to measure it against.

Our quality of life is linked to the degree of gratitude we feel for all that we have been given. It is our awareness of life's contrasts that makes us feel gratitude.

The way we were loved as children produces a learned pattern of behavior.

Very few of us have experienced unconditional love. Most people have been conditioned to believe that they need to pursue achievement in order to deserve the reward of love. This learned perception of love also reflects inwards in the way in which we treat ourselves.

Therefore, when we feel fear of failure it is, in reality, the fear of not being able to live up to loving ourselves. "Should" or "ought to" are dangerous words, as they carry the expectations others have laid upon us.

We don't need to perform at all.

It is a state that we are seeking – a state in which we are able to love ourselves by literally massaging our vibrating body mass when we tune into it using sound.

Energy Centers

When you begin to work meditatively with your sound, you will eventually find that the sound induces a humming energy in your body. The reason for this is that deep and thorough breathing energizes the organism. The largest magnetic fields in the body are situated along the spine. There are seven major fields (chakras) and these are connected by three currents of energy that run the length of – and through the middle of – the spine. In Sanskrit terminology the feminine, inward-flowing energy current to the left of the spine is called the *ida*. The masculine, outward-flowing energy current to the right of the spine is called the *pingala*. The *sushumna* is the spiritual canal, where the feminine and the masculine energies join at the center of the spine.[3]

A deep breath can feel like an internal massage up and down the spine. With the Note from Heaven, you feel as if you yourself become a channel of energy – a connection between the energy centers is created and at the same time the energy collects at the *sushumna*. For that reason, it can feel as if the spine is an open pipe resonating as the wind blows through it via the breath.

Life's influences on us are expressed in our voice. This is because the body's muscles store the compensations and repressions with which we have protected ourselves. In this way, a pattern of tension has been created that affects, among other things, how we breathe.

A massage can relieve muscle pain, but it will not automatically remove the emotional patterns created by deeply buried traumas. Tensions function similarly to bad habits if you have lived with them for many years. Wherever there are tensions it will be difficult for the energy to flow freely, resulting in a constant loss of energy.

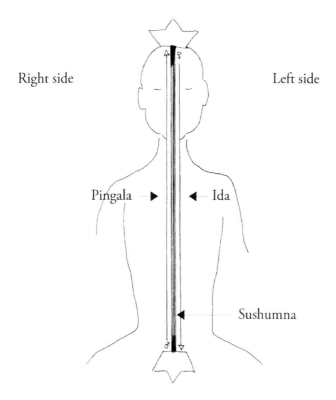

The three currents of energy running in and along the spine are known *as the* sushumna, ida *and* pingala. *Note that the* ida *and* pingala *are reversed in left-handed people.*

Right side

Left side

Pingala ▶   ◀ Ida

Sushumna

Therefore, by listening for your natural voice, you are also seeking a tension-free state. This occurs quite subconsciously as you focus totally on the sensation of the quality of the sound experienced in your body. Our ears are the key to re-experiencing ourselves as whole. Thus, vocal expression is not an isolated phenomenon, but rather an integral part of a greater unity of energy. A totality whose essence it reflects.

Since I will be referring to the body's seven primary energy centers throughout the book, the following is a simple explanation of their functions, especially in relation to singing. These centers have different names in different languages (notably in Japanese, Chinese, Sanskrit and English). I have chosen to use the names that I personally feel impart the greatest depth of meaning. In Sanskrit, an energy center is called a "chakra" meaning "wheel". Right away, this word gives a deeper meaning than "center", because each chakra rotates.

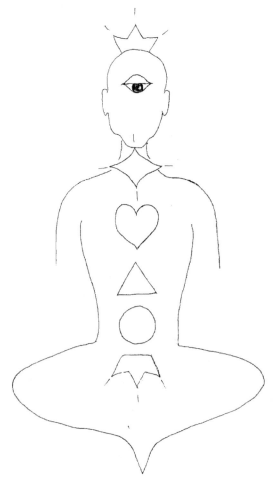

The seven main chakras are located along the center of the body.

Root chakra (*muladhara*)
The first note: Sa

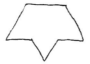

The root chakra is located near the coccyx (tailbone). *Kundalini* is a pure life force that lies coiled in the root chakra. In the event of a total purification of all the chakras (i.e. an unblocking of the energy flow between the chakras), this force can rise up within the body and bring about an experience of cosmic consciousness. Such an experience can lead to illumination, also called "enlightenment".

The root chakra is our connection to the earth. If this center is poorly connected to the others, while the connection between the higher chakras in the throat and head are open, you will need to ground yourself. After all, it is not really all that satisfying to be very spiritual and floating high if you cannot choose when you will come down to earth again.

If you climb a tree with weak roots, you risk the whole tree falling down. That is why the root chakra is the first stone on the path to enlightenment and to a healthy voice.

In humans, the basic note is a rather deep note, symbolizing contact with the root chakra. The deeper the sound is – the more coarse the vibration – the further down in the body it oscillates. Therefore, the foundation for a healthy voice depends on contact with the deep tonal register.

The root chakra represents, among other things, the instincts. The associated sense is smell. The sublimated form is secretion or elimination, and the color is red. Earth is the element of the root chakra.

Sacral chakra (*hara*)

The second note: Re

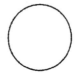

The sacral chakra is located a hand's breadth below the navel. Fertility, sexuality, vitality, balance, motivation, and appetite are associated with this chakra. The degree of strength and power in the voice is dependent on contact to the *hara*.

Tight pants and belts that constrict the waist diminish the connection to the sacral chakra. In this way, people cut themselves off from their own power. Therefore, women who aspire to a narrow waist and a flat stomach risk confirming their stereotype as the "weaker sex".

Every time we inhale deeply, an undulation in the sacral chakra stimulates and massages our inner organs. The same thing happens when, for example, we feel pleasure, have a hearty laugh, sob, or sing devotedly. This activates and releases the energy in the sacral area to flow freely again and interact with the surrounding chakras.

The sacral chakra is associated with energy and the element water. The sublimated form is energizing of various types (note: water conducts electricity); and the color is orange.

Solar plexus chakra (*manipura*)

The third note: Gha

The solar plexus is located in the soft triangle situated where the ribs separate under the chest. Among other things, emotions relating to the ego are associated with this chakra.

This is the most complicated chakra with regard to singing. Linked to the autonomic nerve system, the fear of failure can manifest itself as a tension that locks the solar plexus in a tight grip.

Similarly, most people feel discomfort in the solar plexus area when they are psychologically out of balance. This is because the autonomic nerve system reduces the contact to the chakras below the chest – a survival mechanism that cuts off the energy supply to the digestive system in a freeze-flight reaction.

In a life-threatening situation, where you need to make the right response in order to avoid death, this is an excellent mechanism. However, if you are on stage and become overwhelmed by fear, a tense solar plexus will prevent you from breathing freely with the result that you get short of breath, and can, therefore, only express yourself through a weak and shaky voice.

From my own experience, a tense solar plexus reflects a frightened ego. Uncontrollable emotional reactions like self-pity, fear, jealousy, anger and desperation compress the energetic field of the solar plexus. The result is paralyzation leading to loss of grounding and clear thinking.

In fact, our mind can become overwhelmed by delusions that appear completely real and true. That is how the snowball starts rolling, getting bigger and bigger until we hit a wall and explode in emotional despair.

Awareness of what our physical reactions indicate can prevent such delusions. During a demanding singing situation a tensed solar plexus can be overcome merely by recognizing that it is the symptom of our fear of failure, and nothing more. In any case, the fear diminishes when the singer becomes overwhelmed by the higher state of the music and surrenders to the Note from Heaven.

To release a traumatized solar plexus, by which I mean that the muscles have been tense for years, requires physical stimulation[4] combined with singing. Here a deep emotional release can relax the muscles, when you sing yourself free.[5] Personally, I am not an advocate of reliving traumatic experiences. There is a risk that painful re-experiencing can result in the ego and the emotions overpowering consciousness. With its cool overview and objective outlook, it is consciousness that gives us the best chance of breaking free from the trauma. Therefore, it seems obvious to me that healing of trauma needs to take place on an impersonal level. The Note from Heaven is a tremendous tool for that purpose because it unites us with the Oneness level. When we are one all separation and thus pain vanishes.[6]

The solar plexus is associated with the element fire. Movement (from one place to another) is the sublimated form; the sense is sight; and the color is yellow.

Heart chakra (*anahata*)
The fourth note: Ma

The center of the heart chakra is located in the middle of the breastbone. If you look at the picture of the menorah, the seven-armed Jewish candlestick (also found on the altar in Christian churches), then you will find the heart chakra, the fourth chakra, right in the middle. The menorah image also shows how the other six chakras are paired with each other (for example, the solar plexus chakra with the throat chakra).

The heart is the path. Through loving care and devotion to our fellow human beings we can forget ourselves. All problems disappear. They are simply not present when we sincerely do things for others that make them feel good. This "forgetting of the ego" creates a temporary space for the soul to commune.

The same is true when we sing. When you sing from the heart, something magical happens. All the muscle tensions disappear and the body functions as if it had forgotten all the injuries life has ever inflicted upon it.

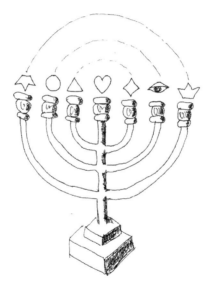

The Jewish seven-armed candelabrum known as the menorah is an excellent illustration of the seven chakras' communal and paired relationships.

It is indeed magical that you can sing yourself into a Oneness state where everything feels whole, where time disappears, and where you hardly remember anything afterwards.

Even more magical is the unmistakable sound of someone singing from the heart. A sense of sacredness descends over the listeners and the singer. You can feel your hair stand on end. A higher dimension of energy is present. The performing singer has conveyed something that cannot be interpreted as a personal achievement, but more as a spiritual experience that fills us with a deep gratitude for being alive.

The experience of release that comes when we sing from the heart demonstrates that we are so much more than just our body. Miracles are a possibility at any given moment.

In the Key images chapter, I will describe a method designed to help you to sing from the heart.

The heart chakra is associated with the element air. The sublimated form is unconditional love, forgiveness and creativity; the sense is feeling; and the color is green, or sometimes light pink with a green border.

Throat chakra (*vishuddha*)
The fifth note: Pa

The throat is the bridge between the body and the brain. In terms of energy, it is a key point as it connects the four lower chakras with the two higher chakras in the head.

The energy centers in the brain including the third eye (the Pineal, hypothalamus and pituitary) rule respectively the endocrine and the nervous system, and are related to the higher consciousness and the soul (the mental aura), which represent our potential for spiritual powers. Since we all have a soul and a higher consciousness, we all possess the ability to connect to them, if our organism allows it. When your throat chakra is more or less closed, it can be difficult to access your spiritual powers. This is not because you are not spiritual (we all are);

it is because the throat is a bridge, and the energy cannot flow freely from the body up to the brain.

There are people who speak in a slightly grating voice. This grating wears the vocal cords and therefore the speaker's voice quickly tires. I have noticed that people develop a business-like, objective timbre to their voice with this kind of abuse.

For example, a doctor might need to convince a patient that he or she has things under control. So, subconsciously, the doctor begins to adopt a slightly grating tone. As well as conveying authority to the patient, this change in tone also subconsciously bolsters the speaker's own self-confidence. Physically, the soft palate behind the hard palate is lowered. It actually feels as if you are closing off the connection to the head by making the palate flat and loose.

In terms of energy, this reaction stems from our human need to have solid ground under our feet in order to feel safe. With a connection to the spiritual centers in the head, the soul is able to take over from the ego. The resulting sensation of an abyss underneath us can be so intense that we freeze in fear because we do not know how to manage this connection. That is why many people close off in the throat chakra by using the voice "inappropriately".[7]

Another form of closing off in the throat can occur when an emotional reaction is repressed. A lump in the throat or tears held back can cause our facial muscles to stiffen into a mask as we struggle to maintain a controlled façade. Crying is a way to clear the throat and solar plexus chakras. The pent-up energy that the muscle contractions have been holding onto is released. If the tears from a traumatic situation are not released or compensated for in another way, then a chronic closure of the throat and solar plexus can ensue. That is why some people suffer, for example, from a feeling of strangulation.

The experience of fear fully taking over during a performance – whether it be in speaking, singing, or another mode of expression – can result in a third form of closure in the throat.

You become "speechless" – the shoulders slide up towards the ears while the solar plexus in the diaphragm contracts like a fist. Subconsciously, you turn your hands and arms inwards. The body stiffens from fear.[8] As previously mentioned, by becoming aware of the purely physical manifestations of fear you can help yourself to view your situation with some detachment, and thus resolve to pull yourself together.

There is a very good reason for doing this. Just a single experience of helplessness in front of an audience can create a trauma. Repeated experiences of this sort of trauma can result, for example, in tone deafness, stammering and difficulty in breathing.

As mentioned before, strengthening your connection to the heart chakra can temporarily dissolve such traumas stored in the body. Since the heart is the center of the whole chakra sequence, and the solar plexus and throat chakras are connected on either side like the two closest planets, it seems obvious that an energy charge in the heart must have a contagious effect.

The throat chakra represents the element ether. The sublimated form is communication; the sense is hearing; and the color is sky blue. The throat chakra is associated with communication, active contact to intuition, the arms (action), and to a state where desires are fulfilled.

The third eye (ajna)
The sixth note: Dha

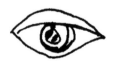

The third eye is located between the eyebrows. The center of the chakra is the uppermost point of a triangle, of which the eyes are the other two points. We touch this spot spontaneously when we need reassurance or to concentrate. For example, consider how when we are worried we cradle our forehead in our hands, or when we are crying we hide our face in our hands, with our fingertips resting on our forehead. Then there is the thinker, who, with fingertips placed on the third eye, intensifies his concentration. An agitated child is comforted by gently stroking the forehead.

When meditating with closed eyes while looking upwards, it is possible to merge into a spot, a light, which at a certain level appears to the inner sight as a violet or blue-colored eye.

Higher consciousness resides in this the sixth chakra. Connection to it calms us by giving us a matter-of-fact view of our situation without the interference of emotional energies.

If you imagine the body as a circle, then the higher consciousness would be located in the center.

Higher consciousness is the fulcrum on which we achieve balance. The same is true of the sound of our voice because the center for the free-flowing sound of the Note from Heaven is located in the third eye. The circle's circumference corresponds to the power source in the sacral chakra and the encircled space corresponds to the body's resonance. If we return to the seven-armed candlestick, then you will see that the sacral chakra and the third eye are paired with each other. When singing the Note from Heaven, the location of the note and the power become one. The circle dissolves and is replaced by a sense of being purely present in the here and now, a state of Oneness in which we disappear.

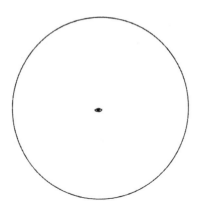

The center and body of the Note from Heaven are placed, respectively, at the psychological and physical balance points – the third eye and the sacral chakra.

The same phenomenon can be seen in Zen Buddhist archery. The archer seeks to merge with the aim, and when he disappears as a person the arrow, as if by magic, always hits the bull's eye. This phenomenon also occurs in other sports. Take the example of golf, where a "hole in one" is a similarly mystical experience.

The third eye represents the inner sound/higher consciousness. The color is violet or indigo blue. (With the two higher chakras in the head, no element or sublimated form is associated with them, since we are moving beyond the physical plane).

Crown chakra (*sahasrara*)
The seventh note: Ni

The crown chakra is located at the top of the head, in the

soft spot of the fontanelle. This chakra is the soul's entrance to the body.[9] Here we have a breathing hole, which we literally use in dreams, meditation, when we get inspired, and when we "disappear" in other ways – for example, when singing the Note from Heaven. This opening is also used for healing purposes. It is through the crown chakra's breathing hole and the hands, respectively, that you receive and transfer light energy. The healing energy feels like fine vibrations. Sometimes during and after singing you can feel a faint quivering on your scalp or chest, and your hands get warm and occasionally quiver as well.

When we sing the Note from Heaven, our body opens up and becomes a channel for a higher power, just like it does for a healer. Therefore, singing the Note from Heaven is comparable to healing.

The higher the note we sing, the higher up in the body the sound resonates. This is how a gradual ascension in the notes you sing will bring you to a point where the sounds are mainly in the head – the point that in classical terminology for a male voice is called falsetto.

Before singing high notes, however, you need to develop the ability to sing low notes with the total support of your stomach muscles. When a high note is created the vocal cords are stretched like a rubber band: the more tense the vocal cords, the easier it is to injure our voices and ourselves. This is like practicing mountain-climbing techniques in a low place before actually tackling a steep mountain. When you have mastered the techniques, you can climb without too much risk.

In the worst of all possible cases, the psychological effect of pure contact with the crown chakra, before having purified the lower ones, is madness. This madness comes entirely from an inability to control one's state of mind. An enlightened person can draw on the infinite knowledge they gain precisely because they can control their state of mind.

My experience is that the high notes you sing yourself

stimulate the crown chakra from within. The voice has a useful cut-off mechanism that ensures it becomes hoarse if you try to force it up too high without supporting it with a grounded breath. In this way you will not be able to activate higher energies in yourself unless you are properly grounded by a full breath. The breath is your omnipresent guard.

As we have seen from the menorah image, the crown chakra is connected to the root chakra. Both these centers are sources of energy, the framework for our life, Mother Earth and Father Sky. A definition of the "I" – a form to relate to.

The crown chakra represents inner light/the connection to Oneness; the color is white or violet.

Before You Start

Environment

If singing is still something new for you, try to find a place where you can practice alone.

If that is impossible, you can sing your way through any concerns you may have about other people's opinions. Singing the root note repeatedly makes the people around you quite quickly lose interest. When others perceive the singing as a form of meditation, it can help you to become immersed in yourself and tame the ego's thoughts about what other people might be thinking.

Finally, it is possible to sing in the car or in Nature. There you can benefit greatly by developing awareness of your breathing, your support (the use of stomach muscles), sensing the location of the note in the third eye, and awareness of the soft palate.[10]

Understand, though, that it is essential to develop your ability to listen within. This must be done in a quiet and closed room.

A room with good acoustics gives self-confidence. Good acoustics can be found in large or sparsely furnished rooms, in front of a window or in the bathroom. Factory buildings and echoing churches can be beautiful to sing in. However, they are not revealing enough for the work of listening. The acoustics swallow the little thorn bushes that we need to weed out. If your only option is a room where the acoustics are not so good, you can intensify your listening concentration by cupping your hands behind or in front of your ears. Another thing you can do is to sit faced towards a window or a wall, which will reflect the sound of your voice.

It is a good idea to develop some small rituals associated with your daily practice. These might include choosing a good fragrance, a bouquet of flowers or a picture of someone you love dearly, lighting a candle, tidying the room before you begin, drinking a warm cup of tea, or pouring yourself a glass of water to have at hand. (However, do not drink milk, as it causes mucus in the throat.)

Such preparations signal that you are now taking care of yourself and your senses, which makes a good start to the practice session more likely. Our senses are entry points to the past. Just think how evocative a smell, taste or melody can be. A flower, for example, can conjure up innocence through its appearance and fragrance.

Warming up the body

Stimulating our muscles influences our energy centers and eases muscle tension. In general, warming up the body is beneficial for singing, because it opens the flow of energy between the chakras. A balancing occurs, we get warm and our mind and body open up, allowing for freer expression while singing.

Some exercises create an overall flow of energy in the body and will strengthen posture and consequently the position of the spine, which, when surrendering to the Note from Heaven, will reach up like a flower towards the sunlight.

It is essential to keep the spine supple, since the body's three main sources of energy the *ida*, *pingala* and *sushumna*[11] run along it. One way to achieve this is through prayer. People naturally bend down while praying and kneel on the ground in a position similar to the fetal position. In religions where the practitioner bends down to pray several times a day, this movement creates a flow in the spine that, combined with the increased grounding from the kneeling position, strengthens the energy flow through the chakras. In this way, an appropriate position and movement support the mind's submission to the divine powers.

Another possibility is to concentrate your exercises on specific energy centers in the body.

If you have tensions in the diaphragm, for example, it would be obvious to work with breathing exercises combined with movement, contracting and releasing the muscles involved.

In case the stomach muscles are slack they need to be strengthened because, no matter how good our intentions, the strength and dynamic of the tone we produce will be governed by the muscles of the diaphragm. Building up these muscles will strengthen the energy in the sacral and root chakras, as well as grounding us.

Tense shoulders and arms and a painful neck will affect our ability to open up while singing. In this case, the principal offender could be the tongue, since its muscle tissue stretches from the back of the throat and all the way down to the chest and the collarbones.

The jaw can refuse to open up enough to say a genuine "Aaar" with a relaxed open mouth. This can be due to an instinctive fear of revealing our teeth and tongue. In order to keep the lips protectively over the teeth, the body compensates with tension in the jaws.

There is a selection of physical exercises described on pages 98-111. Try to do the exercises with ease and in a meditative state rather than with achievement in mind. All you need to do is to choose the exercises that are right for you and your needs.

Singing posture

Sitting cross-legged is a good position for singing because it creates contact between the ground and the root chakra. This position will continually stimulate the root chakra and hold you to the ground like an anchor. If you prefer to sit on a chair (as many Westerners do), you can sit on the edge of the chair for a similar effect. For both positions, it is recommended that you sit on a slanting pad, as shown in the illustration. Sit without a back support, if possible. If you sit on a chair, then plant your feet solidly on the ground pointing forward, a shoulder width apart. The thighs should be parallel to the floor, meaning that short-legged singers can add blocks or pillows under their feet to obtain a correct position.

You can relieve any discomfort caused by sitting cross-legged or without back support by using pillows, blankets, etc. for support. This is especially important, since pain can prevent you from listening inwards.

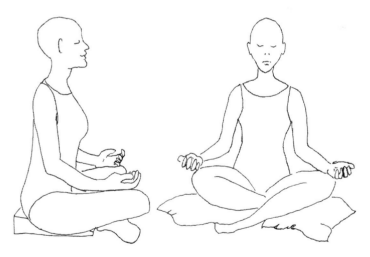

The use of a wedge-shaped bolster sitting cross-legged.

In addition to sitting on a slanted cushion, you can avoid pain in the legs and back by supporting the knees with pillows.

Make sure there is enough room to spread your arms out, so you won't need to worry about hitting anybody, furniture or walls.

Keep your eyes closed as much as possible while singing, as this will sharpen your listening skills.

Breathing

As mentioned earlier, our breath reflects our physical and psychological state. The act of concentrating on your breathing function can, in itself, feel so unfamiliar that you become nervous, and so tension gathers in the solar plexus, restricting the breathing. Therefore, breathing is a delicate matter. If breathing "with the stomach" feels unnatural, you should practice to breathe correctly in your daily life before going on to singing.

Practicing deep and natural breathing is most easily achieved by observing your breath. This means that, at first, your breathing practice is more a matter of concentrating on the breath than on controlling your muscles. Becoming conscious of the way you breathe is in itself the first form of progress.

Our lungs function rather like bagpipes. When filled with air, they inflate like balloons. Metaphorically speaking, that means we suck air into our inbuilt balloons when breathing in. We squeeze the air out of the balloons when breathing out by pressing on the thickest part of the balloons with the abdomen's "laughter muscles", which lie a hand's width down from the navel.

For those who are unfamiliar with deep breathing, the physical exercises 12, 13, 14, and especially 15, on pages 103-105 are recommended.

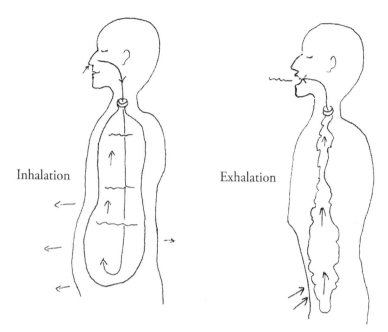

Inhalation

Exhalation

Symbolic illustration of inhalation and exhalation in which the lungs are likened to balloons.

Physical effect of an extended exhalation

When singing the Note from Heaven, your exhalation becomes four or five times longer than normal. A long exhalation actively made from the stomach clears and balances the nervous system and activates the parasympathetic nervous system which has a soothing effect on stress. The prolonged exhalation alkalizes the body, which means that acids and toxins are breathed out.

If you suffer from sleeping problems you can inhale through the left nostril (close the right with your thumb), pause while concentrating on the third eye and exhale through the right nostril (close the left with your ring finger) while singing "Aaar" or a purring sound "Nnnnng". You can also exhale silently if you sleep beside someone. Inhaling through the left nostril activates the ida energy linked to the right hemisphere of the brain and the parasympathetic part of the autonomic nervous system supporting the secretion of noradrenaline. This breathing method is called the Moon Breath.

If you need extra energy do the opposite: Breathe in through the right nostril and exhale as slowly as possible through the right nostril as described above. Inhaling through the right nostril activates the pingala energy, which is linked to the brain's left hemisphere, and activates the sympathetic part of the autonomic nervous system to secrete adrenaline. This breathing method is called the Sun Breath.

In Barbara Wren's book *Cellular Awakening: How Your Body Holds and Creates Light*, she describes how the cells' ability to absorb light photons and to detoxify is dependent on our ability to listen to ourselves and respond to what we notice. Chronic illnesses/stress are interconnected with the dehydration of body cells, which when feeling threatened make their cell walls thicker in order to protect themselves. This restricts absorption of light photons/energy and over the years can lead to illness. The key to stopping this kind of chronic state of emergency lies in the large intestine.

When a person connects to the Note from Heaven, the cells are revivified, which can feel like a tingling in the body. The large intestine is activated, so that the sound is literally expressed from the bottom of the torso via active belly breathing. The singer can become quite moved by re-experiencing old emotions that now are liberated and once again see the light of day.[12] A detoxification at the physical level takes place, which can produce temporary side effects if the transformation has been deep. These can be alleviated through diet, intestinal cleanses, enemas, liver cleanses, vitamin supplements, castor oil packs – all of which support the purification process.[13]

Dr. Mark Sircus, author of the book *Sodium Bicarbonate*, states:

The bottom line is that we can literally create miracles in medicine simply by adjusting the flow of a person's breath. Doctors can be superheroes without all the pharmaceuticals by giving their patients a simple breathing device that gives them a non-toxic, inexpensive, non-invasive, natural way to instantly reduce stress hormones, calm emotions, boost oxygen levels, gently massage internal organs, let go of stress, assist in returning to their centers, relax muscles, detox the body and simply improve the overall efficiency of the organs and body. That's in addition to increasing cell voltage and improving pH.

Key images

Instinctive exclamations like "Ah", "Uuuh", "Oooh" and "Aaar" are genuine sound reactions – spontaneous expressions of feeling without interference from the judging intellect.

"Aaar" is normally expressed when the body finds something very pleasurable or painful. The vibration of this syllable is universal.

To really feel the "Aaar" and encourage a genuine reaction that gives a true expression from the heart, we can consciously guide our thoughts to a place where our body and mind overflow with joy. I call this place a key image.

An experience of a sunrise, a favorite flower and its fragrance, a joyful experience, a dream, the fulfilment of a wish, someone you love unconditionally… The image needs to animate something pure and authentic in you.

The kind of image is not important. The only thing that matters is that it should fill you with pure joy.

Experiment with various images in your practice. The ones that work can be used again and again.

Breathing exercise with key images

- You have now chosen to concentrate on a specific key image. Place the visualization of the image in the third eye and keep it there for a while.
- Express your wish to allow yourself to overflow with

joy by saying, "Aaar." At first, this can feel awkward and artificial. Treat it as a joke and just let your body respond as it wishes. Laughing and smiling is a good sign, because then joy is within reach. The deeply felt "Aaar" can cause half-smothered giggles, red faces and outbursts of laughter, especially when sitting in a group. This means a positive atmosphere is already developing.

- Keep concentrating on the image and move it down to the sacral chakra, a hand's breadth below the navel.
- Inhale through the nose and feel how the air is causing your stomach and flanks to extend.
- Stop for a moment and fix your awareness on the joy generated by your key image as it nourishes the air in your stomach.
- Share this joyful feeling with the world through an "Aaar", and note how the stomach muscles are pressed inwards, pushing the air upwards.
- On the out breath you can imagine that the air current, and the joy it carries, flows out through the mouth. In this way, you are passing the joy on to the world.
- This cycle of breathing can be used until joy takes hold in your body. When the voice, and with that the body, have opened up and the state of joy can be maintained, then you can stop the exercise and open up even more through a total surrender to joy.
- Play track 2 on the practice CD[14] (tanpura and guide song) if you want singing support. Play track 21 (tanpura only) if you can find the root note[15] yourself, which in this case is note A.
- Make the joyful "Aaar" tone ring, and concentrate on keeping in contact with the key image rather than evaluating your sound.
- As your joyful sound gradually takes hold, you can begin to experiment with how to make the sound feel

even better in your body. The main thing is to gradually open, open and open even more with each breath.

If you have difficulty controlling the current of air with your stomach muscles – for example, if the current acts in the opposite way to that described in the exercise – then keep your concentration on the key image and forget completely about the way in which you are breathing. Place your image in the heart chakra (in the center of the breast bone) and surrender to it totally while singing, "Aaar."

Surrendering to joy generally induces correct breathing, because the stomach muscles are brought into use.

Take, for example, laughter. Who can laugh heartily without using the diaphragm?

Students who have difficulty surrendering to the full breath with joy are usually either fearful or intellectually focused on the technical details of breathing. If so, it can be helpful to breathe together with another person while holding a hand on each other's stomach and keeping the same rhythm of breath: Inhalation – big stomach, exhalation – push the stomach actively inwards. By breathing together the focus will move to the other person and this gives place for the natural breath to unfold. It is a very pleasant and soothing feeling to breathe together with fellow human beings while holding a hand on each other's stomach.

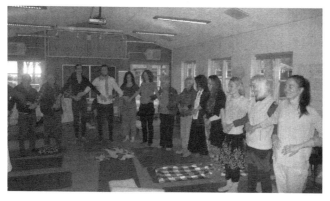

In order to express the Note from Heaven you will have to transcend the barrier of fear by jumping over an abyss. When you know how to breathe from your stomach, close your eyes and jump unconditionally. You will experience that the jump itself is the rescue. Surrender is faith. The moment you feel the wings of your voice you lose the need to be self-controlling. It feels as if it is not you singing; something else and very powerful is singing through you. At that moment you realize that you just need to dare to step aside and let go.

When the ego releases its control, the soul, the divine aspect, takes over.

There is nothing to lose and everything to gain.

Awareness of Tone

In language communication our words account for just ten percent of the expression. The tone of our voice accounts for the remaining 90 percent.

Relating to sound is difficult, because it occurs in the present moment and disappears immediately after being expressed. When you remember a sound, you remember the electrical imprint of the feeling it awoke in your body. Every reproduction of a sound will be a new sound, because the moment will be a different one.

The sound behind the words is a major cause of emotional frustration. We remember the way the words were spoken by recalling the sound linked to the memory of an electrical imprint which left an emotion in our body. By thinking about our interpretation of what happened, we strengthen the electrical imprint of the emotion. That is the reason why thinking about words that, for example, have been said in a hurtful manner will just deepen our pain. Therefore, a tonal expression carrying a negative energy can create emotional confusion, since it provokes feelings that are impossible for the intellect to grasp. You are solely what you think.

In this way the tone carrying a word conveys subconscious feelings, which everyone can clearly feel, but only a few can consciously explain. The closest we come to an explanation could be, for example, "She spoke to me in a derogatory way." However, who knows how I myself sounded, without being aware of it?

Just like a melody loses its true meaning when a single phrase is removed, the same thing happens when we relate our experiences to others. The experiences are no longer completely authentic. They become distorted.

By developing the ability to listen deeply, the awareness of the tonal vibrations that we and others send out and perceive is increased. We expand our consciousness in this way, because something we were not aware of before is now picked up by our consciousness. Listening to the tone of a voice, or of another source of sound, and consciously noticing whether what we are hearing feels good, will protect us from frustrating feelings in the body.

If you get taken by surprise and feel hurt you can sing yourself free of the negative emotional matrix, so that you avoid hurting others. All it takes is to seek a space, where you can sing freely and let the bad energy leave your body.

Objectivity allows us to recognize, for example, that, "She is speaking in a derogatory tone," and thus experience, that it is her problem. Her tone is not sucked into our subconscious by agitated emotions that get our thoughts whirling in an attempt to figure out what just happened. The experience has become impersonal, because our consciousness rather than our emotions is governing our ego. The ego will not, therefore, go on red alert. At most, it will gently nudge the event to one side.

The root note

The main purpose of classical Indian singing is to become one with your self, with your divine essence.

A good singer is "god gifted".

In order to be a divine instrument, the body needs to be used in a way that allows for optimal sound. When it functions like an open pipe, it achieves just that.

We decide, therefore, to open our body up to one note. Imagine a frozen lake. With the help of your root note, it is possible to create a sound hole in the ice. The hole can later be expanded to also include the other notes in the full register. Sticking to one note in the beginning to make a proper connection to the fluid waters below the ice is of the utmost importance.

When establishing the root note, remember:

Start with the note that feels most relaxed and pleasant when you sing "Aaar".

It should be possible to sing deeper than the note you choose as your root note. You should be able to sing "P.a", which corresponds to a fifth below the root note. (The second and third notes in the song: *O Come, All Ye Faithful* shows this tonal interval.)

You can sing the note for extended periods of time without your voice getting tired or sore.
Use the note that sounds most full and beautiful on "Aaar".

Use the note that feels best in your body.

For women, the basic note is located around the note A below the piano's keyhole.[16]

For men, the area of the note is less definable, because there is a big difference in where they feel most comfortable.[17] For some men (basses) the root note is the same as for women meaning that it is placed around the note A. They just sing it in a deeper pitch (an octave below). That is why the root note on the enclosed practice CD is A. Most women and some men will feel comfortable with that note.

It is an interesting detail that the note A was also once the starting point in Western musical notation. The alphabet was transferred to the notes. In the Northern countries, we have partly forgotten this, because there was a writing mistake when the note system was introduced: A monk wrote the letter b rather indistinctly and it was interpreted as an h. That is why Danes still operate with a note system that is: A, H, C, D, E, F, and G. This is contrary to the rest of the world, where the H is named B.

If the root note on the practice CD does not feel good for your voice, you can create your own root note. This can be done either by experimenting with the help of a tanpura app or a sound-source like a piano, or by finding a vocal sound therapist who is educated in the principles of the Note from Heaven.

If your root note is close to A, it is possible to regulate the sound of the practice CD up or down by using a standard recording computer program.

Another option is to get yourself a shruti box,[18] an Indian organ (harmonium) or a tanpura. Female tanpuras tune around A, male tanpuras tune around C or E. Note though, that you need to be able to tune the tanpura, and that the strings can break if tuned too high. The quality of tanpuras varies a lot, so, if possible, let a trained musician check whether the tanpura can hold its tuning (for example A if it is an A tanpura), that it has correct strings, and that the strings will play overtones when you add threads to the meeting point with the bridge. Do not trust the salesmen in tourist areas of India; always ask a musician where to buy good instruments and let them choose the right one for you, if you do not know how to do it yourself.

The easiest is to buy a harmonium or a shruti box, which

sounds rich, and which you can easily learn how to play a drone on. See instruction at page 67. It doesn't need tuning, you can play in any key and it plays loud enough that you can instruct even bigger groups with it.

In London there is a shop called JAS that sells very good harmoniums.[19]

Alternatively, accompany yourself with a musical instrument (piano or guitar, for example). It is easy for a beginner to learn, since you only need to play very few notes, namely the root note and the fifth (seven halftones up from the root note).[20]

You can make it more musical either by including the third and playing a whole chord or just by doubling the fifth and the root note.

"Aaar"

We have expressed the sound "Aaar" since we were babies. This vowel is round with a lifted soft palate and not flat like in "Aaah", where the soft palate is lowered. Classical Indian singing is based on a combined training of the two halves of the brain: partly by training the consciousness in the mutual, vibrational connection between the notes, which is done by working with the note names; and partly by training the senses through a purification of the nervous system by working with the sound "Aaar".

Besides being the spoken vowel that opens the mouth the most, "Aaar" is also the easiest vowel to sing deeply. The body opens to "Aaar". You can experience this directly, by experimenting with different vowels.

In certain yoga systems, "Aaar" represents the sound of the heart. Buddhistic Esoteric philosophy and psychology speak of the physical body as having different energy bodies. The subtlest energy level is called the causal body and the sound connected to it is "Aaar".

Rudolf Steiner's eurythmics involves a system of body

positions and associated sounds. "Aaar" is coded together with a position very similar to the one I learned to initiate healing sessions with. You stand or sit with your arms open and the palms lifted up in the air. In healing, this is done in order to become a channel for a higher energy to flow through. It is useful to do exactly the same thing when singing.

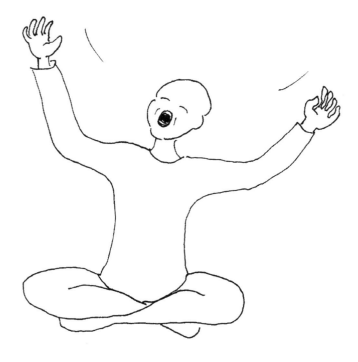

Surrendering to the Note from Heaven leads to a distinct feeling of being a channel for something higher than yourself. Physically, the act of surrender is encouraged by a gesture of submission: the throat is bared, as the neck tilts slightly back and the open hands are lifted up towards the heavens.

It is a human instinct to put up your hands when surrendering.
Peoples from the East dance with their arms and hands lifted upwards. This gives the dancing an ecstatic element, since the

body seems to surrender to a higher power. In Scandinavia, we dance more with our hands in slightly clenched fists, which we box with, while the rest of the body stamps in time to the rhythm. That kind of movement gives grounding.

Some people are unaccustomed to surrendering, with their hands reaching up. If you find this gesture odd, ask yourself what may be trying to hold your arms back when the final surrender to the Note from Heaven takes place. Raised arms with open palms make it easier to let go, as this is the body's way of saying "lift me up". Uplift me?

An additional benefit of this movement is that the lungs get more space in the rib cage.

Especially at the start of this process, you should be aware of the singing guidelines listed in the box opposite.

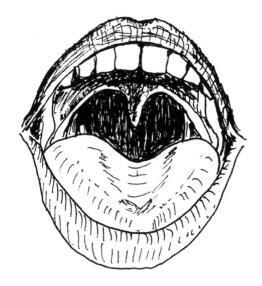

Position of the tongue when singing "Aaar". The tongue lies relaxed at the bottom of the mouth with the tip touching the lower teeth.

1. The mouth needs to be open, preferably too much rather than too little. When the face muscles have been suitably stretched, you will be able to find the open-mouthed position that is most natural for you.
2. The tongue lies relaxed at the bottom of the mouth with the tip touching the lower teeth.
3. When you are tuned into your key image, take a moment to make sure that your breathing is correct.
   If you usually breathe in reverse order (paradoxical breathing), it is a good idea to observe your breathing throughout the day. Repeatedly remind yourself of when the stomach needs to be going in, and when it should be going out. Combine this with one or more of the breathing exercises that you feel at ease with.[21]

These three points will gradually be encoded into your nervous system. The sound itself will reveal to trained ears when something is wrong. For example, you can hear immediately when the support of the abdomen is not functioning (see point 3).

The soft palate

There is a spot in the soft part at the back of the roof of your mouth that is instinctively raised when you are overwhelmed by your feelings. This can occur when you laugh or feel moved, cry or are about to cry and when you yawn. I mention these three examples, because their common denominator is the sound "Aaar", which is a component of the sound we make when we laugh, cry and yawn.

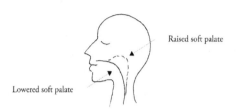

The raised soft palate puts us in contact with the "higher self" (the soul) and adds mechanical pressure on the pituitary.

Picture yourself in these three situations and sense how the space in your mouth expands. The soft palate is raised and the resonating space in the oral cavity increases.

Note how you can get tears in your eyes, whether from joy, yawning or grief, merely by raising the soft palate.

There are healers who consciously raise the soft palate, and with the help of this gesture get in touch with their healing powers. In several sessions with Daniella Segal, a healer in Israel,[22] I always yawned at the end of the healing. It always happened when I was overwhelmed by a sense of deep gratitude to the divine powers, so I felt embarrassed about the yawning, since I felt anything but tired. Daniella explained that it is a normal reaction: we yawn simply to make room for an overpowering feeling.

Similarly, think about why it is we gawp or say "Uuuh" when someone frightens us. In these cases, the soft palate is also raised – the body tries to help us by accommodating the feeling and simultaneously gives us the means of releasing a sound.

As the space in the oral cavity expands when the soft palate is raised, the pressure increases on the nasal cavity connecting the nose with the central nervous system.

The roof of the nasal cavity leads up to the seat of the pituitary closely linked to the hypothalamus and pineal glands, which are in charge of the endocrine system (the third eye/the crystal palace (Taoism)).[23] The body is so ingeniously put together that it stimulates contact to the central nervous system/the center of higher consciousness to help us accommodate overwhelming feelings.

It is an instinctive reaction to breathe deeply before raising the soft palate when we are in the grip of any sort of deeply felt and uncontrollable outburst. Try to breathe very lightly high up in the throat and yawn at the same time. It is impossible.

Note that a deep breath accompanies every real yawn. The same thing applies to a hearty laugh or cry: there needs to be wind to fill the sail. On the other hand, when we work against the body's reflexes, the soft palate is held down and breathing is inhibited. You will, for example, get a lump in your throat if you try to refrain from laughing, crying, or yawning by subconsciously keeping the soft palate down. If the soft palate is raised, nothing can hold back the expression of a true emotion.

Therefore, one of the cornerstones of the Note from Heaven is a raised soft palate, which again is connected to efficient breathing, another cornerstone that supports the roof of the singing temple.

If it is easy for you to sing an open-sounding, round "Aaar" and your voice doesn't tire when you talk for a long time, then take no further notice of this section, because your soft palate is in good shape.

The grating voice that closes up the throat chakra, discussed on page 23, is caused by a slack soft palate. There are people whose soft palate is lowered most of the day. This results in the muscle getting so loose that the voice can no longer sound beautifully in the head, because the loose soft palate blocks the way. Try to say "Aaah" and then "Aaar". Which vowel sounds more free and spacious?

The soft palate is automatically raised when you sing a spacious "Aaar".

If you have difficulty in saying "Aaar" and have a tendency to sing a flat "Aaah" instead, I recommend the following exercise.

Strengthening a slack soft palate

One way to strengthen the muscles of the soft palate is to sing, "Ngggg." Alternatively, you can hold a similar mouth position without actually making the sound; that is, with the back of the tongue pressed against the back wall of the nasal cavity, the tongue tip resting on the lower teeth, the lips gaping. The sound, if you do make it, is nasal, closed and buzzes in the head.

Sing or just hold this mouth position as often as possible. It could be done in the car, while cooking, in the shower... Another possibility is to sing, "Arng-arng-arng-arng..." since repeating this sound makes the soft palate move, so that each "ng" hits the wall of the nasal cavity. This exercise increases your physical awareness of the soft palate. Be prepared to yawn quite a bit.

A third exercise is to throw the tongue backwards and keep it there. That will automatically raise the soft palate.

If these exercises provoke resistance, you may need to take a deeper look at emotional issues, because in energy terms the activation of the soft palate opens the door for unconscious emotions to be released. You can say that singing on "Aaar" creates a bridge up to the third eye. This connection is of great value to every person who wishes to develop his/her spiritual potentials.

If you have no trouble singing "Arng", you can also sing "Huuh" on any higher note that feels good together with the vowel. The soft palate no longer leans on the back of the tongue, but is held up by its own muscles and the flow of air. A slightly lifted tongue supports the soft palate to raise while singing "Huuh".

You could start by rolling the tongue (if you can) and pursing your lips on "DrrrrUuuh" or by rolling the lips (if you can) on "BrrrUuuh".

Try to center the sound in the third eye. When you can do that, your "Huuuh" note will ring with overtones and have a rich, beautiful quality.

Depending how much practice you do, it will take one to three weeks for the soft palate to regain enough strength to be able to arch beautifully on an open sounding "Aaar" or "Haar".

Note that tiredness and exhaustion also affect the voice. The soft palate will get slack. Therefore, sleep and relaxation are the best forms of "song training" to start with.

If you do not sleep properly it is possible to stimulate the pineal gland to secrete melatonin with Hung Song.[24]

The Note from Heaven

The Note from Heaven is true. It is true because our personality/ ego is not interfering with how it should sound. The note comes from above and overwhelms us when we relinquish all control.

As mentioned earlier, by absorbing yourself in your key image you can take a shortcut and experience the Note from Heaven without any sort of physical preparation. The experience of joy creates a feeling of gratitude and those two emotions combine to fill the heart with a devotion that allows us to surrender safely.

When we surrender, the body opens up and functions as if reborn.

The Note from Heaven puts you in a timeless state. When you have achieved this – which takes about ten minutes following the actual surrender – it feels as if you could sing the same note forever. You are being sung and the voice resonates with wholeness leading to the feeling of Oneness with all there is. It feels as if it is not you singing. You get the tangible experience of not owning your own voice. The voice is a wild and uncompromising animal that will always be most beautiful when it is free. Taming the voice in its free and natural form requires the proper bait and a loving attitude. Otherwise, you will conjure up the ego's fear and pretense.

The experience of the Note from Heaven is holy, because it is not constructed with the help of the ego. If you try to sing it in public, it takes quite an effort to stay clear of that little ego troll.

If it is allowed to affect the sound even slightly, the whole thing falls apart on the spot.

Therefore, trained singers need to be aware of previously learned forms of expression. Only a very few singers sing with their natural voice. For example, most singers automatically add a vibrato to their "Aaar". This is true of both rhythmic and classically-trained singers. Such deliberate interference with the sound might bolster their confidence enough to ward off performance anxiety, which every stage performer has to face, but, unfortunately, they will also miss the chance to free themselves from their ego, since it is built into their voice. At worst, the performance will be so polished and professional that it never touches the heart.

A person is most beautiful when stripped down to who he or she really is. Only in that state is it possible to take off with the Note from Heaven.

When you listen within to your sound, you will discover how artificial it is to bolster yourself with voice-makeup. It is just showing off for the crowd. The ego animates the ego in its audience. It may seem like success, but, spiritually speaking, it is the complete opposite.

I recently met a former fellow student from the Royal Academy of Music. I remember she sang opera fantastically and scored top grades in the mid-term exams. Now, meeting her again after fifteen years, she admitted she felt that she had cheated the examiners; that she had been play-acting. She had used her voice like a costume with which to please them. Towards the end of her studies, she gradually lost her ability to sing in tune, without anyone being able to figure out why. Today she still feels unable to trust her own ears; so much so that she decided to give up singing. What may have happened is that she became aware of her dishonesty, but neglected to deal with it and was thus caught between two poles – the ego and the soul. A strong ego can easily lead to success – although that kind of success has quite a hollow ring to it.

The primal sound behind the Note from Heaven

To get the primal sound behind the Note from Heaven to break through, imagine that you are a wolf howling at the moon from a mountaintop, or a gorilla that wants to win respect by showing off his powerful voice.

Deep down most people love to play monkeys. Just try saying "Huh, huh, huh, huh" and scratch yourself under the arms, while bouncing at the knees. Most people really have fun, once they have overcome their shyness. It feels so good to come down to earth.

Finding the strength of your voice

Close your eyes. Imagine that you are an animal or a primitive person.

- Picture yourself setting a boundary. You do this with your voice, which will soon demonstrate the fact that you exist, and that you, being a wild animal, are capable of releasing your overwhelming, pure and terrifying power.
- Breathe deeply down in the stomach chakra, as this is the seat of power.
- Tilt your head slightly back and look upwards behind your closed eyes.
- Concentrate the center of the sound in the third eye. Here it is possible to adjust the sound to be ruthlessly sharp and nasal by adding the "Nggg" sound in the center of "Haaar".
- Spread out your arms in a "daredevil" way and raise your palms upwards, while you release whatever deep sound that feels good for you on a "Haaar". It should feel as if the "Haaar" sound is vibrating through the spine.

51

- Sing as long and as loudly/sharp (adjust the centered "nggg") as you can. Lower your arms when the tone ends.

The sound becomes uncompromising when fully expressed and you can sing for an unusually long time on one breath. It can feel similar to shouting.

As children, many of us were taught not to make noise. Push that aside. It is exceptionally delightful to shout and feel the power singing in the body.

Stop if your voice starts hurting. Check your breathing; do one or more of the physical exercises 12-15 on pages 103-105. You can try singing again when your breathing functions correctly.

The primal sound can be heard three times, a good way into track 2 on the practice CD (with the volume turned down to avoid frightening anyone within earshot!).

The strength behind the weakness

When you know your strength, then you are no longer at the mercy of your weakness.

Weakness becomes a choice. The same principle works in singing. You can express whatever you want when you know your own strength. It turns into a conscious choice, which gives you a feeling of freedom. The freedom to choose to express yourself.

Some people have no problem at all in expressing themselves forcefully – quite the opposite, in fact. The difficult thing for them is to be weak, gentle and empathetic.

Someone who possesses such rigid strength is not truly free. The strength itself has become an entrenchment against the outside world. The heart is wrapped up tightly, because the ego is guarding it. It wants no more pain than it has already suffered.

Difficulty in singing gently from the heart is not due to insensitivity in the person. It is caused by the fact that there is a mental barrier blocking the way.

If you cannot sing beautifully when softly singing "Aaar" on the root note, then you simply have not opened up enough yet. Open, open, open even more, and continue to open, even when you think you cannot open up any more. Make sure that the sound is not "Oorr", but really an open sounding "Aaar". Smile and let the teeth be as they are.

When you smile freely, everyone will see your smile, not your teeth. Get into the habit of smiling unreservedly in your daily life.

Singing the Note from Heaven with strength behind the weakness

With the previous exercise, you made contact with your strength. Now use this strength and feel the Note from Heaven through it. The note will become unusually long and it will feel as if a higher power is singing through you.

- Gradually bring the sensation of your sound down to the heart chakra. It helps to let the torso's point of balance (in the middle of the stomach chakra) and the head's point of balance (in the third eye) join in the heart. You can do that by surfing on the air current, as explained in the exercise to relieve tightness in the solar plexus or throat on pages 11-13.
- Choose a key image that envelops you in a feeling of love or caring. For example, the thought of a child, a pet or person close to you can fill you with that wonderful feeling of wanting to give everything you have to another living being.
- Avoid sentimentality, because then you will be moved and will need to cry, which will close the throat. Look at

the experience as a blessing that sets you free, since all self-importance disappears.

- Sing on "Aaar" or "Haar" and let the sound swell in your chest.
- While you are singing to your imaginary loved one, perceive your voice as soft and comforting, but with the security of the strength that lies behind it.
- With each breath try to open yourself up more and more to an acceptance of your outward sensitivity and weakness, while simultaneously feeling an immense strength on the inside.
- End by singing "Aaar"/"Haar" freely and surrender to the Note from Heaven without any kind of conscious thought.

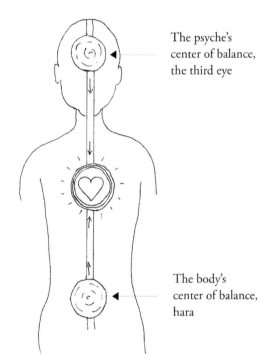

The psyche's center of balance, the third eye

The body's center of balance, hara

With the help of the in breath and visualization, the energy field at the hara is brought up to the heart chakra. With the help of the out breath and visualization, the energy field at the third eye is brought down to the heart chakra. After that, the sound will swell in the chest and it will be easier for the singer to feel devotion and, thus, be more able to express love.

Once your body has opened up and understands the nature of the Note from Heaven, you should be able to freely sing "Aaar"/"Haar"/"Sa" on your root note for a half hour to an hour each day.

Listening with the ears becomes the same as feeling with the body. You simply are.

At this point I recommend that you stop reading and practice Part 1, as it is the foundation of this book.

In the following part of the book, I use musical expressions and terms that readers who do not come from a musical background may have difficulty understanding. I wish to emphasize that, by engaging in the exercises on the practice CD yourself, you will have the opportunity to understand everything in your own way – just as most of what I describe in this book comes from my own experience. The problem with putting this subject in writing is that words can never perfectly convey the real experience of working with the Note from Heaven, since it can only be experienced as a state. The sound speaks for itself.

Should you find these musical expressions difficult to understand or uninspiring, then you have not found the Note from Heaven and need a Vocal therapist[25] to guide you. Whatever happens, the Note from Heaven is a latent opportunity in you, a doorway through which you can unite with Oneness.

Part 2:

Singing with The Note From Heaven

Note Names

Many Western schools use the tonic sol-fa/solfège system of naming musical notes: Do, Re, Mi, Fa, Sol, La, Si, Do. In India, they have corresponding names:

SA   RE   GHA   MA   PA   DHA   NI   ŚA

Both scales correspond to a major scale (refer to track 11 on the practice CD).[26]

Singing the note names helps you become conscious of tonal intervals.

It is easier to attract an animal if you know its name. The cow is no longer just a cow; it is a specific cow, named (say) Bessie. All cows can become specific cows, if we choose to have a relationship with them. The same is true for musical notes; in fact, it is the same for anything we become deeply interested in. By naming the notes, we get a conscious and, therefore, personal relationship to something as intangible as sound.

The location of specific vowels in the body

Since the Indian note names are mostly based on the sound "Aaar", it is healthy to sing them in the speech register, which is the range of notes that mainly resonate in the torso. Do, Re, Mi... "Oooh" and "Eeeh" are related, in terms of vibration, to the throat and head, which means it is easiest to express them with a free-flowing sound in the higher registers (falsetto and middle-range registers).

The illustration represents my experience of how sounds, vowels and body resonate together.

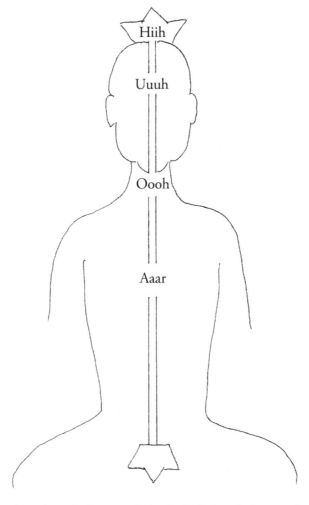

The location of particular vowels in the body in relation to where they resonate.

The deeper and slower a sound vibrates, the lower it resonates in the body.

Men with a good bass are usually down to earth and rarely considered "flighty". A deep voice has a soothing effect because it connects us to our roots, our foundation. "Aaar" is the spoken sound that vibrates most easily in the lower parts of the body, at a lower pitch. "Uuuh" belongs to the root chakra and hara too if you are relating to the over- and undertones of the sound. However, that is another matter.[27]

For our purposes, the preferred vowels are "Aaar" at the bottom, "Oooh" or "Uuuh" in the mid-range and throat, and "Uuuh", "Eeeh" and "Iiih" in the falsetto, the third eye and crown.

The remaining vowels are also useful and necessary in sound scanning, and in the language we use in everyday singing and speech. However, we will disregard them in this first book, since they are more difficult to sing in a relaxed way. The body very seldom uses these other vowels in animated outbursts. "Aaay", "Uehh" and "Eeem" are not usually very powerful and mostly relate to mental activity. "Oorr" is close to "Aaar", but is more closed and resigned in its expression. Some people have difficulty in singing "Aaar" and subconsciously switch over to "Oorr".

Deepening the Voice

In the classical North Indian *dhrupad* singing tradition, there is a rule about not singing higher than your root note for the first five years of practice. My Indian singing teacher, Mangala Tiwari, reassured me with this information when I asked her why she wanted me to sing as low as possible. It was simply in order to deepen my voice.

In ancient Indian singing it is a matter of getting the Ṣa *below* the root note Sa to ring out freely – that is, the note one octave below an already rather deep note.

When you are able to do this your sound can also travel upwards freely. This is because your vocal cords relax completely when you make the deepest sound you can. As the vocal cords become free of tension, they become more flexible. The sound can, therefore, resound more freely when you raise it to the mid-range. The same is true of a rubber band or a guitar string.

When the band or string is stretched, the sound gets higher, and when it is slackened the sound becomes deeper.

That is why it is worth beginning by developing the voice in a downward direction. You might say that we let the voice develop a strong, well-developed root system, which will help it absorb nourishment and grow big and strong.

Stretch your voice downwards at the beginning of each singing session, and especially in the morning if you want to reach really far down. (I touch on this only briefly on the practice CD, because the depth to which people's voices can go varies greatly.)

How low can you go?

This exercise is for training your voice to go as low as possible. However, be careful not to push it beyond its limits.

- Imagine your voice as a rubber band that you stretch in a soft glide from the root note and downwards.
- Find a deeper note to glide down to and repeat the glide until it feels light and good.
- Then stretch it down a little further. Gently massage the deep notes by breathing fervor into them with your song. If it feels comfortable to sing the deep notes for a long time, then by all means do so.
- When you have reached the limit and your voice sounds like a hollow rustling in the trees, stop pushing yourself any further.
- If this depth exercise gives you problems, it could be possible, especially if you are a man, that your root note is wrongly placed at note A. In that case, refer back to the root note section on page 39.

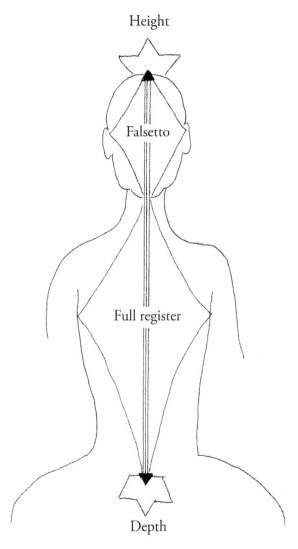

Height

Falsetto

Full register

Depth

The pitch of the tone of a sound dictates where in the body the sound's resonance will be felt. The deeper the tone (the coarser the vibration), the further down in the body it is resonating. The higher the tone (the finer the vibration), the higher up in the body/head it is resonating.

Using the Note from Heaven to build up your voice

On the practice CD first one note is sung (Sa), then two notes (Sa, Re), then three notes, etc., up to nine notes. The idea is to work one track at a time.

For example, sing the combination of Sa and Re until:

1. You are sure of how the note names function in relation to their specific tone.
2. You have experienced the Note from Heaven spreading from Sa to Re.
3. You are able to sing Sa and Re combinations on your own supported by the tanpura (track 21).

After that, you add the next track to what you have already worked with. Give each track the time it needs. Whether that be hours or weeks, do not hurry, because if you do your house will be built on a shaky foundation.

Example of a work method

Sing together with, for example, track 3 on the CD, where the singing of the Sa and Re combination is led.

Repeat this track until the two note names have become second nature, which means the singing and the location of the sound feels natural, then change to track 21 on the practice CD. Sing exclusively to the tanpura accompaniment. If this feels difficult, return to track 3. By singing with the tanpura alone, you can really listen to yourself. It is here that the final expansion of the Note from Heaven, for example from Sa to Re, takes place. The expansion occurs when you sing on "Aaar" and keep an awareness of the note names in the back of your mind at the same time. As with the examples of singing on the CD, this is maintained by alternately singing the same phrases using the note names and on "Aaar".

By gliding from one note to another as slowly as possible,

the opening through which the Note from Heaven reverberates can be expanded. Put yourself into slow motion during this process, because this will lengthen the pathway between the two chosen notes. The longer the pathway, the more details you can experience. The microtones begin to appear during this attentive listening. It is important to let go of the stairway perception of notes. Perceive Sa and Re as two points between which the voice draws an elastic line. The function of the note names is solely to define the working area, from one point to another point.

While working, you move smoothly into a heartfelt, floating state. It can be compared to caressing the notes as gently as you can.

I see the process as similar to making a hole in a frozen lake. The moment when the Note from Heaven breaks through is like pounding a hole in the middle of the ice. After that, it is important to expand the hole by softly melting it with utmost care. If we go too quickly, the ice breaks and we lose control of our work.

Indian Note Names

In the following section, I will give examples of experiences I have had with the individual notes. As mentioned earlier, these experiences have occurred as I slowly and gradually worked my way through the basic scale: Sa Re Gha Ma Pa Dha Ni. In Indian music theory, there are countless versions, and as many interpretations as there are authors, of what the tension values of these notes represent. One system perceives the intervals of the scale, which are always measured out from the root note, as corresponding to different animal sounds; in another system they correspond to different human organs, and so on. I don't think it really matters which version you follow. The main function of these stories is to inspire the singer. Therefore, it can be beneficial to create your own stories or visualizations for each note. By developing a subjective relationship to the notes, you can forget yourself. This is what lifts the music up to a spiritual level.

The subjective relationship is a type of converter, through which the otherwise indefinable sound can be captured and studied. The following description of my note experiences is completely subjective. It is only included to give you an idea of what this is all about. Please do not treat the explanations as rules that need to be learned by heart. The only important thing is that you become inspired to explore your own relationship to the notes. If it is difficult at first, by all means choose some elements from my experiences and draw on these until you begin to get your own ideas. As mentioned earlier, it is important to proceed slowly, note by note.

Sa

In Indian terminology Sa is called "the human sound". Sa is an abbreviation of the name Shadja. Sa is the root note and can be any sound that suits your voice. So it is not predetermined at C, as Do is in the French sol-fa system.

When we establish a Sa, we decide on a starting point (for example, A) and tune the tanpura's strings accordingly. A field representing the ground note is created with the help of the tanpura's drone.

To rest in Sa gives a feeling of being relaxed and well. You feel at home, because you "agree" with the tanpura, since Sa is the tone quality of the tanpura.

If on the other hand you sing other notes, different qualities of tension will arise that clearly do not feel like "home".

In meditation and healing, Sa symbolizes the root chakra and is associated with the color red.

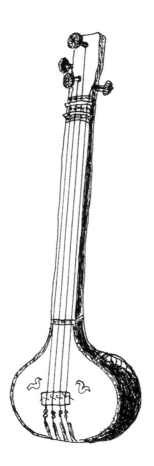

A tanpura is an Indian stringed instrument. It normally has four strings and is made mainly from a half calabash, wood and a bridge of bone or ivory. The first string is tuned to Pa (fifth), the two middle ones to Sa (root note), and the last string to Ṣa. In some ragas/scales, however, the first string is tuned to either Dha (sixth) or Ma (fourth). The tanpura is used as a drone accompaniment by both singers and instrumentalists in enharmonic styles (i.e. where the harmony does not change).
The sound of the tanpura is loaded with overtones, which are created with the help of threads placed exactly where the string rests on the slightly arched bridge.

Re

This is the second note. In the major scale, Re is like the first step away from home (Sa), where everything is safe and peaceful. Re is outgoing, like a traveller seeking new horizons. Still, you are not so far away from home that you cannot immediately change your mind and rest safely in Sa again.

There is an uplifted and timeless anticipation in Re: what is waiting out there in the future?

Re is an abbreviation for the name Rishabha, which means the big second (tonal interval).

In meditation and healing, Re symbolizes the sacral chakra and is associated with the color orange.

Gha

This is the third note. In the major scale, which is sung on the practice CD, my experience of Gha is similar to admiring a beautiful view. Via Re we come to Gha, a magnificent valley in glorious sunshine.

Do not hold yourself back when singing Gha (the big third). Many students hold back on this note. This may be a sign of low self-esteem. It seems as if the student is silently telling himself or herself: "No, I don't deserve the many blessings of life. I will hang my head and hold myself back."

Allowing yourself to believe that you do deserve all the best, the most beautiful, the most wonderful in the world will quickly cause Gha to compete in radiance with the sun. The tone becomes silvery and very moving.

Gha is the determining factor as to whether we sing in major or minor. Gha sets the trend for the tonality of the whole scale. The scale becomes major when Gha is big (*shud*, pure) and minor when Gha is lowered a semitone (*komal*). (The minor Gha komal is always underlined – meaning it is komal.)

In Indian music there are microtones. If you sing Gha in minor and then lower it slightly further, the expression and feeling of the scale or melody changes noticeably. It becomes more serious, heavy, sorrowful.

If, on the other hand, you sing the minor third Gha a little sharper than it normally is in the minor key, then the expression becomes one of a sweet longing or weeping. In addition, the minor third symbolizes the feminine, introversion and the moon, and the major third represents the masculine, extroversion and the sun. A whole scale can become colored by feminine or masculine energy merely from the tension around the third. Gha's important role in defining the tonality of a scale can be explained by the note's symbolic location in our body: the solar plexus, the center of emotions. The color of this center is yellow and is connected to Gha.

Ma

This is the fourth note in the scale and is called the fourth in Western terminology. Ma is an abbreviation for the name Madhyama. In my experience you cannot really rest at Ma. Ma is heartfelt, mystical, a little introverted and aspires both upwards and downwards (notice that it is placed in the middle, just like the heart chakra). The tonal cadence – the three basic chords of harmony-based music (children's songs, pop songs, classical compositions) – is built on Sa (tonic), Ma (subdominant) and Pa (dominant). The combination of these three chords contains all of the notes of the major scale. They are so to say the building blocks of harmonic music. In Indian music theory Ma symbolizes the sound of the heart chakra. Ma is flighty and deep like love; she is our mother, "Mama", and can be connected to the heart chakra's colors, green and pink.

Pa

Now, who would be number five then? Of course it has to be "Papa", daddy, known in Western terminology as the fifth.

The cycle of fifths (our harmonic system) is actually built

on the theme of "mother, child and Father" – Ma (fourth), Sa (prime), Pa (fifth), with the child in the center. It fits wonderfully well, doesn't it?

In Indian terminology, Pa is associated with the throat chakra. Among other things, this center represents communication. Pa is the note that, in terms of resonance, is closest to Sa. Here you can relax. Using the analogy of a field trip, Pa would be the point at which you would stop to eat your lunch. Pa can get a little boring to sing for a long time, though, as it lacks Sa's deep inner calm.

Pa is an abbreviation for Panchama and can be connected to the throat chakra and the colors sky blue and turquoise.

Dha

Dha is the sixth note of the scale and is called the sixth in Western terminology. It is an abbreviation of the name Dhaivata. Dha is also on its way somewhere, while at the same time remaining in the comforting presence of the less tense Pa.

Just as Sa and Pa share some similarities in their chemistry, so do Re and Dha, although I do experience Dha as a little bolder than Re is. If we are climbing a mountain on our field trip, then Dha is the note that gets a whiff of the approaching summit. In its major form Dha is curious and upward reaching.

Dha symbolizes the third eye and higher consciousness. The note and center can be connected to the colors violet and indigo blue.

Ni

Ni is the seventh note and is called the seventh in Western terminology. It is an abbreviation of the Sanskrit name Nishada. As Ni, in its pure form, functions as the note leading to Sa, it is difficult to remain with it. We seek the objective of the field trip, like the person in love longs for their beloved. It takes discipline to explore Ni and not rush through it in a flurry. For some, it can be almost painful to stay with Ni, as it is right next to Sa, the note with which the tanpura/drone instrument continually seduces our ear. Nevertheless, it is a good exercise to stick to your guns and your intentions: "I will keep my focus, no matter how tempting my surroundings may be."

You can even come to enjoy the tension in its own right. When it is finally released on the high Sa, at the top of the mountain, then the sensation is that much more powerful. Our field day has a "happy ending".

Ni is associated with the crown chakra and the soul. Notice that the "ee" sound makes Ni vibrate at the top of the head, where the seventh chakra is located. The color is white or violet.

Writing the note names

The row of note names repeats itself endlessly, both upwards and downwards.

When we write notes that lie an octave below the basic scale of Sa, Re, Gha, Ma, Pa, Dha, Ni, one dot is placed under the note, two dots for two octaves lower, and so on. When we write the notes that lie an octave above the basic scale, a corresponding dot is placed above the note concerned. If we need to write down an even higher octave (which is normally not necessary in this context), then we place two dots above the note in question.

In Indian terminology, the lowering of a tone is called *komal*, which is shown with a line under the note in question, and the raising of a tone is called *tivra* and is written with an accent above the relevant note. Only the notes Re, Gha, Dha and Ni can be *komal* and only Ma can be *tivra*.

In this way, the Indian system is identical to the Western twelve-tone system, except that it is more simply expressed in the Indian single-harmony one-harmonice system? method of writing:

Sa Re Re Gha Gha Ma Má Pa Dha Dha Ni Ni

Benefits of the note names

One reason why it is rewarding to sing the note names is that you become aware of how to express yourself through sound. This training of consciousness is not only effective within the discipline of music; it can improve your whole life in the long term. By learning to be conscious of the note names, you can also learn to be conscious of other mechanisms in daily life. Starting out to develop our consciousness with something as innocent as singing is very beneficial because it takes us into an area that is like a playground. It is quite simply fun to sing. If we choose to stick our head straight into the hornets' nest of personal weaknesses and announce, "Consciousness", we will usually bump into the wall that our subconscious mind has quite properly built to protect us.

In addition, singing on note names is excellent ear training. Knowing how the note names relate to specific tones helps us to write them down and to read melodic passages. Besides that, note language is great to use in vocal improvisation. Here, the Indian note names sound catchier than solfége: (Do, Re, Mi...).

If you try to improvise without being conscious of the note names, the tonal material can get used up long before you manage to establish a true expression of any mood or feeling. By becoming aware of note names, you learn to distinguish the different "wavelengths" from each other, and so you are able to use the available notes more economically.

With practice, you will not need to think any more. At any one time you will "know" where you are in the sea of sound. Your foundation will be the tanpura's constant ground note, saying: "Here you belong, here is your home, take your soundings from me."

In Israel, I had an immensely talented singer as a student. She sang enchantingly from the first lesson. However, this natural talent actually became a problem for her. The depth got lost. She was used to being able to impress people right away.

With the help of the note names, she learned to improvise, and through that, to tell a story. If a scale aspired upwards towards, for example, the high Sà she could now choose to heighten the tension by weaving around Sà for as long as the sensation felt good, before finally surrendering and letting Sà bring satisfaction. That student's singing gave you goosebumps.

We had some fantastic lessons together and gradually became friends, so that the teacher-student relationship eroded. She slid back again and never really developed her talents properly.

Suddenly one day she decided to live as an orthodox Jew. Nobody in her circle of acquaintances was religious and many people shook their heads ruefully. I did, too. Until the day she sang a religious song at a private wedding ceremony.

There it was again! Goosebumps all over. The tears trickled quietly down my cheeks. She had become religious; she had made a decision that went against her surroundings, and had finally found a structure through which she could breathe. A breakthrough had been made. She sang straight from the heart. Oh, what a joy to hear her sing!

This example shows me that true spiritual belief and having a conscious relationship with notes have something in common. It's to do with getting closer to authentic expression, deeper into the music. Away from the ego, into the soul. Finding balance between the chaos of feelings and the dictates of the intellect. Disappearing somewhere between these two states, and growing from that place through the music.

Scale

In this section I will touch on the concept of "raga". To gain a true understanding of the raga, first you need to know the note names and their tonal vibrations in your body. If you are reading this book for the first time and have not yet worked with the note names, then feel free to skim over the sentences you do not understand.

The following explanations about the raga concept are partly meant to serve as an appetizer, and partly as an explanation of the Indian tradition's exceptional ability to link sound and emotion.

The primary purpose of this book is to liberate the natural voice. Therefore, it does not cover the raga concept in great detail. Should you wish to explore the subject more deeply, I recommend that you find an Indian song teacher.

What Westerners call a scale is known as a raga in India. However, the term raga also encompasses an overall form in which there is both improvisation and established melodic elements. The raga starts with an A-lap, which is a free improvisation without underlying rhythm, through which the notes of the raga are slowly presented in delicate slides and ornamentations. There is nothing to say exactly how long the A-lap should last. Its main purpose is to enable the musician to find a way to his or her divinity, and through that, to merge with a higher state. It is that aspect of the raga which this book deals with.

In the raga, the A-lap is followed by compositions and rhythmical improvisations that are technically very demanding. The tempo gradually increases, until the musician cannot play any faster. If the musician is gifted, this form can express a kind of ecstasy.

The vibration of a scale

In Ravi Shankar's book *My Music, My Life*, the raga is defined as "that which colors the mind".

The note is, in itself, a vibration. More notes together create a new vibration, an atmosphere.

Switch yourself on as a listener. You are a sensitive mechanism with billions of nerves, which come into play like small buttons being pushed.

When there is total silence, the nerves are passive, ready

to react to stimulation by any sound. The body is like a white screen. Each note leaves its color, its form. For example, if a raga has five notes, then five different colors are applied to the screen, five different forms that, by interacting, create even more forms. A picture is created with a particular atmosphere. This atmosphere is dependent on how you combine the colors, and in which order you use them. The nerves are incredibly sensitive to tiny nuances. The aim is to express a feeling in as pure a form as possible by working with a scale whose vibration corresponds to, and thus affects, the relevant nerves. If you grope around among the colors in an unfocused way, the screen will become brown. You have to know the way the colors function in order to get them to glow.

So the Indian raga is not just a scale, but also a set of rules on how to treat the notes in order to express a distinct feeling (color).

The source of these rules can be found all the way back in the Vedas (approximately 1500 BCE).

During my studies in India, I asked Mangala what would happen if I sang one of the notes that is not part of the raga (they are called *vivadi*, meaning enemies).

"That is very simple," she replied. "Then it is another raga."

I discovered that the rules give scope for deep concentration. They are hard to learn at first. For example, in a specific raga it is not allowed to go straight to Sa (the leading note must not lead directly to the root note) when you are in the lower pitch. There must be five notes in the ascending scale and six in the descending scale. There are special notes, which in certain situations may need a glissando or a note may need to be sung a microtone above or below it – there are countless variations, depending on which raga you are singing into.

With practice, these rules gradually allow you to create an atmosphere that moves you and feels natural. By repeating a particular pattern of notes until you know it by heart, it becomes a part of you. This very same mechanism applies to the good and bad behavioral patterns that we unconsciously follow every day. We learned them once, but now they are automatic and that is why they feel such a natural part of ourselves.

Learning the feeling of a scale

The raga's *pakad*, or way of singing, is learned by repeating phrases sung by the teacher, and not through analysis and memorizing. It corresponds to a child's parrot fashion learning, which is an extremely quick way to learn languages (refer to tracks 3-10 on the practice CD).

Simply by copying the patterns, with no pressure to sing them well, you will find that they automatically become impressed upon your subconscious. At some point, the patterns will have become so sustainable that you can just fall into them and the musical phrases will pour out of your mouth. Suddenly the raga takes you over and its core essence reveals itself to you through a surprising "a-ha" experience.

It is wonderful to sing, floating around in a raga, to identify with it without being an emotional captive. You are both caught up in your feeling and, at the same time, master of it.

The feeling is legitimate, since it is not attached to any sense of guilt. It is beautiful when purely expressed. Frustrations, rejection, doubt, jealousy – the sides of our life and our self that we do not like – also have quality and can be beautiful. For when feelings are recognized in the raga, their explosiveness is defused and they become harmless.

You can spend your whole life exploring the raga concept, since there are as many ragas as there are nuances of feeling. New ragas (new note combinations) are still being made, in step with the new feelings that developments in society engender.

It is, fundamentally, a heart-searching effort that demands deep reflection and immersion.

The best way to work your way into the raga universe is

to learn one raga as thoroughly and as well as possible. That can take several years of work, or, if you have the proper surroundings and can practice four or five hours a day, it can take less time. Some Indian singers practice for up to twelve hours a day. The song is their *dharma*, a way of life.

The raga, a state

Working with ragas, we learn how to disappear into them. The feeling of sliding into the raga, when everything you needed to learn has simply become the raga's soul and no longer needs to be remembered, corresponds to the feeling of the Note from Heaven. You are led to a sense of being present in the moment.

The question of how many ragas you can sing is irrelevant. What counts is what you are able to express from the heart at that particular moment.

In his book *The Mysticism of Music, Sound and Word*, Sufi master Hazrat Inayat Khan describes a sitar player who always played the same raga when he gave concerts. People were deeply moved and came to his performances again and again.

One day he was asked why he always played the same raga. "Why should I play another raga, when I can play this one perfectly?" he answered.

That which touches the heart is never boring.

We come up against the same truth again and again. It is the essence that is important, not the story itself.

Common Western ragas

The major scale, which is presented on the practice CD that accompanies this book, is familiar to most people in the Western world. The majority of our songs are written in the major mode, with fewer in the minor.

Examples of songs in the major scale: *Row, Row, Row Your*

Boat; Happy Birthday to You; For He's a Jolly Good Fellow; Oh!
Susanna; What a Wonderful World...

Examples of songs in the minor scale: *Summertime;*
Greensleeves; Scarborough Fair...

So the major scale is already familiar, which makes it easier
to concentrate on listening to yourself. On the other hand, the
weakness with this scale choice is that the note language is so
straightforward.

The experience of "being taken over" by a raga in the major
scale can be difficult to provoke, because we are working
without rules while dealing with a scale that does not have that
many levels or facets to explore.

In India, the major scale is called *bilawal*. It is not used very
much in the classical Northern Indian music. When I asked one
classical Northern Indian musician about *bilawal*, he told me he
found it boring.

However, it is used a lot in Indian folk music where the
theme is usually religious as, for example, in *bhajans*.

To compare Western and Indian note language is interesting,
because it says something about our cultures. The use of keys
in the West stays within a moderate number of scales, mostly in
the major mode. The major is positive and we can hold problems
at bay with a happy song. The question, however, is whether we
can solve them with oompa, oompa rhythms and tra la, la.

In India, there are ragas that are suited to the seasons and
to special occasions. They might, for example, use a particular
raga when they need to call forth rain.

Even so, a raga or scale is normally associated with a
particular time of the day. The major scale is associated with
noon, when the sun is warm and high in the sky.

At this time there is no tension between light and dark. The
light, the masculine power, has taken over. In cooler climates
such as in Northern Europe, a preference for the major scale
could therefore be explained by a need for optimism in order

to withstand grey, dark weather. This is hardly true of India, if one's state of mind is to be measured by the hours of sunshine.

Other scales

If you want to set about learning other scales to express different emotions, then I recommend you first go through this basic material. Later, it will be easy to change the scale, because the note names are already integrated. Perhaps you do not feel comfortable working with the major scale. Maybe you harmonize better, for example, with an introverted, intense atmosphere. In that case, the basic work can also be done using the minor scale.

When looking for the small nuances in our sound, we cannot be humble enough. Therefore, it is important to start with a scale that is relatively easy to handle.

The degree of difficulty should be low enough not to impede the sense of well-being we derive from the musical experience.

Scale exercises

This section is for those who wish to develop themselves musically. Practicing scale exercises are not necessary for learning Sound Healing but it is helpful to develop your hearing of tonal intervals.

Do not attempt the exercises outlined in tracks 12-20 of the practice CD (see pages 116-118) until you are ready for them. The basic scale (track 11) is useful for everyone to memorize forwards and backwards at the beginning, whereas the rest of the exercises could be overwhelming for a beginner.

The exercises break the major scale into different mathematical patterns. These are very similar to the exercises that are known in both the classical and rhythmical schools of Western music. Feel free to make up your own combinations, if you want to.

Since we are now moving into the dangerous area of technique, it is exceptionally important to play with – and get into the spirit of – these tonal figures, rather than becoming addicted to a mechanical recitation of note names and sounds. For example, you could imagine yourself verbally explaining something to a person while practicing.

The aim of learning the scale patterns is to stamp them onto your subconscious mind. Then these patterns can be naturally combined and grow into the melodic phrases of an improvised passage.

By singing the note names, you can train your consciousness to recognize the relationship between the notes, while also practicing intonation and attack. Always work at a slow enough tempo that you can work accurately, avoiding mistakes of pronunciation and intonation. The brain is totally naïve in nature – it records all the information that it receives. If we record an incorrect piece of information, this error is hard to overwrite, which is why we tend to repeat the same mistakes over and over. Consequently, it is highly beneficial to work patiently at a much slower pace than we think we can handle.

After 10-20 correct repetitions, you can try to see if your technique holds at an increased pace. If there is just the slightest touch of hesitation in your expression, please return to the original tempo. And when you build up your own tonal pattern, avoid jumps that are too large or difficult between notes. They will be hard to express naturally in an improvisational context later.

By repeating the scale exercises on "Aaar", you will train the flexibility and the intonation of your voice. Just as it is possible to write with a pen without lifting it from the paper, the voice can express a long, unbroken line when it moves between the notes of "Aaar" on an exhalation. It is an undulating movement, which is reflected in the visible up and down movement of the throat. This sliding angle of attack on the notes will, when sung at a fast tempo, result in a vibrato created solely in the throat. In Indian singing, this technique is called *gamak* and it is explained further on page 116.

Part 3:

Creative Music-Making

Improvisation

Improvisation is the natural next step after you have learned to express yourself in note language. We speak in notes. Everyone can improvise – it is merely a question of adjustment and of rejecting the ego's fear of surrendering to the divine.

When we connect to the Note from Heaven in our improvisation, the sounds mingle without interference from the ego. When this succeeds and is recorded, we hear the most beautiful melodies. Usually, the person who sang them cannot remember what he or she expressed, which is not surprising as the most beautiful melodies arise when we are "lost" in the moment. We are "gone" in that state, and afterwards can seldom recall more than that something good just happened. By perceiving improvisation in that way, the improviser is prepared to let something else sing through him or her. To create in the present moment means taking a chance, jumping into an abyss, abandoning all self-restraint, making room for the manifestation and birth of a divine expression. Mozart seems to have worked in this way. He composed as if he were dictating straight from heaven. The incredible number of notes he managed to write in his short life (he was just 35 when he died) supports this theory.

Addiction to notes

I believe that the reason why so many Western musicians, including the most highly educated, feel inhibited when asked to take a creative, improvisational approach to music is that they depend so much on reading music.

When we sing or play melodies from notation, we are seeking to breathe life into what, hopefully, has been the composer's experience of a divine moment. The notes are the skeleton, which we then reanimate with flesh and blood.

The melodies that continue to inspire us, despite the changing styles of music over time, have, much like crystals, a clear and balanced design that somehow does us good. Some melodies make us share the emotions the composer experienced, when the holy fruit fell into his or her lap.

However, if you only play or sing music that has already been written you will not necessarily recognize and find your own divinity.

We tend to idolize fellow human beings whom we perceive to be geniuses. But then we feel inadequate in comparison.

The commandment "Have no other gods than me" is vital in this context. It is all too easy to just give up on yourself and feel incompetent in the shadow cast by a brilliant person. It is like idolizing a guru who has developed a high level of consciousness. You can learn a lot from that kind of person, but idolizing someone else can prevent you from finding the same elements within yourself.

An authentic model of inspiration or guru does not need to be adored. Such a person knows that he or she is just a channel for a higher power and bows down in honor of this divine miracle.

When individuals express themselves, the expression is a mirror of their innermost self. Therefore, it serves no purpose to look at someone else's expression and compare it to our own. Doing that has a stagnating and limiting effect. We end up whispering to ourselves, "I am not good enough," or, "Wow, look how good I am compared to..."

In creative work, we express ourselves through, and thus train ourselves to unite with, the same channel used by the Note from Heaven, and by being inspired we surrender to the present moment and thus to the divine power within us. When a perfectly ripe fruit falls into our lap in the form of a poem, a melody, a painting, an idea, etc., that which, paradoxically, makes us happiest is being moved and stimulated by a divine power. It is the deep-seated driving force behind all creativity – a yearning for divine expression, a yearning to vanish along with our ego and thus experience our soul as complete and from a higher world.

Considering that we all have the seeds of perfection within us, it is amazing how often we put obstacles in our own, and other people's, path.

During my studies at the Royal Academy of Music, I sensed, despite all my many positive musical experiences there, a constricted energy visible in the pale, anemic faces of many of the students. I myself felt I was suffocating. The creative aspect was missing and it is definitely not a priority in most public institutions of classical music in Europe.

Experiencing your own divinity is, for me, to see the deeper meaning of life. It teaches you to be present in your musical expression. You can then fully understand what composers were feeling and the power they were channeling.

Without this understanding, the notes are nothing more than a series of small instructions, which first the eyes obey and then the ears hear: "Did I read that right, it sounded funny, didn't it? Oh, yes, that was correct." We blindly follow the orders and play correctly in order to please the ego, while feeling dissatisfied by any mistakes that we make. The childhood experience of conditional love and the associated fear of failure is given fertile soil to grow in when you only work in this way with notes. Consequently, our entire musical development ends up on the wrong track, and music becomes more of a battle of nerves than a surrendering to something higher.

All this gradually became clear to me when I took two months of sabbatical leave from the Academy and was introduced to Indian singing, where improvisation is the actual challenge and the written compositions function like small islands you can rest on while developing the nature of the raga through improvisation. According to the Indian tradition, the indisputable purpose of music is union with God.

Composition

As mentioned in previous sections, complete melodies can arise in improvisation. These moments of sudden beauty appear spontaneously and unexpectedly. We can all compose, if we allow ourselves the freedom to do so.

A recording is the best witness you can have when improvising a composition. Since the composition arises in the moment and vanishes afterwards, the singer is not usually able to remember it.

Another way to compose is to put text to music. I often use this form of composition with students, since it is clear-cut and easy to do. Everyone ends up writing a song, even those who resist at the beginning.

The interesting thing is that, by saying a sentence out loud, you can sense how to direct the melody. It is a matter of relaxing and letting what comes come, while at the same time noticing whether it feels right.

In order to remember the song, it needs to be recorded in pieces, sentence by sentence. I know from experience that we tend to overestimate our ability to remember melodic phrases. Since they are part of the moment, they evaporate like morning dew. Always record every finished phrase, singing the song from the beginning to see if it "stimulates" the later sentences. Then record the new part that is added and continue like that until the melody is finished. If you play an instrument, it is possible to have a coherent memory of the melody, due to the support from the underlying harmonies.

Sometimes when you are in the middle of some activity, a melody you have never heard before will suddenly come into your head. If this happens, drop everything you are doing and record it right away. If you are good at note language, writing the song down in note names could be an option. If you consider yourself tone-deaf you will need help from a teacher. It is difficult to hold on to a melody when you're not sure about the notes. The teacher can sing or play back the student's melodic phrases, and in that way, the student can correct any tonal misunderstandings.

Tone deafness

Funnily enough, those people who believe they are tone-deaf have repeatedly surprised themselves, and me, by composing some excellent songs. Maybe this is because a self-declared tone-deaf individual has nothing to lose. Therefore, there is no reason to try to impress anyone. This eliminates the ego's influence, which leaves room for suggestions from the soul to break through.

In most cases, a tone-deaf person can sing their own melody in tune, because he or she has created it. Through that process, they have set their own parameters and, therefore, worked without being influenced by preconceptions as to what they should achieve.

As a result, the process of composing strengthens the student's self-confidence and reveals the source of the tone deafness as primarily psychological and fear-based.

Creativity generates a "self" confidence that unfolds through the experience of inspiration, a word that derives from the Latin *in spiritu* – "in the spirit".

Children, Adults and Voices

It is not surprising that presumed tone deafness or feeling inhibited about using one's voice, whether when singing or communicating, originates, in most cases, from childhood experiences.

For us as adults there are a lot more sources of noise than in the past.

In addition to obstructers like the radio, washing machine, TV, stereo, etc., there is an abundance of electrical installations that influence us with radiation of microwaves inaudible to the ear.

Nevertheless, our nervous system picks up all these vibrations and gets irritated by them. The fact that we increasingly work indoors, sitting in front of screens like computers, iPhones and iPads radically reinforces the constant vibrational influence on the body and its energy field.

Then, when we spend time in Nature, far away from all sources of artificial noise, we discover that the body, quite inexplicably, calms down. We breathe a sigh of relief, or maybe even feel slightly uneasy in the silence if we are confirmed city-dwellers.

Our body and energy field suffer noise pollution in everyday life, so our level of noise tolerance declines.

There does not need to be much noise before it almost physically pains us.

Children have a need to get to know themselves. The voice is a wonderful toy to experiment with since it represents the breath and our life force. The adult's understanding of the way the child expresses itself vocally is enormously important, since the basis of the child's relationship to its voice is established in the first years. It is not only about singing in tune. It is also about maintaining a grounded breath and contact with the higher centers in the head, which among other things connect the child to its intuition and self-confidence. If the child is forbidden to use the voice for experimentation, the body will seek to compensate for the blockage in the flow of energy in the throat.

Then, the energy can only flow freely in the five lower chakras and this pent-up energy will try to express itself through bursts of anger, nervousness, crying, violent behavior, apathy, hyperactivity or screaming and yelling, which are the lower chakras' way of communicating. Thus, a vicious circle is created, caused by the adult's misunderstanding of the child's attitude.[28]

Try to imagine that you are doing something that feels good

and completely right, and then someone tells you that what you are doing is wrong.

Let us say, for example, that you have been sitting singing and are totally absorbed in the Note from Heaven and then someone interrupts with, "What are you screaming for?" or "Stop that noise!"

How will you react to that? In many cases, a blockage will occur, because, when you have just surrendered yourself to the moment while singing, you are in a completely soft and open state, like an infant. At the very least, the response will have a negative effect, even though, with our adult intellect, we can rationalize the situation and understand that our hinderer didn't understand what we were engaged in.

Children sing the Note from Heaven spontaneously. Small, healthy, natural voices fill and rip through a room with their vitality. When my sons were young and I had students at home, I could hear them singing along in the distance. Children love to sing long notes on "Aaar".

In the early years, children see their parents as gods and copy anything we do as they perceive it to be the "right" thing. If we tell them to keep their mouths shut when they are in the middle of truly loving their own voices, their self-confidence becomes damaged. What can they trust, if their own evaluation of what feels good is wrong? Experimenting with one's own voice becomes tinged with guilt.

You don't need to just swallow your irritation and let your children be noisy. The idea is to subdue the noisiness in a constructive way by listening to the child's sound and then communicating on an equal footing, if not through language, then through sound.

With regard to the infant years of both my sons, I have experienced how happy babies become when you understand their sounds correctly. A sound based on an understanding of what the child is doing when they scream, is strengthened by the listening work described in this book. You learn to sense and listen intuitively to whether the child is really sad, angry, setting limits... or just playing with its voice. Parents ought to use their instincts, and just take the time to stop and listen attentively to the child's sound, rather than immediately reacting with irritation and trying to quiet the child down. It is all about being present.

The trick is to give the child the stimulation that it calls for.

Calming a noisy child

If a child is screaming for no apparent reason, you can assume that the child is playing with his or her voice. To calm the child down, I would lift him or her up in front of the mirror and try to copy their sound without ridiculing them in any way. By seeking the child's sound, I tune into his or her level of consciousness and, through that attitude, develop a true acceptance of the unfolding of the child's voice. I try to hit the note the child is expressing and after a while draw it up and down in slides with my voice.

The child will do the same, as children love to imitate. When that exploration has been exhausted, you can make the notes break into a melody that the child is fond of and then you are singing a song together, after which the child will very likely become interested in playing with something else.

This method is also effective for situations where the child takes a small tumble and starts crying.

A method for calming children who are able to talk is to let them know that you are sensitive to sound right now, and would like some quiet time. Maybe suggest that they scream outside, but say clearly that you know how much fun it is to use your voice in this way.

In general, singing has a calming effect on people, which is why we sing lullabies. So perhaps doctors and nurses should learn a repertoire of songs to suit different types of patients.

Our son broke his leg when he was two and did not like getting his cast cut off by a noisy, vibrating and rotating knife blade. Both we and the medical staff were worried that a trauma might develop. To cover up the noise and the crying, we parents started singing his favorite children's song with all our strength. The doctor and nurse joined in spontaneously. He stopped crying in sheer amazement at this meeting of his own fear and the festive spirit of the singing. It was a beautiful experience to stand there and sing together with these two people in their white coats. The masks and barriers completely vanished. Our son still whimpered, but the worst of the fear had been warded off by the singing and, in the meantime, the cast was being cut through and removed.

Understanding through imitation

Why do we find it so funny when a comedian imitates a well-known person's voice?

It seems to me that what makes us laugh is that we can so clearly sense the character of a person through the vocal caricature. Children constantly copy voices in the first years. Not only do they learn language in that way, they also acquire knowledge about their parents' personalities. Children perceive a grown-up's "tone" of speaking and integrate it subconsciously into their own personality. It is, therefore, not so strange that in later life you discover traits from your parents in yourself, traits that you thought you had left behind a long time ago. These character traits, which are learned through intuitive intonation, are well embedded in our behavioral patterns, whether we want them to be or not.

Essentially, we learn undesirable behavior patterns through active listening. The good news is that we can also listen them away again. This is what happens when we work with the Note from Heaven.

The Note from Heaven enables us to experience an opening,

a glimpse of ourselves in full bloom. After that, it is entirely up to us whether we wish to express our true self through our voice. When the voice opens up and becomes increasingly natural, active, negative behavior patterns break up while, at the same time, corresponding expressions of sound in the voice disappear. The fewer inhibiting behavior patterns, the more flexibility and freedom can be experienced, both in the sound of the voice, and in the mind and body.

Creative Writing

All inspiration comes from the same source and manifest when you surrender to the Oneness level where present, past and future merge into the "now". As a channel of the Oneness level, the Note from Heaven can be recognized in all creative work. Just as it is valid in improvisation and composition to let something higher sing through you, the same is true for writing texts.

The only thing you need is a certain level of writing ability, combined with an openness to believe in your higher self. Just like singing the Note from Heaven, it is a matter of opening, opening, opening... in order to give space, let go of your need for control and drop every judgmental attitude.

You can capture a particular emotional experience and express it in words that evoke that experience every time you read those words. When the words are also put to music, the effect becomes even stronger. This makes the creative process an excellent tool for self-understanding and self-examination.

You don't need to write a cogent account if you don't want to, although that is one valid approach. You could end up writing a series of images that make no sense at all at first. However, by looking closer, you may find that they reflect your reality, rather like a dream does.

The story itself is unimportant. It is the fact that we are developing our consciousness that matters.

There are myriad approaches. I am suggesting one possible course of action to get you started if you are not used to writing.

An approach to creative writing

- Sit in your singing position. It is important to keep the spine straight so the body's energy can flow freely.
- Have a pen in your hand and a piece of paper or cardboard within reach so you will be able to write as soon as the words come.
- Close your eyes. Breathe air into the sacral chakra (*hara*, a hand's width below the navel) and press the stomach gently inwards with each exhalation.
- Concentrate on your third eye. If there are thoughts, let them remain there. Open the space in the third eye outwards like ripples in water. Let each thought float in its own ring. There is stillness in the center. Try to stay there.
- When you feel peaceful in your mind (perhaps like a silent helicopter with so many thoughts rotating and disappearing out to the periphery and yourself resting in the peaceful emptiness of the center), move your awareness down to the *hara*.
- Let the third eye fuse together with the *hara*. It is as if your body is disappearing between the two centers. It is a wonderful feeling.
- Sense the two centers' collective space. Observe the space. Ask to have some words sent.
- The words can come in the form of images or feelings. Describe what you see or feel. If there is something you want to know more about, ask and wait, observing the space.
- Seize the inspiration when it comes, write and don't hold back. It is up to you whether you do so with open or

closed eyes.

• Take a break when you have emptied your mind.

Later you can go over the material and make any necessary adjustments to ensure it makes sense to you. Usually, you will develop a fuller understanding of the written work during the editing.

If you want to put the text to music, go back to the Composition section on page 86. When processing text into music, be prepared to polish the material further, as the rhythmical relationships between the words are of greater importance here.

Performance

When you find a form of expression that brings you joy, you will naturally wish to share it with other people. This is a spiritual law: joy is like fire. When you pass it on and it is accepted, it spreads. To experience giving yourself and being gladly received is a basic human wish. Such an experience can change our lives fundamentally. It strengthens our self-worth, affirms that we have something to offer to others, affirms, in fact, that we have a mission here on Earth.

Therefore, a successful performance can be a great boost, especially if our relationship to our voice has been warped by repeated unfortunate experiences.

As mentioned in the section on performance anxiety, the danger with performance is that the ego can take control. It craves the applause from which it gains a false sense of self-confidence. An authentically successful performance is, therefore, one in which the soul is strong enough to outshine the ego.[29]

By experiencing situations that call for the best in us (the soul, the higher self, the divine), we can learn to recognize the difference between control by the ego and control by the soul. Above all, when we are governed by the soul, time seems to disappear, the words and sounds flow naturally from our lips, we feel warmed and touched deep in our hearts, and we are overwhelmed by a feeling of devotion, joy and safety. The more the soul has the chance to influence us through such experiences, the stronger its hold on us will be.

That is why it is good to sing the Note from Heaven for hours. The soul will eventually overwhelm us with its irresistible power of love.

Sometimes students drop the Note from Heaven before they have completely absorbed it into their body, and switch to a familiar, well-known song. The voice, which was free-sounding and whole before, all at once sounds meek and fearful. This is because the familiar song represents the world we were born into, including all the old behavior patterns, which are what create performance anxiety and a feeling of unworthiness – "Just who do you think you are?" we ask ourselves.

It is possible to transfer the effect of the Note from Heaven into a familiar melody, but to achieve this you need to have become convinced, deep down in your heart, of your own divine power. We are most beautiful in our natural form. Sing the song as it is without adding artifices and extra frills. Let it live, fill it out; let it lead you to the Note from Heaven. Be the song instead of performing it.

Singing for each other in a group is the very best way to train performance while allowing the soul's message to come through. This audience is conscious of the forces the performer has to deal with – if the ego wins, it is no defeat, because everyone present understands what it is like to deal with the mechanisms of the ego.

You can keep on trying, and when you finally succeed in singing from the heart, everyone receives a great gift. An atmosphere of devotion descends upon the room because everyone present has been deeply touched and, quite frankly, healed. Sacred moments like these are charged with a natural, loving atmosphere and complete calm, which in daily life can only be maintained by conviction and faith – an inner conviction, whose function is to preserve the essence of those moments in which we have felt blissfully whole and well-functioning.

Experiences like that happen spontaneously. They do not arise from talking to others about our inner truth, so maybe we would do better to stop talking and start singing instead. Song is a beautiful way to communicate, because no one is betrayed. Its power is unmistakable and it makes no wars. It gently sprinkles its loving frisson onto us all, cutting across all barriers.

The trees, the snow, the sky, the silence of nature. I, a tree, stretch my arms up towards the sky's milky-white arch and touch a moment of eternity. My heart becomes suffused with gratitude.

Epilogue

Tree *(Song from the CD* Zeros *2015 www.gilalai.com)*

Tree you are me.
I am a tree,
Each of your leaves'
green lights relieve believe in me.
Under your crown "I" becomes "We",
A scepter of love,
A bridge to eternity.

Tree you are me.
I am a smile,
Open to be –
two eyes one sight burning to Thee.
Inside your crown an embryo grows,
A scepter of fire,
A key to divinity.

Tree you are me.
We are one,
A moon and a sun,
a miracle where the end has begun.
Over your crown a union of light,
A scepter of truth,
Balance the day, bless the night.

Githa Ben-David, 2013

Appendix

Physical Exercises

Face

Exercise 1

- Make faces and hold each grimace for a few seconds. Feel free to include the tongue in your creations.

Exercise 2

- Do lip rolls, quick vibrating movements with your lips, so that it sounds like a helicopter or a snorting horse. Make the movement as relaxed as possible, both with and without tones.
- When you have got your lips vibrating easily, it will not be long before other facial muscles become involved. After about five minutes, the nose begins to vibrate. It is a simple way to give yourself a facial massage.
- If it is difficult to do lip rolls, try pressing the corners of your mouth together with the index fingers. Another possibility is to splutter explosively, similar to a baby spluttering its food. You might wish to do this outside in order to avoid spitting everywhere!

Just a few rolls are enough to get a sense of the exercise. Then practice whenever possible. It can be fun to do when driving or cycling, for example.

Sooner or later the jaw muscles loosen up and the lip roll becomes relaxed.

Exercise 3

- Tongue rolls vibrate further down in the throat. Roll your tongue while you sing through the whole register of notes. Be sure that the tongue rolls lightly up against the hard palate. It is easiest to start further back.

Not everyone can make tongue rolls. If you have problems, exercises 5-8 may help.

Neck and throat

Exercise 4

- Head rolls, as done in yoga. The whole exercise is done in a gentle and, preferably, very slow tempo. Tilt the head to the right, then to the left five times. Breathe in deeply with each stretch, and feel the muscles letting go with each exhalation.
- In the same way, let the head go forwards and backwards, five times in each direction. Note that in these initial stretches, you can support your head with your hands, especially if you have a weak neck or back.
- Now turn your head in gentle, slow circles or half-circles, whichever is more comfortable. There are some people for whom it is not advisable to turn their head in complete circles, as this can injure the vertebrae in the neck. Repeat the movement five times in each direction.
- After this, breathe in deeply through the nose. Hold your breath, then while lifting the right shoulder up to the right ear, breathe out. Do the same with the left shoulder. At the end, lift both shoulders up at the same time and release them on an exhalation.

Tongue, jaws and neck

Exercise 5

- Hold the tongue in the right side of the mouth as long as it feels comfortable, relax and do the same on the left side.
- Stretch the tongue as far backwards as possible and hold the stretch while looking upwards with eyes closed. Relax.
- Stretch the tongue out of your mouth as far as possible, while looking upwards with eyes open. Relax.

Exercise 6

- Make circles in the air with the tongue in both directions. Stretch the tongue down, hold the position, then upwards towards the nose, hold. Relax.
- Make the eternity symbol – a horizontal 8 – in the air with your tongue. It is also possible to do this exercise inside the mouth. Relax.

Exercise 7

- Write your full name in italics in the air using the tip of your nose. You can imagine that you have attached a little pencil there. Notice the pleasant sensation in your neck.

Exercise 8

- Massage the joints of your jaw and feel free to grunt and make baby sounds at the same time. The jaw joints, or hinges, can be found by opening and closing your mouth and, at the same time, placing your fingertips in front of your earlobes.

- After that, massage your jaw muscles. Do this vigorously with both hands. Start from the middle of each jaw, then draw the muscle out to both sides – up towards the ear and down towards the chin at the same time.
- Try to yawn. Note that the temples are activated as well. The fine muscles that attach the jaws to each other are to be found here. Therefore, massage these small indentations with your thumbs as well.

Shoulders, neck, chest and spine

Exercise 9

- Stand with your feet a shoulder width apart with loose knees. Breathe in through your nose and stretch your right arm up along your ear and backwards, while following it with your eyes. Allow your arm to continue describing a backward circle while breathing out.
- Repeat with your left arm.
- Roll both arms backwards and let your neck fall all the way back while breathing in through the nose. Bend your knees a little.
- Continue the circular movement as you exhale, while moving your arms forwards and upwards and slowly raising your neck.

Do this exercise as often as you wish. If you get dizzy, bend your head forwards as in exercise 10.

Exercise 10

- Imagine that your arms and head are a heavy burden for

the rest of your body, which in this exercise is a crane. The "burden" is hanging and dangling downwards. Do not overstretch your knees, but be sure to have some feeling of stretch at the back of the knees.

- Hang there and feel gravity working. Do not press your hands towards the floor, but hang totally relaxed.
- Now let the crane pull the load up as slowly as possible. Lift one vertebra at a time, starting from the bottom and moving upwards. The slower you do this exercise, the better it feels.
- When you are standing again, bend the neck backwards while rolling the stretched arms up over your head, and letting them go backwards as far as possible on an inhalation. Continue the circular movement by returning the stretched arms to the front and slowly raising the neck while exhaling (as described in the third step of exercise 9). If you get dizzy, bend your upper body forwards and relax in that position.

Yoga exercise that benefits the eyes, the ability to concentrate and activates the third eye

Exercise 11

The maximal visual angles that our eyes are capable of when they move to their extreme positions can be described, as in this exercise, in terms of the numbers on a clock.

- Look up (12 o'clock) and look down (6 o'clock), five times in each direction.
- Look to the sides (3 and 9 respectively) five times in each direction.
- After that, look to 2 o'clock five times and then to 8 o'clock five times.
- Repeat for 10 o'clock and 4 o'clock.

- Draw circles with your eyes trying to describe a round, soft arc. If the eyes tend to jump, try giving them extra time in those places where they jump. Make five circles in each direction.
- Hold your thumb 10 cm (4 inches) from your nose. Focus on the thumb, and then focus on a point in the distance. Do this five times.
- Warm your hands by rubbing them together and cup them in front of your eyes. Let your eyes relax in the darkness.

Breathing, posture, spine, tense solar plexus and awareness of the *hara*

Exercise 12

- Get down on your knees and bend forwards in the fetal position. Let your arms rest in front of you in a relaxed way. Breathe deeply (preferably through your nose). Try to place your hands on your back (or better – get someone to do it for you). Note how you are breathing in your lower back and sides. Put your hands down again.
- Relax in this position, keeping your attention on the breathing in your back.
- At the same time, bend your tongue backwards, while you look gently up with eyes closed.

Exercise 13

- Do the reverse of exercise 12, by lying on your back with your knees pulled up to your chest.
- Hug your calves with your arms and press your thighs in towards your body. Sense the breathing in your lumbar region again. Breathe out and make the sound "Tssss" or

"Kssss" and note which muscles become activated.

Exercise 14

This exercise is a classical breathing exercise, effective for people who usually breathe in their chest. Do it very thoroughly and with concentration. Stop if you are unsure of when the stomach should go in or out. Clarify this and then continue the exercise.

- Sit on the edge of a chair. If possible, rest your face, chest and stomach on your knees. The arms are hanging limply alongside the legs.
- Breathe in and let the flow of the in breath push you into a sitting position. Hold your breath. Place your hands on your stomach.
- It is important to exhale with the help of the stomach muscles alone. Keep your concentration on the balance point, which is a hand's width below the navel.

Push the air out gradually while singing: "Haar". Sense how the muscles around the balance point under the navel are actively pushed inwards with a slow thrust, as if you were gradually accelerating a speeder.

Exercise 15

Seesaw breathing **(Moshe Feldenkrais)**
The following exercise is very helpful in enabling the Note from Heaven to break through. It activates energy flow in the five lower chakras and simultaneously strengthens awareness of the breath. It can have a releasing effect on a tense solar plexus and breathing problems in general. At the same time, the inner organs are massaged.

- Lie down on your back with your knees bent and feet on the ground. Be aware of your back. Your whole spine is now in contact with the mat.
- Breast: Breathe deeply through your nose, fill your body with air, hold the breath and push all the air up into your chest. Pushing your stomach inwards does this. Activate your root lock by pulling your pelvis up. Activate your neck lock by pressing your chin down, which closes the throat. Notice how the chest muscles are stretched out front and back. Hold the breath as long as you can. Breathe out. Repeat five times.
- Stomach: Now do the opposite, so that the stomach instead of the chest is pushed out. Breathe deeply through your nose, fill the body with air and push the chest muscles downwards in order to make the stomach as big as possible. Hold your breath and enjoy the feeling of the stretched muscles in the stomach and lower back. Close off your throat and pelvic floor as in the previous step (root lock, neck lock). Hold the breath as long as you can. Breathe out. Repeat five times.
- Now the two parts of the exercise are combined. Breathe in through the nose, fill the body with air, close off at the top and the bottom, as before. Slowly push the air from the chest to the stomach area, back and forth in a gentle, rocking movement. Note how it goes up and down the spine, how your organs are being massaged and are very likely making sounds. You may be able to hold your breath for an extremely long time in this position.

When the above exercise can be done easily, you can choose to do the whole exercise, or just parts of it, without air. This means exhaling and then activating the root and neck lock. Doing the exercise in this way is more demanding. It is not advisable to do this exercise just after a meal.

Exercise 16

Yoga relaxation

- Lie on your back with your legs outstretched and your arms by your sides with the palms turned upwards. Roll your feet from side to side and feel how your legs roll with them. Stretch your insteps downwards, hold the tension, then relax. Draw your feet towards your body and press down with your heels, relax. Tense the whole buttock area, holding your breath for as long as you can, then relax.
- Tense the chest muscles, hold your breath, then relax. Tense your shoulders up towards your ears, hold your breath, then relax. Clench your fists, hold your breath, then relax. Squeeze tightly every muscle in your face, purse your lips, then relax. Now open your face wide, stretch your eyes open and stick out your tongue as far as it will go. Relax.
- Stretch your whole body downwards. Chin, hands, arms, legs and insteps are stretched as far down in the direction of the soles of the feet as possible. Hold your breath, then relax.
- Slowly and gently roll your head from side to side. The head is a ball or a bubble gently bobbing in water or on a current of air. The slower you do the roll, the deeper the effect. Center your head comfortably and relax.

Neck, breath, energy flow and suppleness of the spine

Exercise 17

Shoulder stand

- Lie on the floor with your legs together and your hands, palms down, by your sides. Inhaling, push down on your hands and raise your legs straight up above you.

- Lift the hips off the floor and bring your legs up over and beyond your head, at an angle of about 45 degrees.
- Exhaling, bend your arms and support your body, holding as close to the shoulders as possible, thumbs around the front of the body, fingers around the back. Push your back up. Lift your legs.
- Now straighten your spine and bring the legs up to a vertical position. Press your chin firmly into the base of your throat. Breathe slowly and deeply in this pose, keeping your feet relaxed.
- To come down from this pose, lower your legs to an angle of about 45 degrees over your head, place your hands, palms down, behind you, then slowly roll out of it one vertebra at a time. Among other things, this pose encourages deep abdominal breathing, because it limits the use of the top of the lungs.

Exercise 18

Plough

This exercise has the same starting position as the Shoulder stand, but the legs are stretched backwards over the head instead of upwards.

- Support your back with your hands, keeping the elbows as close to one another as possible. If your feet comfortably reach the floor, walk them as far behind your head as you can. Now clasp your hands together and stretch your arms out behind your back. Breathe slowly and deeply in this position. Use the shoulder stand rollout (exercise 17, last step) to come out of the position. It can be beneficial to sing Hung Song (see film link) into the tension while doing this exercise.

Exercise 19

Fish

This exercise is pretraining for the Fish pose and a counter exercise to the Plough and the Shoulder stand.

- Lie down on your back with your legs straight and your feet together. Place your hands, palms down, beneath your thighs.
- Pressing down on your elbows, inhale and arch your back, resting the very top of your head on the floor. Exhale. Breathe deeply while in the position.
- To come out of the pose, first lift your head and place it gently down again, then release your arms.

Exercise 20

Stomach muscles

The stomach muscles play an important role in singing. Therefore, this exercise is invaluable unless you already have a trained body. Many women believe they cannot do this exercise. I too felt that way at first. The point is that the breathing helps you to get up. Without the initial inhalation, you cannot move at all. Note that this exercise is not suitable for people with back problems.

- Lie down on your back with your knees bent and the soles of the feet placed on the floor. The arms are stretched down alongside the body.
- Breathe in through your nose and, in an extension of the inhalation, lift your upper body up and forward while trying to reach down between the knees with the tip of the nose.

- Breathe out and roll back to the lying position. Aim to do this exercise five times, then relax and try to do it five more times. Regulate the number of repetitions according to your physical strength. It is essential to pause in the middle. In addition, women need to do the root lock – pull the bottom of their pelvis up, because of the pressure on the uterus.

A more difficult version of the exercise is to do it with your hands folded behind your neck and/or with outstretched legs.

Exercise 21

Balance, awareness of the hara, activation of the body's energy flow
- Stand with legs slightly apart and note your point of balance, the *hara*, a hand's width below the navel.
- At the same time, fix your eyes on a specific spot in your surroundings.
- Let the two points merge in your awareness.
- Stand on your right leg and, with your left hand, take hold of your left instep. Pull your leg back and up into a horizontal position. This presses the lower leg down, which pulls on the arm.
- Besides the stretch in your thighs, you can also feel how your shoulder blade is pressed inwards. Keep the position as long as possible and keep your focus concentrated on the inner point (*hara*) and the outer point (in the room) the whole time. The free arm is used as a balancing bar. Breathe deeply in this position.
- Change sides. If your ears buzz and everything goes black afterwards, bend forwards with your head and arms, as in exercise 10. If you want an even greater challenge, hold the instep with both hands.

Exercise 22

Opening the chest, relieving pain between the
shoulder blades

- Lie on your right side, bend your left knee, slide it forwards and down to the floor. Put your right hand on the bent left knee. Then stretch the left arm back. The arm will be up in the air for most people. You will feel a wonderful stretch in the chest and the whole shoulder area. Breathe deeply into the tension around the arm. Try to relax in this position. Take your time. You can relax the muscles by letting the arm rest in front of your chest for a moment, after which you roll back into the stretch.
- Lie in the position until the hand touches the floor on its own. Eventually it will, although it may take some time. After that, turn onto your left side and do the same exercise with your right arm.

This exercise is frequently used in yoga and relaxation.

Exercise 23

Sealing off uncontrolled air in the voice

This is a classical glottis exercise. The glottis is the narrow opening between the two vocal cords. When there is a lot of air in the voice, the glottis can become a bit loose. It doesn't close enough when you want to make a distinct or sharp sound. The following exercise needs to be done very carefully and, to begin with, preferably together with a teacher, who can make sure that you are using the muscles correctly.

You start by not actually clearing your throat, but by being just about to do so. Instead of an explosive and unhealthy clearing, there will be a delicate little click. It feels as if you are creating small, crispy bubbles that float out of your throat like pearls. The sound of a creaking door, which is easy to make instead, is much coarser in sound. If you creak, then try to split the sound up into small, isolated bubble sounds.

Do not do the exercise for more than five minutes at a time. It can be done inconspicuously in almost any situation.

The Practice CD

I have attempted as far as possible to tailor the practice CD to each singer's individual needs. As stressed in Part 1 of this book, the idea is to start by singing Sa, the root note, only. This is the principle behind tracks 1 and 2, and later track 21.

When you have worked with a point of the CD (except track 1) I recommend that you repeat for example singing Sa Re alone with the tanpura on track 21. That is the only point where you will be totally confronted by your own sound and, through that experience, develop your consciousness and self-confidence.

If you start by playing the CD and trying to sing along with it all the way through, you will have begun at the finishing line. You are meant to gradually add more points to your singing practice until eventually you are able to use the whole CD.

If you follow the procedure described above, then, by the time you have finished the CD, you will be able to improvise similar sequences yourself without any support other than the tanpura accompaniment.

Once you have learned to sing the note names fluently, you can go on to connect the notes to colors and chakras (see the diagram on page 119) and in that way give your body a Sound Healing.[31] The healthiest way to sound-heal your own chakras is to see them as a coherent energy flow, where a slow vocal gliding between the notes can cleanse the connections between the corresponding chakras. A balanced flow is thus created through which the energy can run more freely. The result is that your voice becomes more beautiful and that you feel more whole as a person. When concentrating sound on a single chakra in isolation, be careful not to do it for more than three minutes at a time.

The range of notes on the practice CD stretches up to a one-stringed A – that is, right up to the place where most women's and some men's voices begin to change gear from speech register to falsetto, which in many instances results in the voice breaking.

I have chosen this pitch mostly because one of the basic premises of this book is that the muscular support needs to be mastered and completely assimilated in the body in the speech register (the lower part of the voice) before you move up to the higher notes. This is where the "space" gets increasingly narrow, making correct location of the note even more important. It is impossible to maintain such full awareness if you are simultaneously concentrating on developing your body support.

A second reason is that you risk harming your voice if you practice the high tones without guidance from a singing teacher. This is especially true for those inexperienced in listening to themselves and their body's signals.

Track-by-track comments

Track 1

Before you move on to anything else, you need the Note from Heaven to break through on the root note. Track 1 is a preparatory guide for singing the Note from Heaven. You can discard this guidance when you have found your own key image and when good habits of body posture and breathing have become a natural way of being for you.

Track 2

Track 2, where I sing with you on the root note, and track 21, where you can sing alone with the tanpura accompaniment, give you an opportunity to practice the Note from Heaven.

I have included my voice on this track as support. The idea is that you sing over my voice using the rhythm of your breathing. You are not meant to sing after me.

Halfway through track 2, I sing the primal sound behind the Note from Heaven[32] three times. The volume of the note has been reduced to avoid startling unnecessarily. You can sing the primal sound yourself, if and when you need to find your power.

You should repeat track 2 several times while you are in the first phase – trying to open yourself to the Note from Heaven.

Tracks 3-10

This is a slow improvisation, where the major scale is introduced in different combinations. Each phrase is followed by a pause so you can repeat the phrase.

The same phrase is always repeated two times, first in Indian note language and then in "Aaar". This activates both brain hemispheres and enables you to learn both the note names and create a beautiful sound.

With each track, another note is added to the improvisation, so that you can proceed as slowly as you wish. Note that it can easily take weeks to learn the note combinations when a new note has been added. With daily practice, it can take a year to learn to sing along with the whole practice CD.

What is important is not how good you are at note combinations, but how well you feel when you sing.

Practice each track by listening to yourself singing alone with the tanpura accompaniment. Do not rush through it, wanting to be able to do it all at once. For example, try to practice two notes (track 3) and then improvise by yourself with the tanpura (track 21). See also the example of a method of working on page 64.

Tracks 11-20

These ten tracks provide outlines of the flexibility exercises to give you an idea of the melodic sequence of the exercises.

Practice these exercises at your own speed with the support of the tanpura accompaniment (track 21).

Track 21

If you are unsure whether you are singing in tune, it is a good idea to turn up the sound of the tanpura. Let yourself be enveloped in its tones and glide into the landscape with your sound. Soon you will come to recognize when you are singing in tune. If you are still in any doubt, ask someone you trust to give you feedback.

Choose a volume level that enables you both to hear yourself and safely lean on the tanpura's supportive tapestry of sound.

Contents of each track

Track 1 – 8:24

Introduction – establishing breathing and concentrating on the key image.

Track 2 – 5:10

1 note: Sa (sound A)

Track 3 – 3:54

2 notes: Sa, Re (sound A, B)

Track 4 – 5:14

3 notes: Ṇi, Sa, Re (sound G#, A, B)

Track 5 – 6:15

4 notes: Ṇi, Sa, Re, Gha (sound G#, A, B, C#)

Track 6 – 4:17
5 notes: Ṇi, Sa, Re, Gha, Ma (sound G#, A, B, C#, D)

Track 7 – 10:16
6 notes: Ṇi, Sa, Re, Gha, Ma, Pa (sound G#, A, B, C#, D, E)

Track 8 – 5:54
7 notes: Ṇi, Sa, Re, Gha, Ma, Pa, Dha (sound G#, A, B, C#, D, E, F#)

Track 9 – 6:27
8 notes: Ṇi, Sa, Re, Gha, Ma, Pa, Dha, Ni (sound G#, A, B, C#, D, E, F#, G#)

Track 10 – 6:45
9 notes: Ṇi, Sa, Re, Gha, Ma, Pa, Dha, Ni, Sa (sound G#, A, B, C#, D, E, F#, G#, A)

Track 11 – 0:51
The first basic exercise is to sing the scale with the note names.

Organize your method of breathing according to your ability. For example, upwards on a breath, up and down on a breath, twice up and down or three times up and down on a breath.

When you can sing the scale twice on a breath with note language and "Aaar" respectively, you can go further.

Sa, Re, Gha, Ma, Pa, Dha, Ni, Ṡa – Ṡa, Ni, Dha, Pa, Ma, Gha, Re, Sa

Track 12 – 0:24
Sa Sa, Re Re, Gha Gha, Ma Ma, Pa Pa, Dha Dha, Ni Ni, Ṡa Ṡa.

Ṡa Ṡa, Ni Ni, Dha Dha, Pa Pa, Ma Ma, Gha Gha, Re Re, Sa Sa

Sing the note names first and then repeat the phrase in "Aaar". Move your breathing according to your ability, but always sing slowly enough to be able to enjoy your singing.

Note that the passages between the quick "Aaars" always flow within each breath, just as when you write with a pen without lifting it from the paper.

To glide in that way, you approach the note by gliding downwards a little and then up again. This glide is quick and imperceptible and fluctuates by approximately a third.

This technique is called *gamak* and is a profound part of Indian singing. It is a movement that takes place only in the throat.

To practice *gamak*, try to say "A-haar", as if you were suddenly realizing something.

On the last part, the "haar", glide from above and downwards within the tone of your voice. Note the effect on your own throat. It should also move downwards on "A-haar".

Try to say "A-haaraaraaraaraar" as a wavy movement.

The technique can be practiced separately throughout the whole scale. It is beneficial to practice the glides in slow motion and then slowly increase the tempo. Notice that the note, your fixed point, is always totally pure. It is like a well-memorized fact in your mind. You can pull at the fact, which is elastic, but, when you release the elastic, it springs back to its starting point.

It is particularly beneficial to practice *gamak* in exercises that use repetition of the same tone. For example, exercise 12 (Sa Sa, Re Re...) or exercises where there are movements in thirds, for example Sa Gha, Re Ma, Gha Pa... (see exercises 17, 18, 19 and 20).

Track 13 – 0:24

Let's sing tones three and three:

Sa Re Gha, Re Gha Ma, Gha Ma Pa, Ma Pa Dha, Pa Dha Ni, Dha Ni Ṡa

Ṡa Ni Dha, Ni Dha Pa, Dha Pa Ma, Pa Ma Gha, Ma Gha Re, Gha Re Sa

Track 14 – 0:25

After that, you can permeate the spine with the same exercise pattern using four notes:

Sa Re Gha Ma, Re Gha Ma Pa, Gha Ma Pa Dha, Ma Pa Dha Ni, Pa Dha Ni Śa

Śa Ni Dha Pa, Ni Dha Pa Ma, Dha Pa Ma Gha, Pa Ma Gha Re, Ma Gha Re Sa

Track 15 – 0:26

Exercise 3 can be done backwards:

Gha Re Sa, Ma Gha Re, Pa Ma Gha, Dha Pa Ma, Ni Dha Pa, Śa Ni Dha

Dha Ni Śa, Pa Dha Ni, Ma Pa Dha, Gha Ma Pa, Re Gha Ma, Sa Re Gha

Track 16 – 0:41

You can do it in both directions:

Sa Re Gha Re Sa, Re Gha Ma Gha Re, Gha Ma Pa Ma Gha

Ma Pa Dha Pa Ma, Pa Dha Ni Dha Pa, Dha Ni Śa Ni Dha, then do it backwards

Track 17 – 0:27

Another classic exercise is to do every other note, which is breaking the scale into thirds:

Sa Gha, Re Ma, Gha Pa, Ma Dha, Pa Ni, Dha Śa

Śa Dha, Ni Pa, Dha Ma, Pa Gha, Ma Re, Gha Sa

Track 18 – 0:25

Or in reverse:

Gha Sa, Ma Re, Pa Gha, Dha Ma, Ni Pa, Śa Dha

Dha Śa, Pa Ni, Ma Dha, Gha Pa, Re Ma, Sa Gha (Ṇi Re Sa)

Track 19 – 0:23

The two previous exercises combined:

Sa Gha, Ma Re, Gha Pa, Dha Ma, Pa Ni, Śa Dha, Ni Ṙe, Ġha Śa

Śa Ġha, Ṙe Ni, Dha Śa, Ni Pa, Ma Dha, Pa Gha, Re Ma, Gha Sa

Track 20 – 0:48

Sa Re Gha Gha, Re Gha Ma Ma, Gha Ma Pa Pa, Ma Pa Dha Dha,
Pa Dha Ni Ni, Dha Ni Śa Śa

Śa Ni Dha Dha, Ni Dha Pa Pa, Dha Pa Ma Ma, Pa Ma Gha
Gha, Ma Gha Re Re, Gha Re Sa Sa

Find your own combinations, write them down and practice
them in track 21.

Track 21 – 9:00

The tanpura tuned to Pạ, Sa, Sa, Ṣa (sound E, A1, A1, A).

In addition, see page 39 on the root note.

Applying the Tanpura Accompaniment to the Piano

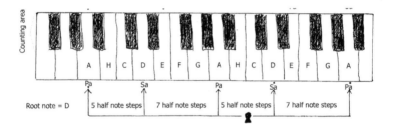

*This is an example of the calculation of the accompanying notes for a
root note in D = Sa.*

*A half-note step is a movement from one note to its nearest neighbor
on the keyboard, whether black or white. It is easiest to count the half-
note steps correctly when you count closest to the keyboard in the
counting zone where the black keys are.*

Chakra Overview

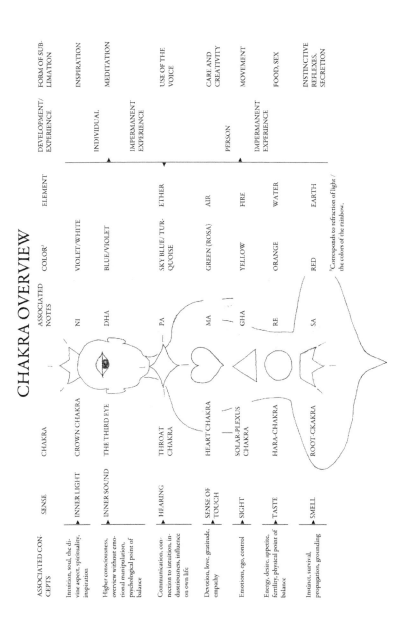

CHAKRA OVERVIEW

ASSOCIATED CONCEPTS	SENSE	CHAKRA	ASSOCIATED NOTES	COLOR[2]	ELEMENT	DEVELOPMENT/EXPERIENCE	FORM OF SUBLIMATION
Intuition, soul, the divine aspect, spirituality, inspiration	INNER LIGHT	CROWN CHAKRA	NI	VIOLET/WHITE		INDIVIDUAL	INSPIRATION
Higher consciousness, overview without emotional manipulation, psychological point of balance	INNER SOUND	THE THIRD EYE	DHA	BLUE/VIOLET		IMPERMANENT EXPERIENCE	MEDITATION
Communication, connection to intuition, industriousness, influence on own life	HEARING	THROAT CHAKRA	PA	SKY BLUE/TURQUOISE	ETHER		USE OF THE VOICE
Devotion, love, gratitude, empathy	SENSE OF TOUCH	HEART CHAKRA	MA	GREEN (ROSA)	AIR	PERSON	CARE AND CREATIVITY
Emotions, ego, control	SIGHT	SOLAR-PLEXUS CHAKRA	GHA	YELLOW	FIRE		MOVEMENT
Energy, desire, appetite, fertility, physical point of balance	TASTE	HARA-CHAKRA	RE	ORANGE	WATER	IMPERMANENT EXPERIENCE	FOOD, SEX
Instinct, survival, propagation, grounding	SMELL	ROOT-CKAKRA	SA	RED	EARTH		INSTINCTIVE REFLEXES, SECRETION

[2]Corresponds to refraction of light / the colors of the rainbow.

Sing Yourself Free:
Regressive Cell-Singing

Dedicated to Péleh Ben-David

Introduction

My second book on the Note from Heaven focuses on a method I have developed called regressive cell-singing, in which you can sing yourself free from traumas that have their origin in this life, the womb or previous lifetimes.

Emotional stress affects our whole organism and causes it to go out of tune. We are all born in tune, with a beautiful composition in our cell structure, a matrix which contains our full potential and which is reflected in our voice.

In regressive cell-singing the Note from Heaven is used as a tuning fork to retune cells to their former harmony.

My view of trauma is as a tension that blocks the free flow of energy in the body, a blockage that weakens the life force and thereby, if left untreated, causes imbalance and illness.

In regressive cell-singing any notes, sounds or outbursts that genuinely express the Note from Heaven can release blocked energy imprisoned in the singer's body as trauma. The process starts a cell-dance, which reorganizes the body into its original balanced matrix.

The method can work alone or in combination with any other kind of therapy. Essentially, when you sing yourself free you spit out the poisoned piece of apple and return to life, just as Snow White did when the prince kissed her and woke her from her deep sleep in the glass coffin.

Part 1:

Collective Traumatization

There is no sin. It is you who make sin exist...
Gospel of Mary Magdalene

Collective Traumatization

Dear reader, in order to bring to your attention one of the biggest collective traumas in the Western world, I will refer to a number of quotes from the apocryphal writings, especially from the Gospel of Thomas. These writings, which are an expression of Gnostic wisdom, were banned in 324 CE by the church fathers who selected the texts that we know today as the New Testament.

When the Gnostic scripts were found hidden in caves in the mid-twentieth century, scholars surmised that some of the authors had probably been disciples of Jesus, and that their writings reflect his original message: a teaching based on self-knowledge and self-development. Orthodox Christianity's dogmatic use of sin, shame and judgment seems to misinterpret this message of love.

We humans are much more influenced by our historical, religious and cultural roots than most of us realize. Orthodox Christianity conditions us to feel that we are "not good enough" and to cultivate false humility, which limit our belief in our own essence. This perception immediately rules out the Note from Heaven as a possibility because we do not feel worthy of the light!

These collective religious traumas lie deeply stored in our subconscious mind and act as the main gateway in the process of release. If a person is in contact with his or her inner divinity, then it is usually easy to find resonance. If the gateway is closed, then as a healer you can at best scratch the surface a little. "I carry my burden with a smile." If a person doesn't want to throw off their burden, then no healer can wrest it from them.

For centuries, Christianity and other religions have suppressed the feminine powers. These include holistic thinking, compassion, intuitive knowledge and wisdom, and a natural tendency to cooperate. Religious authorities have also undermined the sacredness of eroticism through condemnation and punishment, making believers feel guilty for the sexuality that we are all born with. The fact that more and more people are now rejecting these controls is for me a sign that we are ready to open ourselves up to a higher level of consciousness which can only be reached by unfolding the feminine divinity within.

Overcoming the historical traumas, however, is a challenge, for fear is all-encompassing. A woman who has become traumatized after being attacked by a man may find her trauma reactivated by contact with any other man reminding her of that man. Similarly, our experience of any form of religiousness and, therefore, spirituality is affected by these universal, archetypal religious traumas. I believe that spirituality is an expression of the intuitive abilities we all innately possess. However, the historical traumas have stunted our self-development and undermined our confidence in our intuition and innate divinity. The traumatized cornerstones that our cultural heritage is built on must be dug up and brought to light. The most effective tool for this purpose is from my experience to unfold the voice through singing.

The path
You must burn in order to shine.
Lars Muhl (Author, spiritual teacher)

Our destiny can feel like a bumpy ride on a dirt road full of potholes, but when we look back on our journey the higher meaning of all the trouble becomes clear. It turns out that the dirt road leads to a very beautiful place, which we have been destined to reach from the beginning. Some people have high ambitions, they get famous and we think they have accomplished everything. But, in fact, worldly success does not count on the other side of life. What does matter is that you find your path, and that you gain the courage to pursue it with dedication.

We all know people who seem to have found their calling: a wonderful kindergarten teacher, a waiter or sales clerk who has just the right feel for the customer, effortlessly sensing what they need and how best to serve them, a checkout assistant at the supermarket who gives you a smile that sends you home feeling good. To encounter people in their right element is pure joy.

When your light shines, you activate the light in others, and help them to remember that they are complete beings.

Anybody can shine! It is a matter of choice. If you wish to set your light free, then you need to unfold your wings. Let the wind carry you, and be prepared to land on both feet so you can fulfil your destiny on earth.

Dull birds. The cage door is open and you do not even dare to fly. I am scaring you in order to make you fly.
Gitta Mallasz (*Talking with Angels*)

The pain body

The pain body gives us license to project unacknowledged emotions onto our surroundings. It is the ego's mouthpiece and the shadow's storage space for emotions.

You may be wondering what it is that keeps us from walking our path on Earth, and why many of us subconsciously prefer to remain in the shadows.

The key to understanding this behavioral pattern can be found in the pain body.[33] We all have a pain body that in a stressful emotional situation offers us an amnesty, which temporarily puts our adult self-knowledge on hold. Wounded, we isolate ourselves in the pain body to recover our breath and restore ourselves. Here everything is black and white, as we regress to the level of a small child and dwell on a self-justifying, "Pity me!"

The pain body's function can be compared to a big black umbrella that we can open for protection against a sudden storm. Sheltering under the pain body umbrella, the mind gets time to compose itself and figure out how to regain control of the situation.

Temporary use of the pain body as described above is healthy and natural. But it can become a chronic and unhealthy habit. We can end up permanently hiding in a safe, secluded, deep, dark lake, where we drown our light in a soothing abdication of life's demands and responsibilities.

By staying continuously in the pain body, a person identifies with the role of victim and achieves a negatively charged status that separates them from the surrounding world, which they blame for their situation.

When people isolate themselves from their surroundings, they simultaneously exclude themselves from the Oneness level. They justify their pain and their self-perception as victims through a judgmental attitude that says, "I am here and you are there." The "pain" confers a special status around which they base their identity as victims. They complain, but do not want any help.

The four primary archetypal feelings that bind us to our pain body are:

- I am not good enough (I am not lovable).
- I do not belong.
- I am not allowed to be here.
- I do not wish to be here.

These negative thought patterns prevent us from taking part fully in life. They are caused by the fears of the ego and are usually already integrated as a part of our identity in the womb or in early childhood.

The pain body is our challenge, the wood for the fire that will raise our consciousness.

Will you be swallowed up by the darkness or be lifted up towards the light?

It is all about taking responsibility for yourself.

Adults, subconsciously trapped by choices made as infants, are not able to take full responsibility for themselves until they realize what programming they are suffering from.

Without being aware of it, we shackle ourselves to a post and move around in a circle like a chained dog, moaning and groaning or quietly whimpering as we cast longing glances at the horizon, sadly gazing at all the lovely things that are out of our reach.

The best tool to break the chain that links an identity to its pain body is awareness. The awareness is a matter of choice: will I be conscious, or will I not? Will I stay in prison or will I break free? Do I fear freedom? Who do I want to see in the mirror – the familiar little self or the unknown higher self?

Fear of the unknown causes most of us to prefer the pain we are familiar with, because we know what we have, but not what we could get.

Those who acknowledge their own shadow see the light.

A dark cloud can be experienced from two perspectives: you can remain inside it and become blinded and overwhelmed by despair, or you can see the cloud from the outside and recognize that it is merely temporarily hiding the sun.

In order to lift yourself outside the cloud, the consciousness needs a moment of stillness. This stillness will appear the moment you stop panicking, take a deep breath and embrace your pain body in total acceptance.

"I am ugly, I cannot sing, I had a terrible childhood, nobody likes me..." By repeating such mantras, you blow great black clouds in your own sunny way, and the pain body illusion manifests itself in reality. It is true that *"you are what you think"*. As our perception of life will always be an illusion and we can think whatever we like about ourselves, why not create a positive, sunny illusion and let that manifest itself in reality?

Plus power

The higher and lower selves can be seen as two separate parts: shadow and light. This perception causes pain, because it divides the whole. The whole self is unified: where there is light, there is shadow. In that way any minus can be changed to a plus by adding a single vertical line to it.

In the plus sign, the horizontal line symbolizes the dualistic world of good and bad. The vertical line symbolizes the Oneness level (fire – consciousness), which you can reach by lifting your "self" up above the horizon level (water – feelings). Embrace your emotional condition and seek a moment of stillness; this will bring you to the center of the cross, where you can raise your level of awareness.

In the rebalanced "plus" you see the positive part of the negative and can contain both parts within you: the pain body is fully accepted, because your consciousness observes everything from a higher perspective.

The small self (the pain body/ego) and the higher self (consciousness/the soul) are symbolized by two separated dots on either side of the horizontal line in the minus symbol. In the plus symbol, the two selves are connected and merged into oneness. The ego (master of the underworld) and consciousness (master of the upper world) collaborate, with the result that the heart literally opens its red velvet curtains in the middle of the chest.[34] And who appears on stage? The true you!

Every human being on earth is able to create Oneness in their life, to change all the minuses they have experienced into pluses, simply by singing themselves into Oneness. When your heart opens, your whole organism becomes aflame with enthusiasm and passion – a passion for walking your path in life.

Seek and ye shall find.
Matthew 7:7

When all is said and done, it seems meaningless to dig into the past again and again in order to find the reasons for one's lack of self-confidence. At a certain time, everyone must take responsibility for their own life.
Carl Gustav Jung

When I take responsibility for my own life, I stop looking for someone else to blame for my suffering. The responsibility opens my eyes to the possibilities that I alone have.
Anselm Grün

Rise up, take your stretcher and go home.
Mark 2:11

How to truly listen to your self
Blessed be the one who hears the call from the minaret of their heart.
Hazrat Inayat Khan (*Gayan, Vadan, Nirtan*)

When you hear you use only your ears, but when you listen attentively you use all of your senses.

By training your ability to hear microtones, over- and undertones, you are fine-tuning your sensitivity at all levels of your organism. Your awareness of careful listening is the only true master. Through listening to the feeling in the color of a voice, you develop your intuition and start to pick up messages that you were not aware of before. You sense people's energy and feel what is good and what is not good for you. Besides this, you improve your ability to be present in the moment.

When you sing yourself free of a trauma, the Note from Heaven will sound spontaneously the very moment you sing at the right frequency. When it appears, hold on to the sound that expresses the Note from Heaven until the physical tension connected to your trauma is released. If there are any other traumas or tensions in the body, just focus your attention on the affected cells and glide slowly up and down with your voice until you catch the Note from Heaven again. Let it guide you, just as you would follow a beam of light.

Preparing for Regressive Cell-singing

The essence of all life is vibration. When you strike a tuning fork tuned to 440 Hz, any other tuning forks in the room that have been tuned to the same frequency will also start ringing at an audible level. This effect is caused by resonance. If you stop the sound of the first tuning fork it will fall silent, but the others will continue to resonate.

This simple example demonstrates one of the most profound laws of nature: all vibrations in our universe influence each other. So when a frequency finds resonance in your body, it will set the resonating part of your cells in motion.

The question is, what is happening when a sound resonates in our body? Are the cells dancing? Is it our bodily fluids resonating? Is it a kind of electrical process, triggered by a sound impulse?

Even though the voice can affect us in the most ingenious ways, appeals to our senses, works from within us, and is far more sensitive than the most sophisticated computer, it has still not been thoroughly and scientifically investigated. And none of the research that has been carried out has been accepted by mainstream science or brought to the attention of the general public. The main explanation for this is perhaps financial –

the healing effect of the voice is a free medicine that cannot be monetized. Also, each person's voice is unique and the workings of the voice are so complicated that present-day scientific instruments can only measure a limited range of its frequencies. So we can only rely on our own practical experience.

Trust your senses by listening attentively to even the smallest signs from your body, and be aware of the particular circumstances in which they occur. Respond to your body's signals. You know better than anyone else how you feel, but you might not have given yourself the necessary attention because our world values the external over the internal.

When you act on what you feel, you listen to your "self" with the result that your "self"-estimation grows.

By listening to your whole self (including the ego's acceptable needs), you project "self"-respect into your surroundings and they will, in turn, respect you.

A sower went out to sow his seed: and as he sowed, some fell by the wayside; and it was trodden down, and the fowls of the air devoured it. And some fell upon a rock; and as soon as it was sprung up, it withered away, because it lacked moisture. And some fell among thorns; and the thorns sprang up with it, and choked it. And others fell on good ground, and sprang up, and bore fruit in hundredfold. And when Jesus had said these things, he cried: "He that has ears, let him hear."
Parable of the Sower, Luke 8:5-8

Through physical exercises, eating healthy food and respecting your basic psychological needs, you can ensure the Note from Heaven is sown in fertile ground. Through faithful listening to the self, you care for the seed and give it the right amount of water it needs to grow.

The soil symbolizes your pain body, the shadow. There is a lot of potential energy hidden there. You can see traumas as bank boxes that can only be opened by a specific key in the form of a certain frequency. The moment you open the box, the energy becomes free and available for use.

A heavily traumatized soil will have so much energy stored in it that it can be compared to pure compost. Only a limited range of plants will be able to grow in it. So, in order to normalize the soil the traumas must be opened and transformed one by one. At first, potatoes will be able to grow there and in that way the core trauma is transformed, then the next step is to grow squash, signifying the healing of the wounded heart that gradually reopens. Only then is the ground ready for more delicate plants like carrots, beans, salad vegetables, parsley and peas.

Some people who have been in therapy for years may have managed to open their trauma-boxes but not succeeded in withdrawing the blocked energy. In such cases, regressive cell-singing can work like a miracle: all the energy will be withdrawn in one go. The Note from Heaven unites the energy and opens up to its flow, as it casts its beam of resonance into the darkness. It can feel like striking oil or winning millions in the lottery. Some people even experience a spontaneous remission of serious illness when this kind of release happens. The inner experience of resonant sound "knows". God is sound.

You can only truly believe what you have perceived through your own experience.
George Harrison

Your ability to believe is equivalent to your ability to listen unconditionally.

Belief is not a foundation or a state within me. Belief is motion and mobility. God as voice and the human as ears.
Jesper Blomberg, priest in Udby, Denmark

Faith is a vibration that moves our body and soul. Fear causes atrophy and opposes faith.

Everything is given. All that has been hidden will be exposed. And that day is NOW! The illuminated consciousness is NOW and forever.
Lars Muhl (*Grail*)

The Note from Heaven – a gateway to Oneness

In recent years my work with singing has provided me with an increasing number of opportunities for personal development. The Note from Heaven is the key factor common to all of them. My personal understanding of the concept of the Note from Heaven is continually expanding and changing, because contact with that state of mind is a constantly unfolding process which seems to stretch all the way out to the quantum physics of the infinite universe. The Note from Heaven is a doorway to the "moment".

The disciples asked Jesus, "When will you reveal yourself to us, and when are we going to see you?" Jesus replied, "When you take your clothes off without feeling shame and when you take your clothing and put it under your feet and step on it, like small children. Then you will see the son of the living and you will not fear."
Gospel of Thomas, log. 37

Once someone has experienced the state induced by the Note from Heaven breaking through, they will usually search for it again. The path through the undergrowth to the awakening Sleeping Beauty needs to be trodden many times before a permanent pathway is established. Then the Note from Heaven is yours forever. It will sing through you and influence you in far broader perspectives than you can possibly imagine.

Grounding

The human body is an electrical system. It is able to transport an electrical charge with a strength that is carefully adjusted to the resistance that nerves and glands are equipped with in relation to electrical currents. The stronger the body is physically (the meridians' state of purity), the greater the electrical charge it can handle.

Dr. Stephen T. Chang (*The Complete System of Self-Healing*)

For an electrical system to be able to function safely, it needs to be earthed. In the same way, being grounded is also a prerequisite for the body's electrical system to be able to support an influx of energy.

From experience with sound scanning[35] and regressive cell-singing, I know that the stomach, hips, legs and feet correspond to our roots and those deep tones/undertones resonate well here. The higher up in the body the sound moves, the higher the tone, the finer the amplitude, the stronger the electrical current. The way to work safely with strong electrical currents is to have the means to discharge them through grounding.

When the voice cracks and won't function at a high pitch or you get sore from singing, it's a sign that you may have lost your grounding – physically and or energetically.

The voice protects us, like a fuse, ensuring the organism doesn't get burnt.

The soft tissues, keeping our intestines in place (hara), have been determined scientifically to be an independent organ called the mesentery, which is able to store energy. Therefore both the hara and root chakras are crucial for grounding the sound. Contracting the abdomen during exhalation activates and balances the organism's energetic support system and avoids the body having to compensate by tensing the muscles of the chest and throat.

A person with weak grounding should not be exposed to

high overtones without preliminary grounding.[36] This applies to people suffering from stress, for example, as well as those in crisis and highly sensitive souls. Therefore, it is a good practice always to start by working at the deep end of the vocal pitch, as that helps to ground the body and mind.

The experience of being sung by a higher power

Anyone who experiences the Note from Heaven will know what it feels like to "be sung". Below are some typical comments made by participants in my courses:

"It feels as if it isn't me singing!"
"I thought it was everyone else's voices, but it was me."
"Where did that sound come from? Was that me?"
"I could have kept on singing forever."
"Don't you have to breathe?"
"It felt as if I was an open reed, a channel."

Here is an example of a longer feedback:

It's hard to describe, but the way I experience it is that the release which took place at the course in regressive cell-singing just kept going and going… I still have the sensation of volume that I felt in my hara chakra while singing… maybe not the whole time, but I can return to it when I consciously think about it. I don't think I have ever been present in that part of myself before, if you know what I mean… suddenly I was three-dimensional. There was a little white shiny tube sitting in the center of my hara chakra that went up through my throat and switched on a light on the top of my head… and I felt a sense of grief for having hidden my power and my light away for such a long time… And then the grief just disappeared and I was pure sound.
Response from a course participant (Liselotte)

Contact with the Note from Heaven

The ego will not surrender before it recognizes a higher power.

Ramana Maharshi

You are advised to open your voice according to the instructions in *The Note from Heaven* Book I before you practice the following sections.

When you sing yourself free of deep traumas, you should work with a "listener". A listener is a kind of midwife-therapist who supports the singer in the process of regressive cell-singing. In my International Education in The Note from Heaven, the students are trained to be good listeners.

The first thing a listener must do is support the singer in breathing correctly.

Breathing and the Note from Heaven

The vocal expression of our soul can only come into being as movement of air through our respiratory passageways.

Dr. Audun Myskja MD (*Music as Medicine*)

Our breathing is inextricably connected to our psychological state. When we get a shock, we gasp and the amygdalas in the brain turn on the alarm[1] starting an immediate response in the hippocampus. When we find ourselves in a dangerous or stressful situation, our muscles tense, our senses become heightened and our breathing becomes shallow, part of the innate fight-or-flight reflex. Peter Levine describes in his book *Waking the Tiger* how the gazelle instinctively stiffens and plays dead when a lion drags it away as its prey.

Surrendering to its fate creates a potential opportunity for the gazelle to get away the second the lion lets go of its "dead" prey and maybe looks the other way in a moment of distraction. When, and if, the gazelle does escape, it will then react by violently shaking itself, as if it is shaking the experience off.

Afterwards the gazelle is, apparently, not traumatized.

Although this response is incredibly useful in an actual emergency, for many of us it becomes chronic, which causes problems. When we tense up, we almost completely stop breathing. Our fight-or-flight mechanism instinctively cuts off the connection to the digestive system for the purpose of gathering as much energy as possible to be able to run away and survive an emergency.

A lot of people walk around with a frozen breath like tense gazelles that never ran away and never shook off the tensions from their traumas.

During a complete inhalation, the lungs are filled to the maximum. The organs are, therefore, pushed down to the stomach, which then bulges out. The stomach is a big gift. Don't make it smaller than it is.

During an active exhalation, the diaphragm and stomach muscles are pushed inwards, and the organs are pressed up towards the lungs, which are emptied of air. You can, of course, empty the lungs of air without using your stomach muscles, in a sigh where you "let the air out of the balloon". But for effective singing and emotional release, you need to activate the "support" from your stomach muscles.[37]

Your body's "accelerator pedal" is located in the area under the navel. You can feel it like a slanting plate that slopes from the beginning of the lower abdomen and up under the navel. The "fuel tank" is located in the *hara*, the stomach area. To send energy out into the body's circulation system, you have to press the accelerator pedal – the abdomen and stomach muscles.

Everyone carries shock or trauma of some kind. A traumatic experience in our past can cause an instinctive reaction that results in shallow chest breathing without active use of the diaphragm.

When you do not feel that you are good enough as you are, then you naturally try to change yourself: the full breath is restricted, the shoulders are pushed way up to the ears, breathing is superficial and confined to the chest and throat, while tensions in the solar plexus act as a check.

In an attempt to compensate for the feeling "I am not allowed to be here", you breathe superficially to make yourself as small as possible.

As children, many of us were told to be quiet when we were just about to test our full breath by shouting. Children love to shout, because they feel their strength when the breath unfolds completely and functions optimally.[38]

Very few adults recognize or appreciate a child's vocal sound quality when it naturally and with great vitality opens up with the Note from Heaven. The majority of grown-ups have themselves been scolded for making loud noises and, therefore, consider shouting to be undesirable. Thus the pattern is inherited, and happily and unconsciously passed on in the name of good parenting.

Women may feel the need to conform to the idea of "the weaker sex". We push our bust up and hold in our stomach. But by doing this, we cut ourselves off from our power.

Breathing uneconomically is like driving a car in the wrong gear – you end up using twice as much fuel as you need to. In Indian philosophy, life is measured according to the number of breaths we take. If the breathing is the best it can be, one lives optimally and the organism is strained as little as possible.

The breath testifies to the inseparability of body and mind. Every thought sets a process in motion in our physiology. Every physical stimulus influences our psyche.

Shallow breathing reinforces feelings of inferiority: we are never good enough, because we feel we are hiding something away. To hide our true self is to deceive. Imagine, what if someone finds out? How disgraceful! And so the vicious circle continues.

Living a lie can sap our energy and in most cases we don't

even know the cause or identity of this falsehood. A full breath is like a liberating sigh: "I give myself permission to be who I am."

The challenge in taking that step can be overwhelming if you are one of those people who is like a car that is only getting a few miles to the gallon. Being asked to inhale "correctly" deep down into the stomach can feel totally disorienting. Fortunately, the body has maintained the function. A shortcut to experiencing the full breath is to "let go" in the moment, to leap, to live out your emotions by surrendering into Oneness.

When we are overwhelmed by genuine feelings or when we yawn, the full breath functions the way it is meant to. It is like an oasis, where you can be yourself. Many of us breathe deeply when we sleep regardless of the quality of our breathing during waking hours. However, I have come across people whose trauma has infiltrated so thoroughly that their breathing reflexes do not function properly even during sleep.

How a listener can support the opening of a traumatized breath

- Invite the singer to hold his or her hand on your stomach while you at the same time put your hand lightly on their stomach, if that is okay with them. Breathe simultaneously. In the role of listener, show the singer how the stomach moves out on the in breath and is pressed gradually inwards while exhaling. This tactile and sensual experience through touch can do wonders.[39]
- Guide the singer through classical breathing exercise 14 from Book I (see Book I, page 104).
- Stand behind the singer. If they permit you to do so, support the singer's neck with your right hand (this soothes the autonomic nervous system/reptilian brain) and place your left palm *lightly* on their forehead (this

activates the anti-stress points in the forehead). As the reptilian brain/the brainstem, which governs instincts, heartbeat and breathing, and is associated with the flight-or-fight reflex, is helped to relax, the singer will breathe a sigh of relief and lean their head slightly backwards as the breath starts to open. If the stomach breath is working well you can urge the singer to open their arms and express whatever sound feels comfortable. When the Note from Heaven breaks through, the breath is fully unfolded.

How a singer can work alone with a traumatized breath

- Concentrate on a physical tension and seek to express the feeling of that tension with your voice.
- Lie in a fetal position and breathe, hum quietly and comfortingly to yourself and note how your breathing gradually gets deeper. Undertones and low tones... sing what feels good.
- Perhaps take a teddy bear or some other soft thing and imagine that it is you when you were a baby. Hold it close to your heart and sing to it. Have fun with it. Notice that your breath becomes deeper. Eventually take the teddy bear with you wherever you go in the house so you can nurture yourself.

Images and the Note from Heaven

In the first years after I explored the Note from Heaven, I taught singing with the aim of bringing the singer into contact with his or her natural voice.

I usually cheered the singer on when their voice started to open up to an authenticity that touched my heart.

It was during this type of teaching that I once came across a highly educated woman with an unusually strong resistance to opening up. She had a determination that was difficult to tackle.

From childhood I have seen images flowing through my mind when I relax. I never took much notice of them, as I always thought they were a kind of dream or flight of my imagination. When I was getting nowhere with this particular woman, despite all my efforts, I noticed some clear inner images appearing every time I listened to her voice with my eyes closed. It felt like quite a big step for me to share these images as I had never before talked to anybody about them. But finally I asked the singer, hesitantly, if she wanted to hear what I saw. She agreed.

I described to the singer the image of a woman slowly walking down the aisle of a large cathedral with her unusually long hair let down, trailing behind her like a gown (the course participant had a short page hairstyle). At the altar she meets a priest who orders her to put her hair up.

The priest addresses the singer directly through me and asks her if she would agree to put her hair up in that situation. She replied emphatically, "Heavens no! Why should I submit to the priest's demands for piety?"

The imaginary priest then calmly explains that it will be much easier for her to open her voice, if she puts her hair up. The Singer then agrees to roll up the whole lot of it onto the top of her head.

The very moment the singer imagined the woman with her hair all set up on top of her head, the Note from Heaven broke through.

I clearly remember this episode, because it opened up completely new avenues for working with the Note from Heaven. The story and use of images in relation to the singer's sound expression led me to devise the vocal release format, which later evolved into regressive cell-singing.

We Are Tone-Deaf

I established regressive cell-singing during the Christmas season of 2003. Several tone-deaf people had participated in my Sound Healing and singing courses. One day, one of them called me and told me it had been nice to experience that her sound could be healing, but she also wanted to be able to sing along to Christmas carols without feeling embarrassed. "Can you make a course where we learn how to sing in tune?" she asked.

I had previously had good experiences with one-to-one singing lessons for supposedly tone-deaf people. While surrendering to the Note from Heaven, they experienced moments when they forgot themselves and sang completely in tune. It was already one of my hobbyhorses: everyone can sing. Tone deafness is a blockage that can be removed. I had no idea how, but I firmly believed that it was possible.

Before I knew what had happened, there was a group of five totally tone-deaf people. I had no idea how to design the course. One thing was for sure, though: no more than five participants. Three days before the course, I received the revelation that to this day is still the core of regressive cell-singing:

- A blockage is stored in the body's cells.
- Cells can be energized and purified by sound.
- By activating the emotion that has created the blockage, the appropriate cells are contacted.

The unresolved emotion is reactivated through *code words*: particular thoughts, images, sounds, words and expressions that touch the traumatized person emotionally.

The moment the emotion is activated, it is transformed into a sensation and affects the singer's physical state in the form of tension, pain, discomfort, difficulty breathing... symptoms of the suppressed discomfort that a trauma or shock have caused.

The outward, physical symptoms are the therapist's only

way of measuring the degree of release taking place during regressive cell-singing. When recited at the end of the session, *the code words* that caused discomfort at the beginning of the session should now be demonstrating no, or at least only minimal, physical reaction.

When a person's tone deafness or other trauma originated before he or she started speaking as an infant, playing with baby sounds can bring the adult human back to a bodily experience of that preverbal state.

The sounds can easily spark off reflexes such as sucking, kicking, crawling and grasping, especially if the practitioner is lying on a mattress on the floor. The singers should be encouraged to give free rein to these responses; perhaps by being nursed or maybe even tickled a bit.

Parts of the tone-deaf person's identity have been kept on coat hangers in the pain body's dark closet. Some of the outfits are for formal and official use – for example, "I can't sing in tune, so I will keep my mouth shut" – but there are also moth-bitten clothes lurking in the recesses of the closet as forgotten hopes: "The teacher told me to stop singing, maybe he was mistaken?"

As the listener, I am fully convinced that the teacher was probably right that his student was singing out of tune at that moment, but at the same time I know he was wrong to leave that student alone with their self-perception, "I can't sing." My antidote to that is: "Yes, you can sing! No matter how hard you try to convince me that you can't, I won't believe you. I know you can! What you are suffering from is a certain type of trauma, which is a frozen sense of powerlessness that has become a reflex. This means that every time you are about to sing, the 'chained dog' inside of you starts howling, telling you that it is pointless to try."

The day of the course came. We played with the body's sounds and in that way slowly got closer to the five participants' blockages. After we had worked for four hours, finding and vocally releasing the blockages at the root of their tone deafness, and looking at each individual's specific difficulty, I sat down at the piano. We had not practiced singing in tune at any time. I'll never forget that moment. I thought to myself, they must realize that this is an experiment; if even one of them manages to sing in tune, I'll be more than happy. I played two notes. The whole group repeated them together. Each one of them could do it. It continued like that. In the end, I went so far as to sing children's songs with them. Yes – they could even hold the tone when I added in a second voice. So we threw ourselves into singing in canon. The atmosphere was thick with energy and several had tears in their eyes. We sang and sang. Finally, each of the participants plunged into singing solo. They each chose a particularly cherished song that they had dreamed of being able to sing their whole life. I remember one woman in particular who sang, "Edelweiss, Edelweiss..." without going off track at all. She and all the other participants achieved what is normally considered as "singing in tune".

This experience became a decisive turning point. If singing therapy could dissolve blockages of tone deafness,[40] then surely it could be used to dissolve other types of blockage too.

Footnote

1. You can sing Hung Song on the amygdala and rebalance them, if the shock is establishing a chronic condition. See film link.

Part 2:
Regressive Cell-Singing

Principles and Practice

Jesus said: "When you bring forth that in yourselves, this which is yours will save you; if you do not bring forth that in yourselves, this which is not yours in you will kill you."
Gospel of Thomas, log. 7

In regressive cell-singing, the listener supports the singer in singing his or her cells free of the energy trapped inside them. When the energy is liberated it reveals itself as the Note from Heaven.

In order to listen to a singer empathetically, you need to accept their state completely.

Sound is mere being. No judgment exists here.

The deeper you are able to listen to another person's sound, the stronger the presence, the greater the sense of safety and human intimacy that can arise.

In regressive cell-singing all feelings are equally valued, because, in terms of sound, they all have energetic potential.

The purpose of the process is to set free the specific frequency that every true emotional expression embodies, to acknowledge and express these sounds and let them ring, so the earth shakes. Those listening are delighted, uplifted by the energy, and wish for more – more. Sing more for us.

A suppressed feeling is an emotion. A feeling is "felt" in the body.

An emotion is transformed into a feeling when it is acknowledged.

A feeling is transformed into an energetic state when it is fully accepted and exempted from judgment.

Listener and singer

In regressive cell-singing, the person singing him or herself free is called the singer. The responsible therapist is called a listener. The listener's main purpose is to listen carefully to the singer's expression of sound and reflect or mirror what they hear; partly through practical advice about the sound and the physical aspects of its production, and partly through encouragement and passing on useful intuitive input and/or images.

Overview of a one-day course in regressive cell-singing

First contact between listener and singers

When someone registers for a session or a course, I ask for a few general details, but a minimum of personal ones. Occupation and education are the usual factors that bind a person to an old identity. Therefore, it is best that no one knows in advance who each person is. This will avoid prejudgments based on people's status.

In the case of heavily traumatized course participants, it is nevertheless important for the listener to know briefly what the case is about by privately discussing it with the singer.[41] Avoid going into too many details about the trauma, as that can weaken the effect of any subsequent "storytelling" (see page 187). The listener should reassure the participant that it is possible to take part without having to reveal which trauma is responsible for the sonic release. If embarrassing situations come up in a singer's story, never ask for an explanation or response. This discretion ensures that the focus stays on releasing the trauma. The actual nature of the trauma is of secondary importance.

Anyone can participate, except for people suffering from a delusional mental illness.

Course participants who are taking medication are obliged to inform the course leader in advance. Antidepressants and psycho-pharmaceuticals place a "lid" over the crown chakra, making it more difficult to get in touch with feelings.

Course structure

- Introductory interview (primary feeling, wish, code words, body tensions)
- Contact with the inner child through sound and/or movement
- Breathing exercises
- Surrender to the Note from Heaven
- Regressive cell-singing
- Relaxation
- Sound Healing/healing

What to expect during regressive cell-singing

- Storytelling (the listener sees images and shares them with the singer)
- The singer sees colors/images
- Regression to past lives/ancestors' experiences
- Regression to the spiritual state between lives
- Healing by the spiritual realms
- Sound Healing through the listener/group
- Supportive singing from the listener/group
- Changing of the story behind a trauma
- Others in the group can be deeply touched and respond to the singer's expression
- The singer's body reacts with spontaneous movements of the sphincter muscles
- The singer is confronted with a choice and has to take a decision in order to move forward
- The singer receives a symbolic tool to help them in daily life
- The singer comes in contact with the spirit of a dead

person
- Forgiveness
- Contact with a master/spiritual group that can clarify important issues
- Secretion of mucus which the singer needs to spit out in a glass

Providing a comfortable environment

During regressive cell-singing, the energy in a room always becomes intensified, no matter how big the space is.

Therefore, remember to air the room during breaks and agree with the participants that they are free to open and close the windows as they wish. Everyone is responsible for his or her own well-being. This means that if you are in a draught, don't just sit there and suffer while looking complainingly in the direction of the person who just opened the window. Swap places. Or close the window again. Or borrow a blanket, if that isn't enough. We are on a course to release the pain body, not to cultivate it.

Most people get warm when they are singing themselves free. Quite a few articles of clothing get thrown off during the process. Afterwards the singer can feel cold, so it is imperative to have blankets ready. These have a symbolic protective significance. Blankets also make people feel cozy after having been "on the spot". So the conditions of the room have to take account of widely differing needs.

Sensitivity to the density of the energy in the room varies. Everyone must take responsibility for him or herself and let the others know if they have difficulty in breathing or develop other problems.

If the course is taking place in an urban environment where the vocal activities may disturb other people, then the windows will have to remain closed. The best thing you can do in that case is to notify the course participants that the energy will get heavy and that the room will be aired between each release. If someone needs air, then they should feel free to leave the room for a while.

An expression of feeling from a singer can cause breathing difficulties for a fellow participant if their cells resonate with that particular problem. If a person's cells begin to sing along uncontrollably, this can arouse fear and cause tension in the throat or solar plexus.[42]

The most suitable location for a course in regressive cell-singing is somewhere isolated. For a singer to have the courage to totally surrender to their sound, they need to feel confident that no one outside the room can hear them.

The listener's role

To listen is to let go of oneself and surrender to a voice that is talking to you. It is to be open to being told a story.
Jesper Blomberg, priest in Udby, Denmark

The listener's role is to support the singer in finding an opening in the sound of their voice through attentive listening.

The following tools are useful, but do keep in mind that no two situations are completely alike and sessions may take place where the opening occurs in a new way, which is the only possible way to overcome that particular singer's fear and self-control.

When a person develops their ability to listen, the ability develops on all levels. For instance, their intuition will be refined and sharpened.

There are methods of treatment that are good and necessary to have as a platform, but intuition, compassion and love for your fellow human beings are the most important qualities of all. These are the qualities that develop through working with the Note from Heaven. A natural consequence of the work as a listener is that "belief" is overtaken by "knowing". This "knowing" fills your heart with gratitude and happiness and urges you to serve the Note from Heaven dedicated with the deepest respect and humility.

If you will come towards us, we will bend down and lift you up.
Hazrat Inayat Khan (A Sufi Master's Pearls)

The amount of energy a person can bear is dependent on that person's ability to step aside and trust fully in a higher consciousness. If the singer is able to rise above the personal level, then they will not have to expend their own energy when singing. On the contrary, the singer will become recharged through the expression of the Note from Heaven, which gives access to an unlimited energy source.[43]

Love for our fellow human beings, humility and gratitude are naturally awakened through work with the Note from Heaven. They are gifts that appear spontaneously and they keep the listener and singer in ethical balance.

While listening closely, the listener becomes aware of the singer's feelings through their sound, and opens up to the singer's world: I hear you. I understand you. You do not need to isolate yourself with your feeling anymore.

When listened to unconditionally, the Singer feels safe and opens up even more. In the purely listening state of consciousness there is no judgmental attitude, since all feelings are expressions of our humanity.

We are all equal and a part of the same whole.

If the listener is able to view the singer's outbreaks of emotion as archetypal, they will both be lifted above the pain body.

If, however, the listener becomes personally affected by the singer's problem and starts to feel pity, contact with the Note from Heaven will be lost.[44]

Meditative vocal work with the Note from Heaven naturally develops the abilities the listener needs. Regressive cell-singing can be carried out responsibly only by therapists who have listened to themselves thoroughly and, as a natural result of that, have purified themselves emotionally to such a degree that they can recognize the archetypes in themselves. This means that they can, at any time, rid themselves of restricting emotions like anger, fear and powerlessness by surrendering to the Note from Heaven. This opening stimulates the development of clairvoyance, clairaudience and clairsentience. When used with humility, these tools can in many cases be instrumental in pricking a hole in the festering boil and get the energy moving and ready to be released.

As a listener, it is an advantage to have knowledge of regression and other associated therapeutic tools, because these can support a singer in relieving traumas from earlier incarnations.[45]

Another advantage for the listener is familiarity with working in "between life" states.[46] These can arise during sessions and it is great to be able to recognize them.

Sound Healing and other types of healing can be necessary if the singer gets stuck or needs help during the process.[47] All sessions of regressive cell-singing finish with Sound Healing, administered either by the course leader or by the course participants who take turns to give each other Sound Healing. The purpose of this is to restructure the emotionally released cells with light and to reinstate the protective energetic field around the body.

Important qualities and skills for the listener

- Ability to express the Note from Heaven
- Intuition developed through work with the Note from Heaven
- Listening without judgment
- Awareness of physical navigation signs[48]

- Experience with the methods of Regressive Sound healing
  - Regression Therapy
  - Sound Healing
- Respect, humility and ethics
- Love, compassion and presence
- Humor
- Authority, responsibility and vigor

Ethical considerations

Full confidentiality. Do not treat people with serious psychological problems/delusions. If your client has abused anybody there are three points that must be fulfilled in order to keep you from contacting the authorities:

1) The client should regret and feel sorry about what he/she has done.
2) The client should be able to feel compassion.
3) The client must be in professional treatment for his/her abusive nature.

The singer's voice must not be pressured to express more than the organism can handle, either physically or psychologically.

Crude provocations that cause the singer's instincts to go into emergency mode may break through the body's natural defences. If an emotion in this way is chased out of its protected hiding place, it has not genuinely been released. The singer's voice will be marked by desperation, anger and rage that are not the result of the release of a trauma, but instead are the body's reaction to being provoked. **Pressure creates more pressure.** If we violently yank at the chains that bind us to the pain body, we will cause deep wounds. It is better to allow the chains to be bathed in the light of consciousness. Sooner or later they will fall to the ground.

The fruit falls when it is ripe. It should not be shaken off the tree.

Forcing out emotions risks re-traumatizing the body. For example, I have heard of another singing therapy where people's spines are hit to prod out deep-lying emotions. This I would never contemplate doing.

In regressive cell-singing, the listener, like a mother bird, leads the singer to the edge of the nest, but the leap to freedom must be made by the singer alone.

The listener can cheer them on and encourage them, "Come on, let go, jump!" But pushing the singer into the abyss before they are ready to use their wings will never lead to any good.

Although most people do make contact with the Note from Heaven during a one-day course, there are also some who do not. Those people, and especially those who carry the trauma of having been ignored very early in life, will have to remove carefully one protective layer at a time. The breakthrough will come unexpectedly one day, like a gift from heaven.

As a listener, you develop your intuition through confidence in working with the Note from Heaven, but you must still stay on your guard. The ego is always poised to enter the arena. The more skill and knowledge you acquire, the greater the temptation to take on the role of a guru and consider yourself superior to your clients.

The taste of power tempts the ego to boast and use the Note from Heaven for personal advantage: "I am born with special clairvoyant abilities and am never wrong." That is when everything falls apart.

The Note from Heaven serves the healer as long as the healer serves the whole.

Anyone who abuses power sinks down to a lower frequency, where their ears become deaf to the ring of truth.

It is natural for some people to see images, because they have easy access to the astral planes of consciousness. That does not mean that the person is grounded or that what they see is useful.

It may seem simple to sit and sing on one note with a group of people and pass on what you, as a channel, see. The problem is that if what you see or sense derives from your ego, then you are an abuser of energy – not a listener.

The key to becoming a good listener is the preliminary, personal, deepening work with the Note from Heaven. By training your ability to surrender, you will stay grounded by the *hara*, which functions like an anchor. This grounding is what keeps the listener's ego in check. The sound speaks for itself: once you have experienced the Note from Heaven, you will always recognize the state intuitively. It is therefore pointless to use the intellect to analyze the power and information that you can access through the Note from Heaven.

The message has to find resonance in the singer. When a sound resonates, its effect is the validation of its truth. When images, messages, symbols, and stories activate a healing vibration in the singer, they are truthful.

Resonance is truth.

The divine is constantly embracing us and is at our disposal at any given moment. The question is whether we are resonant with the moment. I usually say, "Take what works and forget the rest."

Truth and falsehood do not exist at the Oneness level (see below). There are no polarities there, only being.

Listeners may convey intuitive messages, for example in the form of images, to touch the emotions hidden in the singer's pain body. The moment the listener passes on a divine message whose deeper meaning only the singer understands, a miracle takes place. Belief becomes knowing.

The miracle is the spark of trust – a trust that can open the gate and allow a release to take place. Belief and trust in the divine can pierce any armor.

If the singer has a deep spiritual experience, and is able to take it in and integrate it into their life, then they can make a great leap in a matter of seconds.

The Oneness level
Poor is the one who does not acknowledge being enriched.

The Oneness level is the blissful state to which the Note from Heaven leads us. A plane where we are all part of one greater, higher being and become overwhelmed by a deep compassion, love and gratitude for everyone.

No one is alone. We are all part of the same source and belong to a shared power. There is no death, in that we are a connected whole. There are many names for this higher plane – the *akashic* field, *nirvana*, the zero-point field...

When we are in touch with the Oneness level, we can feel so wrapped up in love energy and so integrated that we experience ourselves as enlightened.

The Note from Heaven leads you to a plane of consciousness where you are illuminated, because your energy level is raised and your light therefore becomes stronger. "I am enlightened," the ego can now proudly cry out – but with this, the light bulb shatters and from the Oneness level you plummet down to earth.

We are enlightened when we are illuminated. When the light is switched off, we are no longer illuminated. We are darkness, we are light. We are what we are.

To look for boxes to put ourselves into and labels to give ourselves is an expression of fear. What if you were enlightened and didn't know it? What if you thought you were enlightened and were actually in darkness? The light is given to us. You can't tie it down or capture it. Look for it in humility and maybe, then, you can stay there for a while longer. Who knows?

Trust and faith

True faith is independent of reason.
Hazrat Inayat Khan

Faith doesn't begin with a person needing to think or make something up. No, faith is like when we were children and we listened to a story: "Once upon a time..."
Jesper Blomberg, priest in Udby, Denmark

The process of regressive cell-singing normally starts with the participant making a wish, giving the higher energies permission to work. This declaration is important, because neither the listener nor the power of the spirit has the right to infringe on the integrity that the singer establishes through this initial wish.

Before the formulating process starts, it is useful to establish where the singer's true trust lies.

Does the singer feel secure leaving their wish as "the release of what is most important right now", implying that they trust in an all-knowing power that knows best?

Or does the singer choose to control part of the process and express their own specific wish?

Most participants have no doubts. Some will have complete confidence in the higher plane, but the majority will feel more comfortable formulating a personal wish or prayer.[49]

The degree to which the singer trusts the listener will depend on how much contact the listener has with the Note from Heaven. Can the listener support me if I fall and need to be picked up? What characterizes a good listener is that they have full confidence in the Note from Heaven.

The experience of the Note from Heaven will dissolve any fear of the unfamiliar and supernatural, because the higher powers are integrated as a natural and positive part of our consciousness. We are never alone. Help is always available. The higher powers are cherishing us and we can contact these powers at any time. They are our superstructure, our Internet.

Before a singer's consciousness can expand, his or her pain body must be ready to let go. I have seen several examples where course participants have had heaven placed at their feet, but they were not ready to embrace it.[50]

But the kingdom is in your centers and is about you. When you know yourselves then you will be known, and you will be aware that you are the sons of the Living Father. But if you do not know yourselves then you are in poverty, and you are the poverty.
Jesus, Gospel of Thomas, log. 3

Once the ego is flexible enough to relinquish control to the soul in total devotion, the Note from Heaven can work without the limitation of the participant's wishes. This lack of expectation makes the singer truly receptive.

Beauty is wholeness.

Any flower loses its beauty when dissected.

The resurrection of a torn flower reveals the miracle of its wholeness.

Before the dissection we didn't see the innate miracle, but the resurrection opens our eyes.

The flower's parts must be gathered together again before this can happen. Similarly, the Note from Heaven doesn't lead us "forward", but always back to our original self, so that we, from within the shadows of the lost, can see the light and retrieve our whole self.

Only through the process of separation can the veil covering the face of divinity be withdrawn. A soul is born into the dualistic world and its longing to return to the Oneness level awakens the consciousness, which can view its origins only through such separation.

There arises the possibility of a conscious reunion – a conscious moving between the two worlds. Two notes unite and a new note is born from their harmonious resonance. Wholeness is duality as well as Oneness – to be a point and a wave at the same time.

The placebo effect

Placebo, "I shall please" from placeō, "I please", is a simulated or otherwise medically ineffectual treatment for a disease or other medical condition intended to deceive the recipient. Sometimes patients given a placebo treatment will have a perceived or actual improvement in a medical condition, a phenomenon commonly called the placebo effect.

Wikipedia

Most illnesses are caused by a general weakening of the organism. The petals of the flower are lying spread all over the floor, the stem is broken... what a mess.

Placebos are usually referred to dismissively with a skeptical smile. "He took a calcium tablet, which he believed was such and such and got well." Belief is invisible, but it is belief that makes the connection to self-healing powers. Belief gathers all the petals back together. The immune system's ability to rebalance the body is nurtured by the patient's *belief* that he has the possibility to get well.

Medical doctors have taken on the role of priests in most of the Western world. They radiate authority and the patient gives a trusting sigh of relief: thank goodness, the doctor will know how to treat me. Sick people crave authority to give them hope and pull them out of the pain body's black waters. It is no wonder, then, that witch doctors in tribal communities have a role that covers both doctor and priest – for the one who can activate divine powers can also heal.

Angels exist only if you believe in them.
Gitta Mallasz (*Talking with Angels*)

The Internet works only if the computer is hooked up to the router. You have to turn the television on before anything appears on the screen. You have to knock on the door for it to be opened.

In its meeting with the Note from Heaven, the soul is healed as the participant's trust in the higher self grows. This trust activates the placebo effect, which contains every belief's sparkling and healing strength – a power that at all times strives to regain wholeness for the body and soul.

Wishes and Primary Feelings

A session of regressive cell-singing starts with the singer uncovering his or her primary feeling in order to formulate a wish in writing.

By directing focus to the singer's primary feeling, the listener can help the singer to understand the core of an emotional problem or pattern to formulate a precise wish. During the formulation process it is the listener's responsibility to prevent the singer from spilling out their whole life story – first, because it is not energetically wise to do so, and second, because too much background knowledge given in advance can weaken the effect of any intuitive images or stories that the listener might receive.

Bear in mind the following considerations when working with primary feelings: Painful and negatively charged emotions like hate, anger, jealousy, aggression, suppression, self-pity and so on can only act as primary feelings because they are connected to the individual's self-identity.

Emotions usually arise from the subconscious as feelings of powerlessness, as a result of our personal boundaries being violated. In reality they represent frustration with our inability to command respect:

Why am I being treated with disrespect? What am I doing wrong? Why do I let it bother me at all, when it must be their problem that they are so rude? Or is it me? Why didn't I say the right thing? Why didn't I set a limit? Why did I cry? Why did I lash out? Why wasn't I able to control my emotions?

Seen from a higher perspective, primary feelings are linked to a survival pattern in the reptilian brain: to be abandoned by the tribal community means death. You cannot survive as an outsider. Arvin Larsen, scientist and *heil* practitioner,[51] calls a primary feeling "the neurological template". Bruce Lipton calls it "programming". This programming is set in the first seven years of childhood when the child instinctively submits to the environment's demands by copying all that is said and done by the parents as the "truth".

So our primary feeling is the foundation upon which we form our perceptions about life and death; which means that if we need to change it, we also need to replace it with something else. By exposing our primary feeling, we awaken our awareness of its existence. From self-reflection, we can gradually dissolve the negative, damaging parts of our programming and substitute it with a positive, healing replacement.

The four primary feelings

1. I am not good enough

Indications

I feel ashamed, insecure, lacking in self-confidence. I fear failure, being exposed, being inadequate. I am scared of my own power.

I am not lovable. I am ugly. I am stupid. I am wrong. I can't live up to what's expected. I feel anxious when I need to perform. I find no joy in life. I want to be admired. I want to be perfect. I am not good enough to be the light – not worthy of joy and happiness. I'm not anything special.

Commentary
These kinds of thoughts run in circles incessantly like toy trains on a track.

We all have a potential master within us.

For the light to reside within our bodies, we first need to let it in. If we feel unworthy, we keep ourselves in the shadow.

Positive implications
In your attempts to fit in with your surroundings, you can develop an understanding for your fellow human beings. As a result of your insecurity, you need to try out identities that are not your own. When you land back in your own shoes again, you are able to see through other people's clumsy attempts to be good enough. The fact that you have been there yourself gives rise to care, compassion and empathy. You will be the last person to take advantage of someone else's lack of self-confidence. Power games and controlling behavior are just not part of your repertoire.

2. I don't want to be here

Indications
I want to escape. I want to hide. I don't belong. I feel powerless. I am jealous that everyone else has an easier time than me. I feel hurt. I lack grounding. I long for another dimension and I don't feel at home here on earth.

Commentary

This primary feeling is often experienced by people who have been abused in childhood, where their soul has been at the mercy of an overpowering person and the child has found a way of coping by escaping into a psychological nonexistence. A classic example is when a neglected or ignored child dreams him or herself away.

Another case is the beautiful and rich child who has been given everything a heart could desire, except for true love and attention.

The implications in "I am not good enough" and "I don't want to be here" are quite similar. The difference between the two feelings is nevertheless striking.

The former is all about staying and doing your best to fit in, which entails an endless effort to be good enough. For who is going to decide what is good enough? Who has the right to decide, if not you? You lose your integrity by letting other people define your limits.

The latter is about escape. You don't want to be here, because you don't fit in. The implication is that you'll fit in somewhere else, so you'll wait for an opportunity to get away. You keep your integrity and define your limits.

Positive implications

The instinct to "run away" – spiritually as well as physically – is essential in life. By spiritually running away from a harrowing experience, you remove yourself psychologically and thereby reduce the pain and dampen down the trauma.

On the surface, you are good at protesting defiantly. It's an expression of a frayed and vulnerable, yet persistent self-respect that you will fight for to the end. Somehow you know that there is another world somewhere else, because that is where you have a refuge. This knowledge can be used in connection with spiritual work.

Jesus said: "Blessed is the man who has toiled, he has found the life."
Gospel of Thomas, log. 58

3. I am not allowed to be here

Indications

I don't feel welcome. I try to make myself invisible. No one listens to me. No one sees me. No one notices me. I am nothing. I don't mean anything. I don't want to give anybody any trouble. My parents, my children, my husband/wife – I am here for their sakes.

Commentary

People who have this primary feeling may have felt ignored or unwanted as children. They may have felt abandoned by their closest relatives and left to their own fate. Siblings may have arrived on the scene, leaving them feeling marginalized. They have difficulty noticing what they feel.[52] Delusions of grandeur often go hand in hand with self-effacement.

If the feeling of abandonment is associated with the death of a parent or sibling or another loved one at a young age, this can also result in feeling, "I don't want to be here."

Positive implications

You are good at avoiding drawing attention to yourself. From this hiding place you can observe the world without being disturbed. Therefore, once you can feel entitled to be in your environment, you will have the advantage of understanding it well and it will be easy for you to see through the games people play with each other.

He who understands everything but himself understands nothing.
Jesus, Gospel of Thomas, log. 67

4. I don't belong here, I am different

Indications

I don't fit into society. I feel alone. I yearn for something I cannot express. I'm afraid to show who I am. I feel like an outsider. I'm afraid of my power, because it can reveal who I am. I wish I could be like everyone else.

Commentary

These feelings are often a sign that a course participant has made good contact with their spiritual abilities. To confirm whether that is the case, the listener can inquire if the person had experiences as a child that would conventionally be regarded as abnormal. Be aware that the participant will probably consider these experiences to be normal. So it is the family members' response and reactions you have to ask about.

In regressive cell-singing, participants with this primary feeling are often shown glimpses from past lives: witch-burning, hanging, torture, stoning... the ways society showed its fear and distrust of people who found their own way to the light.

When dealing with such violent traumas, it is essential that the singer is exposed to his or her agonies without getting emotionally lost in them. To do this, the listener should support the singer in surrendering to the Note from Heaven, so that the singer's soul can rise up to the light and be healed there. From this higher perspective, the singer can be shown their path here on Earth and with that come to understand the meaning of life.[53]

Positive implications

You know how to wait for the right moment and are humble in relation to power. The fear of revealing who you are causes you to hide behind different roles. The pain of recognizing this self-betrayal leads you deeper into loneliness. If you can acknowledge the loneliness as a positive teacher, this will lead you to the awareness that we are all separate (living in duality), as well as connected (united in Oneness).

Loneliness can lead to the recognition of unity.

The mote that is in your brother's eye, you see, but the beam that is in your own eye you see not. When you cast the beam out of your eye, then you will see clearly to cast the mote out of your brother's eye.
Jesus, Gospel of Thomas, log. 26

Formulation of wish and primary feeling

The purpose of the articulation process is to come into contact with feelings in the body. Without expressing your emotions, without making a cry for help, you cannot be heard. The wish needs to be felt in the body. In some cases, the client is already so moved during the articulation phase as to be close to tears. As becoming moved and overwhelmed by a feeling can lead the sound directly into the cells, the listener, if possible, should push everything else to one side and urge the client to sing him or herself free right there and then.

In some cases, you really do only get one chance. If you don't seize the opportunity when it's there, you risk losing it. It's like fishing. You have to reel the fish in when it takes the bait.

If a feeling in the singer is ready to surface, you may observe physical signs such as shiny eyes, red spots on the throat and cheeks, restlessness, lips pressed together, a thick, throaty voice.

Rely on the slightest hint from your intuition. Don't wait, but act on your impression. Ask the singer, "Can you sense a feeling inside you?"

If the singer whispers yes or is moved even more, then you must add wood to the fire: "Where is the feeling located in your body? Go into it, sing it out! Let go! Every sound is welcome… in this space everything is allowed. Nothing can scare me. I want to hear all that you are! I love to hear your voice!"

In this situation, the listener is welcome to be as enthusiastic as they wish! During the articulation process, the singer should be made aware that you get exactly what you ask for. Some course participants are under the impression that the articulation process is an opportunity to get as many presents as possible in their "Christmas stocking".

This is not the case. You usually get pretty much what you ask for, but not always in the way you expect and never more than the voice (the soul) is able to carry home from the "Christmas party".[54]

When you formulate a wish you can ask the highest spirits for help. If you could ask Jesus, and he was standing in front of you, how would you formulate your wish? Vishnu, Buddha, Mother Mary or Allah? You deserve the best – the spirits that reflect the highest energy level in yourself.

It is important to ask to dissolve/eliminate/release the main cause/the root cause of your problem, otherwise the problem can return again.

Examples of formulating wishes

Each participant brings his or her unique set of life experiences to the course and so the list of possible wishes singers may formulate is endless. However, the following is a guide to the kinds of wishes a listener will most commonly encounter.

Wishes to alleviate physical problems

- I wish to have the root cause of the pain in my left shoulder released.
- I wish to have the root cause of my life-threatening disease released.
- I wish to dissolve the root cause of my headache and become pain free.
- I wish to dissolve the root cause of my bronchitis/my tinnitus/my reduced hearing...

Wishes to alleviate psychological problems or undesirable life patterns

- I wish to dissolve the root cause of the feeling of not being good enough.
- I wish to dissolve the root cause of the obstacle standing in the way of my trust in God, the universe and myself.
- I wish to dissolve the root cause of my feeling of being different.
- I wish to dissolve the root cause of my feeling of not wanting to be here.
- I wish to dissolve the root cause of my feeling of not being allowed to be here/not being heard/having to be invisible.
- I wish to dissolve the root cause of the pattern that is preventing me from realizing my dreams.
- I wish to be able to sustain a relationship and have the root cause of the pattern that prevents me from doing so released/dissolved.

Wishes for personal development

- I wish to serve a higher consciousness and to dissolve the root cause of the barriers that prevent me in doing so.
- I ask for what is most important, right now.
- I ask for my feminine and masculine powers to become mutually balanced.
- I ask for help in defending myself less and daring to show who I am.

Musical wishes

- I wish to dissolve the root cause of my performance anxiety when I am on the stage.

- I wish to be able to express myself fully when I sing or play.
- I wish to dissolve the root cause of my need to control and to become able to surrender to the music.
- I wish to dissolve the obstacle that makes me tone-deaf.
- I wish to find the natural pitch of my voice.
- I wish to sing better in the high/low pitch.

Code words

In the process of articulating a wish, the listener notes down code words and or tonal expressions that trigger strong emotions to come in to play. An emotion always causes the muscles to tense up in some part of the body. It is the listener's role to observe and note down these physical tensions and the specific code words that trigger them.

The code words are not necessarily part of "the wish", but are excellent initiators for the listener to use if the singer gets stuck in performance mode when singing. It is important to use the singer's exact wording, as it is this specific composition of words that provokes a reaction.

For example, I had a case in a seminar where a woman's code words were, "You are just like Ruth!" This sentence wouldn't have worked if I, as a listener, had said, "You are similar to Ruth."

The code words really got the woman's voice going so effectively that the other participants were laughing their heads off while she sang herself free. Nobody knew who Ruth was or what the background story was, but the code words worked and the woman (who was not named Ruth) experienced such a release that tears rolled down her cheeks from both weeping and laughing combined.

As the listener, I added wood to the fire by repeating the code words until their effect wore off. In the end of a session of regressive cell-singing, I always repeat the singer's code words to see if they still have effect. In this case the words no longer caused tension in her body. She smiled gratefully and gave me a hug.

During the process of singing free a trauma, the listener uses prearranged code words designed to help the singer get in touch with genuine emotional reactions.

At the end of the session, the listener enquires about the areas of the body that were noted and that had reacted to the code words before. If the body still tenses up when the associated code words are recited, the singer is urged to sing into that area again. If listener and singer conclude that the trauma has more than one layer and needs to be released over several sessions, a new appointment is set.

The expression in the singer's voice can tell you whether he or she has had enough.

The listener may intuitively decide to attempt just one last contact in a new way. Frequently, an unexpected breakthrough occurs when the singer has already given up and, with a shrug of the shoulders and no expectation of success, tries one last time, despite believing "the voice is finished".

If the tensions have disappeared after the singing and have been replaced with warmth, tingling and relaxation, a healing has occurred in that particular location. In such cases, the singer's face is usually radiant, the eyes sparkling, and seriousness is replaced by ease and a readiness to laugh.

The pain may have disappeared and the singer feels a blissful peace and sense of well-being. In some cases, a permanent healing takes place. In others, the pain returns after two to ten days. The reason for this is that the body produces pain-relieving endorphins during devoted singing, which can continue to be effective for several days afterwards.

After a process of release, the singer usually needs to sleep for a couple of hours. If there are detox symptoms the singer is advised to relax with a castor oil pack on their liver. The singer is asked to continue the process on their own by singing the Note from Heaven devotedly in their daily life. Perhaps the listener and singer can arrange a program together to continue the work.

Examples of code words

Wish: I wish to release the root cause of the pain in my left shoulder.
Code words: You feel powerless. You are not worth anything. You are not good enough. You are not worthy to contact the divine powers.
Physical reactions: The singer's arms get heavy; there is a pressure in the head, pain between the shoulders.

Wish: I wish to release the root cause of the feeling of not being good enough.
Code words: You are not worth loving. You are afraid to be revealed. You should be ashamed of yourself.
Physical reactions: The throat tightens up, speechlessness, a hard tension in the solar plexus.

Wish: I wish to dissolve the root cause of the feeling of not wanting to be here.
Code words: You have nothing to contribute. You can't be part of this group. Everyone hates you. Who do you think you are?
Physical reactions: The throat tightens up, the body stiffens, shortness of breath, tension in the stomach and lower abdomen.

Wish: I wish to serve the higher consciousness and have the blocks released that are preventing me from doing this.
Code words: You are afraid to show your true face. You are afraid of others' reactions. You can't stay centered. You are not like us.

Physical reactions: The throat closes off completely, a sense of strangulation, tensions in the solar plexus. Cold hands may be an indication that the singer was burned at the stake in an earlier incarnation.

Navigation signs

A navigation sign is just as important for the listener as headlights are for a car driver on a narrow country lane in the dead of night. *Navigation signs tell you whether you are on the right track or not. They appear as physical reactions that vary from person to person, and are a precious tool.* A listener therefore merely needs to be aware of certain physical reactions in their own body.

My green (i.e. positive) navigation sign is a kind of "heart orgasm" where my heart expands and I surrender with a sigh. I feel moved and overwhelmed with gratitude. I yawn and gasp. If you have the same navigation sign, I suggest you explain to the singer in advance that when you yawn it means something good is happening, not that you are bored! My eyes often water during the yawning, especially the left eye.

So, for me, a "heart orgasm" tells me I am on the right track and that I should continue and be patient. The meaning will be revealed later.

My red (negative) navigation signs are heavy arms and a feeling of powerlessness and fatigue across the shoulders.

When I feel these signs of exhaustion, I know I need to stop, because I am no longer on the right track.

To find your navigation signs, follow these three basic steps:

1. Ask to have your navigation signs shown to you. Green light and red light.
2. Pay attention to the fact that the green light will be shown through your physical reactions when you or others are in contact with the Note from Heaven.
3. At a larger Sound Healing course for therapists, several

of them found that tension in the neck was their red navigation sign.

Some clients are difficult to get through to. There may be lots of images coming to you, but the singer can't relate to them. There just doesn't seem to be any resonance. "How long should I continue? Am I heading in the right direction?" Those kinds of questions pop up in the listener's mind. It is good that they do, because a listener can never be completely sure that what they see or sense is pure. And, even if it is, if the singer can't receive it, then it makes no difference.

If I receive a green navigation sign, I continue with confidence, even if the story seems totally absurd and is not having any noticeable effect on the singer.

In cases like this, what sometimes happens is that the singer lets his or her guard down for a few seconds. In that moment, the connection in the story will "ambush" them with such conviction that they will suddenly start to feel trust and, with that, open up to the Note from Heaven.

If I do not receive any navigation signs, I silently pray to be shown the way. In some cases, the story then takes a completely different turn. In other cases, it's necessary for the whole group to provide support and sing with the singer. Maybe a certain way of touching the singer will cause the barricades to fall – especially when dealing with experiences from infancy. Or the listener may need to use his or her voice in a way that speaks to the singer as a small child. Or maybe the singer needs Sound Healing.

Riding on Feelings

The driving force in regressive cell-singing is feeling. The feeling rises just like a big wave, and must be caught at the right moment in order to be able to surf it all the way to the shore.

In brief, the process is: you awaken the emotion, catch the feeling, ride it ashore and in that way liberate the cells.

When a feeling is revived, the body's memory of a given moment awakens and the suppressed reaction to an old, unexpressed emotion will be poised and ready to surge through the organism.

Many of us have clogged up our throats and find it hard to express strong feelings. The essence of the Note from Heaven is deep peace, love and gratitude.

Before we can get to that point, the bottleneck needs to be cleared, so that the excess pressure of carbon dioxide in the shaken fizzy drink can be released.

Regressive cell-singing is a quick method of release, where things can change dramatically from one minute to the next. When long-repressed feelings are released, it often happens with a wild, penetrating force. This may take the form of screaming or angry shouts, often accompanied by corresponding physical gestures.

Although dramatic, the process is profoundly liberating for the singer, so there is no reason for onlookers to be alarmed. However, they may still feel uncomfortable, not out of concern for the singer but because of Resonance with Domino Effect (see page 277).

In cases of screaming and other intense reactions, I have one golden rule: *it takes one to two minutes at most for the excess pressure to be released.* After that, it is the listener's responsibility to lead the singer's expression up into the light for it to become musically beautiful as the Note from Heaven's nourishing energy transforms and celebrates the return to life of what was hidden.

If the singer is allowed to wallow in their feelings for longer than those two minutes, there is a great danger that they will, out of habit, surrender to the pain body and get lost in the trauma. If that happens, the feelings can become stuck and turn into a kind of self-perpetuating floorshow that can be very difficult for the listener to stop.[55]

How to lead a singer up to the light

The listener listens intently for a strong sound in the singer's expression of feelings and emphasizes this sound by singing along with it. In this way the listener pulls the singer up onto a life raft in the middle of the surging sea of feelings. Turbulent feelings can be transformed effectively through "cry-toning" (see page 184), where the tones coming through in the crying are reinforced and sung out.

If a singer in catharsis refuses to follow the listener – and accuses the listener of disturbing them – it is almost always a sign that their pain body has taken over. I have been accused of re-traumatizing a singer, because they had wanted to scream in front of an audience and I had stopped them. The singer tried to get the other course participants to feel pity and draw them into a power game. The result was that everyone present was sucked dry of their energy. In such a case the listener's navigation sign will be flashing red, and the listener must take responsibility to stop the process immediately by stating the truth: "You are expressing your pain body – not the Note from Heaven."

Expression

We need to express what is within us to make it real. And we also need the right kind of response. When our expression is rejected, it feels as if we are being wiped out, annihilated – we become unreal.
Audun Myskja, Professor in Musical Medicine

From the earliest age, we are conditioned to restrict the expression of our feelings. We have learned that it is wrong to yell, scream, be angry or hysterical. Boys are often told that it is embarrassing to cry. Feelings are held in check and tucked away in emotional boxes that are stored in the vaults of the pain body.

Children as well as adults sense the unspoken and unexpressed in the atmosphere that surrounds them: the air is heavy and breathing is withheld. People feel ill at ease when they are prevented from flowering as human beings. As a means of avoiding disapproval or censure, children learn to adapt how they express themselves according to the restrictions they are subjected to. If the adaptation happens early on in a child's life, it will become an integral part of his or her developing identity and that child will learn how best to attract love.

It is vital that a child's expression receives an open response, because true expression connects the child to the higher self. If adults continually reject the child's expression because they "know best", the child will stop listening to their own feelings and lose self-confidence.

Let any expression of the self through vocal sound, truly and spontaneously, be legitimate and praiseworthy. An easy way to meet children's need to express themselves freely is to encourage them to cleanse themselves through sound. Where can the emotion be felt in the body? What does the feeling sound like? Sing it together with the child.[56] As cleansing through sound comes naturally to most children, they usually feel much better straight after the outburst.

When adult and child join together in sound, they create an atmosphere of intimacy and presence. The child feels completely heard, while the process may also allow the adult to release hidden emotions from childhood. Deep love emerges, whereas aggression, irritation and telling the child to "shut up" (so the feelings can't come out) would have spoiled the day.

When accepting someone's expression of an emotion, you help that person to regain balance.

Imagine for a moment a crowd of people going berserk. This reaction could be incited by their football team losing, a perceived injustice, racial hatred or opposition to the government. According to the pain body, it is always *someone else's fault.* Just a single spark can be enough to ignite our bone-dry emotional kindling; the pain body's fuel is self-pity, provocation, projection and suffering.

When the pain body is activated and turns its black, foaming inner side outwards, all hell breaks loose.

However, through conscious vocalization of our feelings, we can regain self-confidence and shine light onto the pain body and heal its wounds.

When a feeling is expressed through sound, a surplus of pure energy is released.

The rocket is fired off, but not aimed at anyone. It's more like a vibrant firework display. The energy fills the room and enriches everyone present with joy. They purify themselves in the moment by surrendering to the sound, singing up to the heavens and freeing themselves and their fellow human beings from the grip of emotions.

Unfortunately, there is a tendency to label people who relieve their feelings through sound as crazy, because they seem to be out of control emotionally. In the worst cases, they get admitted to psychiatric care, where they are heavily medicated and rendered harmless before they can activate too many unexpressed feelings in the "normal" people's pain body.

For eons, tribal societies have instinctively released stuck emotions by making vocal sounds. The Sami, for example, go out into the wild and sing themselves free of surplus anger, joy and grief.

It is just as natural to cleanse yourself emotionally as it is to wash your hands when they are dirty. Holding back reactions for a long time is undesirable, not only for the individual but for society as a whole.

Repressed emotions tend to affect us differently depending on whether we are predominantly extrovert or introvert in nature.

Extrovert expression-pattern

An extroverted person will, sooner or later, need to release the pressure caused by pent-up and festering emotions. The lid blows off and the pressure is relieved through an explosive expression of distorted, deformed feelings. This may manifest itself in, for example, obscure complaints, anger triggered by trivial matters, unjust and inappropriate aggression or physical violence.

Introvert expression-pattern

An introverted person will exude reticence and will be difficult to figure out or relate to. Audible as well as inaudible bad vibrations become "rancid" through being kept hidden too long instead of being addressed as soon as they occur. The result is a slow, leaking expression of repressed emotions that are projected onto the person's surroundings through instances, for example, of bitterness, irritation, anger or psychological violence/psychopathic behavior.

Public recognition of the impact emotions have in our society could save humankind from a lot of its suffering. Just imagine if there was a public sound room in every city for the purpose of clearing out inappropriate feelings! "Go to the sound room and let your emotions out, instead of snapping at us..."

All feelings are worth their weight in gold. The bad ones as well as the good. When you express a feeling openly and it is acknowledged, you can surf on it, gliding like a whale rider and, through the expression of your voice, escape from unnecessary burdens. It happens all by itself in a space where we can make unrestricted sounds in joy and safety. Emotions only do harm when they are imprisoned in the flesh.

Free-flowing water carries all of the vital nutrients around in the body. Movement is life. Still-standing water gradually becomes stagnant. In order to survive we need to drink clean, oxidized water; drinking polluted water can kill us. It is the same with feelings.

Freely expressed feelings enliven the organism. Trapped emotions poison the body.

Cry-toning

As a listener, it is possible to harness the power of crying to help a singer to release pent-up emotions, because the weeping brings out tones that resonate with a given emotion. The art is to get the singer to hop onto the wave of weeping at the right moment: just as the weeping starts the singer consciously strengthens the sounds and in a way dramatizes them by singing on long "sobs".

How to stimulate cry-toning

The moment a singer is moved by a feeling, the listener needs to sustain contact with the emotion, because most people have been taught to hold back their tears. Let intuition and sensitivity rule here. The goal is that, if possible, the volcano should erupt and the excess pressure be released.

It feels good to throw out our arms in a devil-may-care manner. To begin with, if the singer is dealing with pent-up rage, he or she may clench fists. Later on, the listener can invite the singer to open their hands and turn the palms upwards. In that way, the body becomes receptive to an exchange of energy with the higher planes.

Participants who are scared by the inner forces that are breaking through may clench their teeth (a natural defence). This considerably reduces the power of the voice and the chances of crying. While singing on the vowel "Aaar", the tongue must be relaxed and lie forwards in the mouth, with the tip resting on or just behind the lower teeth. With deeply felt cry-toning there are usually no tensions in the tongue.

If the singer struggles with their crying, it is the listener's task to catch the most penetrating and clear tonal gifts that the crying brings out. The listener can briefly emphasize and sing along, "crying" on the notes, to inspire the singer to give in to the cry-toning.

Once the singer experiences the liberating, exuberant power that cry-toning awakens in them, they will be able to keep going.

It feels simply wonderful to release the weeping in a fire of song. After just one or two minutes, maybe less, the serious atmosphere is replaced with one of absurd comedy and opens into euphoric bliss, maybe even hearty laughter. No singer will be allowed to break down in tears. With cry-toning you sing on the crying tones, which releases much more energy than normal crying.

In cry-toning there is no self-pity.

You enjoy the weeping as a long-awaited downpour and use it as a gateway through which to access the Note from Heaven.

Cry-toning in action

For one female participant, weeping was a well-known and safe territory. She cried in the session like a little child who wanted to be heard and yet was not quite sure if it was really allowed. No really clear tones came forward – her voice whistled around in the weeping, like a swirling wind that couldn't quite collect itself to produce a powerful gust. Light puffs of wind don't get the fire going. If you observe the singer's breathing in that kind of halfway-crying, it will be gasping and short, instead of long, deep and dynamic.

At this point I, as the listener, needed to reflect back what I was hearing. The woman's role as "the little one we should feel sorry for" felt safe because she had been playing it for years.

If the weeping is tearless, then the singer is almost always playing out an unconscious, learned role.

The listener needs to be non-judgmentally honest. "What kind of crying is that? Can we get some feelings out in the open here? It's not good enough to hide behind sniffling, I want to hear genuine sound in your crying."

People are used to negative reactions when they cry. Here it is a party. The weeping is a gift. And when the weeping gathers force it is immediately expressed by singing. If the cry-toning is authentic, the feelings remain and now we can get the fire going that will burn the cells free of physical and psychological trauma.

This singer stated that it was a conscious choice for her; she allowed herself to play up her feelings and let the weeping flow so freely that it could turn into sound.

Not everyone is able to do that. As the listener, you will then have to gamble and give the singer a little push so they can make the run-up and take their leap. In most cases it works, but if the person is not ready to let go of their role there is a danger that they will close off instead of continuing.

The singer is faced with a choice. Do I want to passively watch the embers come and then go out or am I ready to actively take the step to consciously blow life into the embers of the trauma and go through the fire of transformation? Am I afraid of my powers? That precious fire, will I let it go out?

A transformation can happen immediately if the singer dares to let go.

Cry-toning can be used for acute personal clearing out of accumulated painful emotions, as demonstrated in the following account.

While out driving with my then husband, we started arguing. Our son, four years old at the time, had a sensitive disposition and wasn't used to conflict. When my husband angrily stopped the car on the shoulder of the freeway and went to the side to urinate, my son and I also got out of the car. Our son was obviously as upset as I was. We opened the trunk, stuck our heads inside it and cried and screamed out our frustrations. Our son thought it was fun. We yelled out full blast on long tones.

My frightened husband came running back with his pants half open. He stood there for a moment and looked at us. Then he stuck his head into the trunk as well and screamed.

We were all in a better mood for the rest of the journey. The air was still shaken, but cleared.

If you want to test cry-toning yourself and there are other people in the house, it can be done into a pillow in the bedroom or, even better, find your own secluded cry-toning place or take a trip in the car and express your cry-toning there.

Cry-toning works so well because the body's instinctive reactions are brought into play. The breathing muscles open up and do everything right, if the weeping and expression of feelings are genuine. You can clearly hear and sense when the real expression comes through. Cry-song is a prayer from the bottom of your heart. The energy is unmistakable. If you are in doubt, then the Note from Heaven has not come through. As humans, we can instinctively recognize the energy that manifests through the Note from Heaven. The power enhances us and makes us happy.

Although the expression can seem very intense, you don't run any risk of psychological or physical injury, because a genuine cry always comes from the pit of the stomach. This means that the expression is grounded and secure.

Storytelling

As earlier mentioned some listeners see inner pictures when a singer expresses him or herself vocally. You can develop these images into stories and tell them to the singer to encourage the release of blocked emotions. The ability to see inner pictures develops gradually, as your trust in your intuition grows stronger. If you see colors, that is also good.

Storytelling reflects the subconscious mind, where the singer can be liberated from the wicked fairy's curse of petrified princes and princesses – in other words, traumas. Traumas are energetic impressions of events. Like footprints in the sand, these energetic impressions are blotted out when consciousness shines its light on them.

The particular benefit of stories is that they can slip past our defence mechanisms unnoticed as, like dreams, they seduce us into forgetting ourselves and thus pave the way for the light of consciousness.

The plot can lead in numerous directions. Almost all of them lead to heaven/a deep understanding, but before this destination is reached, the singer can be led down into the dark recesses of the subconscious mind in the form of regressive experiences in this life, the embryonic stage, or past lives. Maybe they sing themselves to states between lives and get in touch with a spiritual master and receive healing there. It is also quite common to receive a parable that is full of symbols.

The listener is not supposed to try to understand or interpret the meaning of the story as it unfolds, but solely to rely on navigation signs (see page 177). The reason is, that the listener's ignorance preserves the singer's integrity and thus the story's validity and impact.

During the storytelling, the listener can ask the singer whether the story means anything to them if it's not obvious whether the singer is reacting to the images. The singer often nods slightly, completely absorbed in their song, and the listener takes encouragement from this, even though they don't have a clue what's going on.

Story examples
The following stories are all genuine, but due to my professional confidentiality I have excluded distinctive characteristics and specific personal statements.

Story 1: Back to nature
Here is an example of a story in which the sound expression was so overwhelmingly pure that the atmosphere in the room

turned completely devout.

Gender of the singer: Female
Wish: I ask to be shown my path in life.
Primary feeling: I feel different. I yearn to belong. (I don't belong here.)
Code words: You are not good enough to work with sound. You can't find your way. You are fragmented.
Physical reactions: Pain in the lower abdomen and right hip.

The story

Everything is white. *The sound opens up.* There is drifting snow. Strong wind. Eskimos. *The sound becomes melodious and sorrowful. The singer's face lights up.* A leather sled with a child tied to it. The child is wrapped in furs. The man is fighting his way through the mounds of snow. He and his boy have been out hunting and were surprised by a sudden change of weather. *The voice is fighting stoutly and bears witness to images of strong, beautiful nature. The Note from Heaven has come through. Survival. The images are unusually clear.*

Thanks to the man's good sense of direction he makes it home. He is worried whether the child has survived the journey. Everything appears white and impenetrable, but then a crack in the rock appears. The man and child enter through a curtain in the form of several hanging furs. The feeling of relief at meeting the tribe in the long, deep rock cave. The warmth. The child is handed over to the women. The feeling of unity. Acceptance of nature and the will of the higher powers. Song of thanks.

The song is more beautiful than ever. Where before it was powerful, it now glows softly with gratitude. The men around the fire. A clear division between the genders. Laughter in the corners. Children, odors of people, dogs. The smell of food. Finally home.

What happened next

The singer was deeply touched and said that she had always been fascinated by Eskimos. She was only visiting Denmark. Normally she lived with her Native American husband on a small island in western Canada. Her lower abdomen and right hip were now free of pain.

The unusually beautiful song expression in the séance described above inspired me to record a CD of regressive cell-singing. My intention was to produce something that would help the singers and would also be a supplement to this book. The course participant kindly agreed to travel several hours to my home a few days later. I had prepared a studio and wired up. The same code words, the same wish. The woman's pain in her lower abdomen had been gone since the course. The expression in her voice sounded different now.

This time the images I saw were extremely blurred at best. We were both affected by the recording circumstances and "performing" gradually took hold of the singer. Even though her singing was still beautiful, the expression was no longer authentic. Slightly disappointed, we had to acknowledge that the release had already taken place.

You can only express what you are.

An expression of feelings is unique and can't be repeated.

On a later occasion, I tried to capture sound expressions in the moment of release. With the participants' consent, I installed the studio on the course premises.

The course went well and then I started editing the recordings. I felt uncomfortable with this. Some of the participants had come through more clearly than others. Was I trampling on holy ground? When I shared my misgivings with the participants, they urged me to continue. So I decided to keep my promise and complete the project anyway.

When the editing was almost finished, the hard disk in the studio went down and all of the recordings disappeared. That was the first time such a thing had ever happened in the whole existence of the studio. Since then, I have never dared to record regressive cell-singing.

Story 2: Strengthening Faith

Gender of the singer: Female
Wish: I wish to release the behavioral pattern that is preventing me from forming a long-term relationship.
Primary feeling: I am not good enough.
Code words: You're jealous. You're not sure if you want to have children. You're frightened of being rejected. You feel powerless.
Physical reactions: Tensions in the solar plexus and heart.

The story

A woman with her hair wrapped up in curlers. *The vocal expression is going back and forth and isn't making much headway.* She ties a scarf around the old-fashioned curlers on her head. *I say, "What is the woman doing? Take me there with your voice."* She is weaving. There are baskets of wool in the room; she is spinning her own yarn. She is weaving and weaving.

I wonder what all this weaving means and therefore pray to the higher powers to lead us to the core issue. The voice opens up a little bit more. The Note from Heaven has not yet broken completely through.

The weaver now goes out to a little yard to feed her sheep. The sound opens up a bit more. A change of scene: the woman has dressed up and brushed her curled hair. She is cooking and setting the table for two. A man walks through the gate into the yard. He has fair hair, steel spectacles and is dressed in dark trousers, jacket and white shirt. A young priest, a student? The woman is uncertain of his intentions.

They eat and she tries to catch his eye. She senses that he

hardly hears what she is saying. He is shoveling the food into his mouth. The others in the parish must not find out about this. He was late, because he tried to avoid being seen. The woman winces at the feeling of his not wanting to acknowledge her. After the meal, he sits on the sofa and reads the paper while she clears the table. Afterwards, the woman also sits on the sofa, but on the edge and at a proper distance from her guest. She feels uncomfortable. Suddenly the man throws himself at her and kisses her hard on the mouth. He tears at her clothes. The woman resists and gets enormous strength. *Now the Note from Heaven breaks through.*

The woman stands up, pushing the young man away so that he falls to the floor. She runs out into the yard, through the gate and looks for help. Just then she sees a man with a cap and big wooden clogs covered in clay come striding across the fields in the direction of her farm.

The man clearly leads an outdoor life, he must be a farmer or something similar. The woman is crying and the man comes willingly towards her and asks what has happened. He comforts her. He carries her resolutely into the house. They know each other.

I have always wanted to have children with you, he confides. Will you marry me?

This question opens up a choice situation[57] that the singer has to respond to. So, as the listener, I ask her directly: "Do you want to marry him and have children with him?"

The singer answers that she feels it is too soon after what she has just experienced (the young man is gone now), but she can see that the farmer is kind and open. Nothing is held back. "The man wants to dance with you. Do you want to dance with him?" The singer replies, "Yes."

What happened next

Afterwards I was still unsure whether the big release had taken place.

The singer already had a good voice and even though the Note from Heaven broke through, she was still not sure whether to continue her relationship with the farmer. It looked as if she needed more time.

After resting, the singer, slightly shaken, explained that she did weave, that she kept sheep (not on a farm, but in her garden) and had spun the yarn herself and woven with the wool. The young man seemed to be an image of her former boyfriend and the farmer was a gardener she knew who was her weekly dance partner. He had recently told her just what the farmer said in the story: that he would like to have children with her. They had not yet become lovers.

Story 3: Dissolving a social phobia

Gender of the singer: Female
Wish: I wish to get into contact with myself.
Primary feeling: I don't want to be here.
Code words: You've lost your expression. You're afraid of being noticed. You panicked when you had to speak in school. You're afraid of any kind of social contact. You don't feel you belong here. You want to get away from here.
Physical reactions: The whole body stiffens. Throat contracts.

The story

A dead woman is hanging, naked and mutilated, by her neck on a big hook as an example and warning to the local villagers. *The singer agrees to go backwards in the story to dissolve it.*[58]

Now the woman is being tortured by the men of the church. Her two children also, so that she finally admits to being a witch. *We go quickly backwards, only pausing at the violent scene long enough for the singer to make contact with the cells that are bound to the trauma. I sense from the singer's sound and reaction that it's not the violence itself that is the main source of the trauma.*

I ask her directly what she senses the trauma is about. "The feeling of being let down, not the torture itself," she replies.

It's the villagers. She had been their wise woman. It was to her they had all come when they had a problem. She had always been there for them. Being let down – the feeling of being totally let down. Their evasive glances. They bear witness against her. The help she had given them now turned into accusations of witchcraft. Was Jesus Christ perhaps involved? She had been associating with the devil, that's for sure, according to them.

The singer's feeling is clear: I don't want to be here on earth. I want to get away from here. I don't want anything to do with you all. The Note from Heaven rings through the air like a sword. The singer totally manifests her power through her sound. I ask if she would like a tool[59] to help her rediscover the power she is now in touch with. The singer agrees. "Close your eyes and ask for a tool. The first thing that comes to you is your tool, no matter how absurd it seems." The singer gets a flower.

The singer decides that she wants to change the story[60] and, with that, the trauma's energetic imprint. I give her suggestions which she accepts or rejects until the story is just the way she wants it:

The woman is taken off the hook; we rewind the story as if it were a red carpet being rolled up. We come back to her whitewashed house with the beautiful garden full of herbs. She walks in her garden in a light-colored dress. The children are playing. The woman is reborn. The villagers come by one at a time and ask for forgiveness. They bring flowers to her. A man offers to be her gardener. No, she will take care of the flowers herself, but he can help with the vegetable garden. When the villagers have gathered and are all kneeling in a circle and full of remorse, the woman forgives them.

She doesn't want anything to do with the priests, but she wants the church premises preserved. A spiral energy form sucks the priests up and they disappear forever.

To avoid the fear of new, possibly hostile priests in the church, we put an open-minded priest into office. His attitude to the woman and her work is gentle and full of love and respect. He sees that she is a pious woman, who with her good deeds is following Jesus's true message.

What happened next

A week later, the singer, who for years had been retired because of social phobia, informed me that during the past week she had sensed her body in a whole new way and that she now experienced the world differently, much more positively: "This is the most releasing treatment I have ever experienced."

Situations the Listener Must Be Prepared For

The storytelling element of regressive cell-singing can throw up a number of situations that the listener must handle with particular care to avoid impeding the singer's emotional release.

When a choice needs to be made

Almost all stories lead to one or more situations where some kind of choice needs to be made. At these points the singer has to decide how they want to continue – if they want to go this way or that, whether, for example, to forgive, embrace, defy, fight, answer a question…

When these situations arise, the listener must always interrupt the story and ask the singer what he or she wants to do, even if they themselves have a clear sense of what would be best for the singer. By all means discuss the options if the singer is unsure. The listener can give good advice and weigh up the potential consequences of this or that choice, but should *never* make the choice for the singer.

Example

A singer comes to a halt in the development of his or her expression when the story takes them to an old white house. The expression just goes round in circles, becoming monotonous and evasive. At the same moment, the images stop. The sound expresses the singer's insecurity about going into the house. "Do you want to see what's inside the house?" the listener asks.

This is a gentler question than "Do you want to go into the house?" and it helps the singer to recognize how they are feeling. "I'm afraid to go into the house. I can feel my throat tightening." They go on: "The house isn't important; there's something behind the house in the garden. I'm afraid to go there."

The singer starts to shake and cry at the recognition of the emotion beginning to surface. This creates an opening for the Note from Heaven. Situations that present a choice often lead to such openings in the energy field, so the listener really needs to have a sure instinct and good ear for these moments. As no one is out in the garden behind the house and the sound shows no trace of the Note from Heaven despite the opening, the singer appears to have evaded the issue with this maneuver. The listener then rephrases the question: "I would really like to see what's inside the house, would you like to go inside with me?"

The singer still doesn't dare, so an adult comes walking by to accompany the singer into the house. This can work particularly well if the singer's persona in the story is a child who needs to be released from something frightening – they will feel much safer if they have someone to hold their hand.

"A hunter is passing by, is it all right if he goes inside with you?"

"No, I want to go inside with my uncle. I feel safe with him."

When the path to a trauma has been cleared, the singer must

be ready to meet the trauma. When faced with such a choice, anyone would be uneasy about opting for the dangerous path. So, as the listener, you must remove any "land mines" in advance. If bodyguards are needed, provide them.

When other feelings obscure the primary feeling

There are several layers of emotion bound to a person's issues. In some cases, however, one emotion can be so prominent that you can't get around it, even though the course participant seems to have asked about something completely different.

For example, a woman came with a wish to have some heavy traumas from her childhood released. But grief about her dear old dog Spot dying a month before was uppermost in her mind. She hadn't mentioned the episode, but the little tail-wagging, black-and-white spotted dog was the very first image that appeared. This started a veritable hurricane of emotions.

The singer told how the dog had been mentally ill and its illness had filled most of her life. The image of the dog functioned like a needle piercing a hole in an abscess, so the infection could finally flow out.

We just managed to get a glimpse of a big black thorn wrapped in pink robes, before the hole closed up again: there had also been mental illness in her childhood home.

When a singer wants to tell their life story

A personal interpretation of a problem can become so integral to someone's identity that it prevents contact to their primary feeling and bars the way to any fresh insight.

For example, a person who has suffered from abuse may have retold their story so many times that they become trapped in the role of victim. This role entitles them to an attention, which sustains and reinforces the trauma because it gives others the right to feel sorry for them and to feel superior. No one chooses such a role. It gradually becomes integrated into the pain body and the person is taken over by it, and becomes dependent on it.

In this situation the listener needs to break the pattern and stop the singer before they assert this role in the group. As previously discussed, in regressive cell-singing the less the listener knows about the singer's personal life, the greater the chance for the therapy to have a releasing effect.

The listener will need to use intuition to draw the line between information that is important and information that will inhibit the process of release.

Issues of confidentiality

The listener and group members must respect the confidentiality of all participants.

In cases where a singer has been subject to serious abuse in this life, it is advisable for the listener to be briefly informed about it in advance, especially if the cell-singing is taking place in a group. If the singer feels insecure at the thought of singing in a group, the listener must consider whether it would be beneficial for the person to be released in front of other participants. If they decide it would not, a private session should be offered.

Sometimes I have had clear pictures indicating that a singer has been abused, without actually knowing whether this is the case. At times like this, it is especially important to take care not to overstep boundaries.

Listeners can really set the cat among the pigeons if they are not careful. A singer might, for example, begin to suspect on the basis of the listener's images that they have suppressed the memory of abuse in their childhood.

I have known course participants who have received this type of information from clairvoyants and who walk around with a dreadful "secret" that they dare not tell their aged father or mother about, a secret that can very easily get mixed up with other, totally different problems they are already struggling with. Close relationships are easy to poison.

- A listener must at all costs avoid empowering the singer's pain body.
- Negative thoughts tie up a person's energy.
- Pent-up energy is poison for the body as it imprisons the affected cells.
- The listener's knowledge of the cause of a singer's trauma is only important if it supports the process of release.

To protect a singer's confidentiality and avoid inadvertently revealing embarrassing details in front of other participants during storytelling, it is important that all the participants are aware in advance that the listener's images and stories are to be understood as symbolic, archetypal dreams.

I normally merely hint at any images relating to delicate subjects. If the images keep coming, I discreetly enquire about the theme or wait until I can do so privately.

If the listener is in doubt as to the story's meaning or validity, ask the singer to describe their own experience.

Example

Once in a story, a woman was so strongly attracted to another woman that she deserted her husband-to-be in the middle of their marriage ceremony. The story was set in the Middle Ages. The two women then made passionate love.

What can one say to that? The singer sang just as passionately and let go completely… I asked carefully: "Can it be true, that it is two women?" The singer nodded and seemed to become even more aroused in her singing expression, despite being happily married to a man. We never delved deeper into those details. The images led to a release in the voice and thus served their purpose.

The advantage with regressive cell-singing is that the stories, just like dreams, can be interpreted symbolically or as past lives. They camouflage reality, so only the singer is able to draw on the essence of the story. That gives total freedom.

A Few Common Symbols

Animals

Birds

It is quite common for birds to feature in regressive cell-singing stories. I encounter birds of all kinds: eagles, swans, storks, pelicans, parrots, seagulls, owls, pigeons, falcons and small sparrows. Sometimes I see a bird with distinctive features but I have no idea what it is called. In such cases, I describe the features for the singer.

Birds act as messengers between heaven and earth. Sometimes they symbolize a person known to the singer, who passes over and gives advice. Sometimes it is the singer who becomes a bird and experiences the freedom of flight. For someone who is trying to go up towards the light, what could be better than to have a set of wings?

Riding animals

Pent-up powers can appear as horses or other strong animals like dolphins, whales, bears, lions, tigers, elephants, rhinos, hippos, gigantic spiders that break out of their captivity. In that moment, one doesn't know if it is the story or the Note from Heaven that comes first. The Note from Heaven liberates the animal and the animal sets the Note from Heaven free. The type of animal depends on the type of trauma and on the singer's inner experience.

For example, a singer faced a challenge (or so I thought) when she was invited to sit up on a gigantic, black, hairy spider. Without a murmur she mounted the spider and rode it happily through the world while singing and exuding strength. "I have always perceived the spider to be a sacred animal of power," she said afterwards.

In Hinduism, every aspect of God has its mount (called vahana). For example, Ganesh has a mouse, Sarasvati a swan, Shiva a tiger. It is interesting that these mounts also appear again and again as archetypes in regressive cell-singing. The animals carry us onwards from one state to another. They strengthen us with their trusting approach to life.

Embracing animals

When self-confidence is low, having the courage to embrace a formidable or repulsive animal can change everything. Kiss the frog and redeem the enchanted prince or princess. Beauty and the Beast. We all have fairy tales inside us.

Here is an example from regressive cell-singing:

An Indian is standing outside a dark forest. The sky is dark grey and there are no leaves on the trees. The earth is frozen and covered with a fine layer of snow. The Indian is reluctant to go into the forest. Fear. Then he hears shots coming from the forest.

The sky becomes red. *Now the singer's voice sounds warmer.* The hunters mustn't shoot the Indian's beloved animals. He finds a big stick and, filled with anger, goes into the forest. The shots stop, the Indian is in the middle of the forest and feels the fear creeping over him once more. The anger is replaced by frustration at not being able to find the hunters.

Suddenly he finds himself in front of a huge, furious brown bear. The stick would break like a matchstick in its mighty paws. The bear is up on its hind legs in the semi-darkness with its yellow-white teeth glinting. *Here the singer must make a decision: "Do I meet the bear head on or do I try to escape?"*

In the event the singer chooses to run away, but now it is the listener's responsibility to point out that running away may signify death whereas meeting the bear head on, looking the beast in the eye, may represent the singer overcoming and releasing her fear.

201

The singer needs to be persuaded, but as soon as she decides the Indian should stand his ground, the Note from Heaven breaks through. At times like this, when great courage is needed, the other course participants and/or the listener can sing their support.

After hesitating for quite a long time, the trembling Indian takes the first couple of shaky steps towards the angry bear. *You can be sure that's what's happening by the expression in the singer's voice. You would be able to tell if she were pretending and just telling you, "Yeah, yeah, I'm doing it" – the whole organism has to be engaged.*

When the Indian is standing up close to the bear's body, it embraces him tenderly and he surrenders to the mighty beast. *The singer's voice expresses a fullness of power in its grateful unfolding of the Note from Heaven.* The Indian and the bear melt together in a column of light.

The sound moves us all and it gives the woman clarity about her path here in life. Now she has the strength to withstand her fear.

Thinking about the image of hugging the bear will always give her a feeling of power and wholeness. By recalling how her body felt in that moment, the woman will be able to contact the Note from Heaven whenever she wants.

Crosses

Crosses symbolize balance between water (horizontal line) and fire (vertical line) and usually carry religious associations. They often occur in classical stories set in earlier times (for example, regressions taking place in monasteries, churches or during the age of crucifixions). Many singers' stories culminate in release before a church altar, with a cross (or Jesus, God, Mary, Mary Magdalene, the Divine Mother...) leading the singer up to the light.

Union of ego and soul

A heavy drawbridge must be taken up to prevent a threatening and heavily armed army from forcing its way into a monastery.

A group of monks succeed in hauling up the drawbridge at the very last moment. *The singer's voice has low undertones, which continue.* Now they are safe. The enemy can't get in. A priest is clearing up. He dresses himself in a fine cloak, puts a pope-like hat on his head and goes in to pray in the vestry. A big, heavy cross is lying on the stone floor in front of him, upon which a bluish, bald, naked figure is lying, unable to move. It looks like an alien.

As the priest is about to pray, the blue creature opens its eyes. They glow with a blend of precious stones and magnets. They are good eyes.

"Priest, you must unite with me," the bluish, hermaphrodite figure says. After all the priest has gone through, only to be faced by this! Not quite what he had planned. Rather reluctantly, the priest tries to sing strength into the figure without success.

"Take your cloak and hat off, so we can meet in purity," the blue figure says.

As the priest stands humbly and without the trappings of his power, the beautiful blue creature rises up from the cross at the floor. *The Note from Heaven breaks through with its marvelous, luminous overtones.*

The singer experiences total acceptance of the soul (the blue creature) by the ego (the priest). The blue figure unites with the priest. The cross now stands upright, pure and penance-free.

Freedom from an austere upbringing

A young woman is standing by the sea on a bridge. This is the time of Columbus. A merchant ship is approaching the shore. A young man rows out from the ship in a small boat and picks her up. He takes her with him back to the ship. Her parents and brother stand on a cliff and wave goodbye *(it turns out later that they represent the singer's own family).*

The woman sails off to find adventure. She resolves to marry the young man, but not primarily for love. The ship lands on an island, where the couple go into an imposing, square house with columns. They enter a high-ceilinged hall in the middle of which stands a large cross.

"You must dance with the cross," a voice tells her. *I am surprised when the singer's face at once becomes tearful.* As the woman dances with the cross, it comes alive, its contours soften and it transforms into her fiancé. Now she can love him... the light breaks through and the cross gets its own place in the room, while the two lovers dance around freely.

Deeply moved, the singer later revealed that she grew up in a religious family that belonged to an austere Christian sect. She had left the sect as an adult. This had cut her off from her family, but her rigid upbringing still weighed heavily within her. That is why she had to dance with the cross, to soften it with her own hands and make it her own, in order to be set free.

Revealing the Light in a Singer's Voice

Light symbolizes contact to the higher, healing energies. Therefore, the moment in a story when the Note from Heaven breaks through fear's armor will almost always be accompanied by some form of illumination – for example, dark clouds pierced by a healing ray of light causing the sky to become increasingly bright.

Light may also break through as a shaft in a closed room or before a church altar. It may bathe two lovers or a child reunited with its mother and or father, in love, forgiveness, etc., etc. As the listener, ask the singer if they can sense or see the light – they usually can.

Sometimes, though, the singer has so little sense of self-worth that they can't experience how beautiful their sound is. In such cases, the singer may just shrug their shoulders at the story, even though it's obvious to everyone else from the singer's vocal expression that the Note from Heaven is shining through. The singer doesn't dare break free from the pain body. It's nice and safe to be a nobody, who is no threat to anyone and will be left alone, and may even find consolation in the bittersweet taste of feeling like a martyr.

This means the self-unaware singer can't see, hear or feel the light in their sound, even though we all are overwhelmed, and perhaps even moved to tears, by their singing.

"Well, no, it's nothing special."

In such cases, I often ask whether any of the other participants would like to be Sound Healed by the singer. With everyone having been so affected by the light in the singer's voice, there's usually no shortage of volunteers. Otherwise I put myself forward.

The singer will now experience their light and sound reflected in another person in the Sound Healing situation. They will forget themselves, because the one receiving the healing becomes more important, which fits perfectly with their pattern. Through the exchange of energy, the singer will be forced to listen to him or herself, because it's necessary to listen for resonance from the Note from Heaven during Sound Healing.[61]

Afterwards I ask them to sing the light down to themselves again. "Do you feel the light now? Do you hear your beautiful overtones?" Usually the singer's face is now totally radiant and the answer is a resounding, "Yes!"

"Hamster in the Wheel"

When a singer performs melodramatically, it is because he or she is trapped in their pain body. Their vocal expression has become stuck in a groove that can remind one of a hamster in a wheel.

When they scream, yell or cry for more than one or two minutes, their emotional expression has become indirect. Instead of being energizing, the sound will be empty and draining for those listening. A melodramatic performance is exhausting to listen to and will awaken only negative feelings. The singer may be crying, but there are few tears, or even none at all, and the crying doesn't arouse any genuine feelings in the listener's heart.

The same is true for a singing expression that feels stuck and empty of feeling. The singer can sing for hours and whether they recognize it or not, they need help in order to move on.

From experience I have found that in all cases of melodramatic performance it's best to interrupt the singer as soon as possible. Be sensitive and wait until the singer pauses in their breathing. Give tactful, but honest feedback: "You are caught like a hamster in a wheel, let me help you out of the cage. We need to try another way." Or, "I do not feel your expression in my heart." Or, "I experience that you are caught in a childhood pattern, am I right?" "Come and sit down on the floor and let me hold you." "Would you like us to give you attention?" "Do you want Mummy to give you milk?" Whatever fits.

As a listener of course, you should only say things like that if you can identify with the mother/father role in a natural way without ridiculing the singer. Most people caught in the hamster wheel are in a state where they will react like a child. The child is happy to get a response wherever they are at that moment. In any situation, a good laugh can activate the *hara* and set authentic expression in motion.

If the singer is showing signs of hysteria, ask him or her to sing high notes. The high notes are narrow, and represent the pure child in us all. Keep calm as a listener, and express yourself with authority. It's a power game. Do not fear, listener.

The aim is to identify and satisfy "the child's" needs, so they will dare to open up to their true feelings. In this way, an authentic expression can be reached.

In rare cases you may come up against heavy resistance, even be verbally attacked when you try to guide a singer away from their melodramatic performance: "I'm just about to be released." "You've got it all wrong." "You're destroying my process." "You aren't being therapeutic." "I need more time."

You have to be prepared for aggression from a person whose ego is fighting tooth and nail to avoid acknowledging dangerous feelings. Remember, the longer the singer is allowed free rein, the greater will be their embarrassment – and annoyance – when they are interrupted.

When the listener's navigation sign shows red, he or she must act quickly and aim without flinching. I have experienced melodramatic performers who, unconsciously, crave the limelight. Here the "performer" has an opportunity to milk energy from their audience. "Energy addicts" have an overriding need to draw attention to themselves. A child who yearns for his or her parents' attention, and only gets it in a negative form, through misbehavior, may bring this pattern with them into adulthood.

If the listener allows it, a melodramatic performer can cause the session to go round in circles like a hamster in a wheel. For example, the singer may endlessly argue over some trivial matter. The therapist also needs to be aware that the singer's pattern of self-protection may consist of projection. For example, the energy addict may use criticism to try to knock the listener off course and force them to defend or justify themselves. Never bring yourself down to the personal level. The question of whether the listener is good enough is non-negotiable. Anyone can make a mistake, but do not evaluate these with the participant. As soon as the listener's authority is undermined, the stardust will instantly vanish from all the miracles of that day.

The best way to avoid that kind of manipulation is to recognize the melodramatic behavioral pattern in advance by informing the group about "hamster in the wheel" before anyone sing themselves free. Tell them that if a situation like this will appear, we're dealing with compensation for genuine love. It's a learned pattern from childhood. It doesn't benefit anyone if a whole group is sucked dry of energy.

In a worst-case scenario, the listener should be prepared to erect a wall (see page 214) and allow the participant to wear him or herself out, rather than provoke them further by interrupting their need to exploit the situation.

A genuine outburst of anger can contain an opening to the Note from Heaven, so the listener must at the same time try to concentrate on listening to the sound within the rage and cheer the singer on when a strong sound is expressed. Do not stoop to the personal level. Keep yourself floating above the situation by listening intently to the quality of the sound. Praise the person for the real power that is finally breaking through and releasing the pressure in the room. The aggression that the singer had previously expressed will be dispelled by the appearance of the Note from Heaven. All genuine expressions of emotion are a welcome part of the process. They only become harmful if the listener takes them personally and judges the participant.

The state of consciousness behind listening for and noticing the sound in another person's voice lifts the listener like a balloon above and beyond the range of any artillery.

To be able to keep one's consciousness in a state of love elevated above the personal level is the overriding goal for a listener.

Care and physical contact

One purely physical way that a listener can help a singer to surrender to the Note from Heaven is to lay one hand lightly on the singer's forehead and use the other to support the neck, so that the singer can safely lean their head slightly backwards (a bared throat facilitates surrender).[62]

When a singer delves into experiences from early childhood, he or she will invariably respond well to being held or touched. If it feels natural, the listener can play the role of father or mother expressing unconditional love and care, but remember the golden rule: always ask the singer for permission to touch them. In case of abuse touch might be an unsafe solution.

In some cases, caring behavior like this can hinder the process, because it implies that the listener does not trust the singer to manage for themselves. When it is time for the participant to stand up to something, they will need to do this on their own. Just as, when the singer is confronted with their ego or their fear, it is he or she who must take the step to embrace the beast, forgive, agree to change their story, etc.

If the singer hesitates for a long time, the listener and the rest of the group can offer support with singing. The choir can build up an almost ceremonial atmosphere, which supports the singer without taking over their process.

Then the listener recites the code words that, at the beginning of the session, triggered strong feelings. If they still cause tension in the body, then there is more to be sung out. Before ending the session, the "baby" is led back to their real age, which means being able to *stand on their own feet when surrendering to the Note from Heaven*.

One other thing. You risk disturbing a good transformational process by being too caring – for example, the listener must refrain from wiping away a singer's tears as they sing themselves free. Put a tissue in their hand so they can do it themselves.

Don't ever feel pity for a course participant. To have pity arouses pain. To have compassion awakens light.

Tears are a sign that release is occurring or just about to. Tearless crying is a sign that the singer is not yet in touch with genuine feelings.

When the listener touches the singer, they must use their sensitivity and only do what feels natural. If the listener's heart is not awakened by love for the "child", it is because there is no need for those feelings at that moment. If the listener pretends, then a true release will not occur. The child that is calling for care needs the real thing and, interestingly enough, most course participants working with the Note from Heaven are able to respond quite naturally in a caring manner.

Don't just put your hand on someone's forehead or neck because I've told you that it works.[63] It should be something that you do naturally through a process. Please be aware that every thought, every fear you have is registered by the other person.

Encouraging openness about sexuality

Unfulfilled sexuality is often the underlying cause of physical imbalance and, therefore, disease. Surrendering to the Note from Heaven releases bound-up energy in a manner that has orgasmic characteristics and which compensates for releases that could have happened in another way. When there is resonance and unconditional love between the partners, sexual union provides undreamt-of opportunities for spiritual development. Working with the Note from Heaven opens up the way to this kind of spiritual elevation through erotic union.

In my experience, when I put my cards on the table and find a free, natural and light-hearted way to discuss a taboo subject like sexuality, the course participants breathe a sigh of relief. Sometimes two of them will look at each other in amazement: "What? You haven't had sex for ten years either?"

Today's sexual freedom, and the breaking down of traditional gender roles, has, to a great extent, resulted in apathy between the two sexes. Just as the positive and negative poles of the Earth are getting weaker over time, the differences between men and women are gradually becoming equalized. The subject is so extensive and important that it deserves a separate book.

The listener has to rise above his or her own sexuality, so that the client feels comfortable sharing embarrassing details they have kept to themselves for a long time. I might share my own general sexual experiences with the client if I judge that this will help to liberate them from feeling wrong, ashamed or guilty.

A wound has to be uncovered to be cleansed, tended and healed. By removing the boundaries of conventional "decency", we also remove the fear of being punished for discussing sex and sexual fantasies. We all have fantasies, since we are all in contact with the astral plane.[64]

When eroticism is elevated to full-blown love, it is raised up to the higher level of the astral plane, where fantasies are unnecessary because dream-like images appear on their own and often cause deep emotional reactions, especially in women. It is very important that a man sees a woman's crying during an orgasm as a great honor, akin to the transformative reactions generated by singing on the Note from Heaven.

If you bring beauty, truth, health, light or joy into the world, you are doing the right thing.
Shaman Olga Kharitidi

Shared themes

It often happens that the participants in a group have a theme in common. On one course, four out of five participants had difficulty standing up for themselves and all of them were dealing with a similar problem with their mothers; another time, nine women out of twelve had hip problems and had had, or were about to have, an operation for cysts in their abdomen; and yet another time every participant had been subject to sexual abuse, although only one had mentioned it in advance.

There are also mixed-theme days, but it is striking how often there are coincidences, even though the participants are not screened beforehand. Usually, no one knows each other in advance, as it can be problematic for close friends or family members to participate in the same group. A clean slate, where you can be yourself without anyone reflecting habitual roles back at you, is an advantage in the surrendering process.

Getting locked into tonal patterns

In regressive cell-singing some singers unconsciously repeat certain tonal intervals again and again like mice constantly running the same route up and down the stairs inside a cage. They can't break free from the tonal pattern. It's as if the phrase is programmed into their brain.

These repeated vocal patterns usually come from a singer's "training", projecting that they have learned an identity that is "nice", amenable and well-behaved. The patterns are carved like deep rivers in the electrical brain patterns. New patterns can only be done by a conscious choice to try something new.

It can be difficult to let go of an old tonal pattern because it may represent a lifeline to those we hold dear. "If I don't do what is expected of me, then I won't be loved." Conformity can be a protective armor, and it must gradually be dissolved. In some cases, the armor is so strong that the singer, try as they might, cannot get in touch with any kind of feeling. Like in a mollusc, the emotion lies well protected under decades of deposits that have become flinty shells. Here we must rely on patience. If we are lucky, storytelling, with just the right code words (see page 174), can winkle the emotions out.

Sometimes the emotional awakening happens spontaneously when the singer's defences are down, as it does in Resonance with Domino Effect (see page 277).

When a question is practical

Many people are cautious about opening themselves up emotionally. Consequently, they come with a simple wish or a practical question.

For example, one woman asked, "What should I do to get rid

of the fungal infection in my lungs?" She thought her asthmatic bronchitis was caused by fungus.

She got a clear answer when she began to sing with a weakened voice (note that the story has been reduced to its essence – it took almost 25 minutes to draw her voice out): "A sick man is lying down in a little cabin on a ship, which is sailing without a steersman. The journey starts on an icy sea and ends in Hawaii. The ship lands there and the sick man is served by attractive, half-naked women richly decorated with flower wreaths around their necks. They carry him down to the beach on a stretcher. He relaxes here while the women are at his beck and call." The answer was very simple: take a vacation in a warm country, relax and let yourself be spoiled.

Another example. A woman asked to be able to sing high notes. She gradually sang herself higher up via a story and, much to her surprise, experienced being able to sing high, melodious notes. We didn't get an explanation. Straightforward wishes often lead to straightforward outcomes.

Manifestation of Jesus

During a session in my International Education a young man in his twenties had a wish to dissolve the root cause of his fear. When asked if he had experienced violence in this life he humbly answered: "A little bit," and quietly explained that five times he had been brought unconscious to hospital, after being beaten up by gangs in his neighborhood. Beside this his father had beaten him and his brother daily. The young man explained that he passively had the attitude to be patient with his father until he was finished. "I am not for beating, I never liked to fight," the young man said. Instinctively I, Githa, asked for help from Jesus, and said: "You have passed the test, you did the right thing." These words awoke deep feelings in the man, who broke into tears. While singing on the cry tones the Note from Heaven manifested, and I saw the image of the young man being crucified for not wanting to fight for the Romans. When changing the story, Jesus took him down from the cross and blessed him. After the healing from Jesus, the young man started healing his fellow course participants. One of them regained normal sight and did not need to wear glasses anymore.

The Wall

If you say, "I cannot," you don't want to. If you want to, you can.
Hazrat Inayat Khan

Out of several hundred regressive cell-singing sessions, I have experienced only few cases where I needed to build a wall, which I describe in the two case studies below. Despite its rarity, this phenomenon is an extremely relevant subject in order to feel safe and protected as a listener. Building a wall is an important defence mechanism for the listener, because a sudden release, of a singer's withheld anger, can be tricked and surprise the listener. A furious outburst of anger that hits in the personal level can fundamentally traumatize a listener's confidence in the Note from Heaven.

As a listener you imagine a stone wall protecting you against the anger, and invite the singer to expel their anger on this unshakeable wall, while you listen for the Note from Heaven to reach through. Like a tennis ball the anger will jump back to the owner until the sound will clear up and the energy will heal everybody in the room. You can build a wall in a second if a singer attacks you with aggression, criticism or drains you (the listener) and the group of energy. The wall is built solely by the conscious thought: "I build a wall, which the singer can attack without hitting me personally. The wall makes me untouchable."

Example 1: Nooo, I don't want to sing!

When a young woman who had been subjected to many years of incest in her childhood registered for a course in regressive cell-singing, she deliberately hid her major social problems. She lived an isolated private life, had no boyfriend and, in general, felt no desire to live life here on Earth.

In this case, it was quite an advantage for me as the listener to know a little about her background. None of the course participants received any information about the young woman.

During the warm-up the girl refused to sing or make any sound. I accepted her reaction as healthy and dignified. She needed all of her strength and this strength was bound up in being able to say no.

That had to be the point: to get her to say no. And to whom else could she say no other than me? I gave her some time. I approached her carefully with singing for a couple of rounds, accepting her increasingly obstinate refusal. The point at which her anger would be influenced by the others' reactions came nearer. The great balancing act for me here was to judge the right moment for a final confrontation with the girl. The stronger her anger, the greater the discharge; but, on the other hand, if she were pushed too far she might decide to leave the course, and there would be no way back for any of us. The young woman would feel defeated and the atmosphere in the group would plummet so far down that it would be difficult to lift it up again.

I took a chance and asked her to express her "No" more forcefully: "NNNNoooo!" The image of building a wall appeared, so that I was prepared for her attack: she could fire away at me without doing me any harm.

"More 'Nooo', I want to hear more!" The girl let out a deafening scream! She screamed and screamed. The other participants put their fingers in their ears and I did as well. (You are fully within your rights to protect your ears if the sound from a participant is painful to your ears or heart.) The power was indescribably strong. "More, more, we want to hear all of it, out with it!" I had to yell through her screaming.

To give promptings when a singer takes a short pause during

a catharsis is not a good idea as it can bring the process to a halt. For example, saying, "Yes, you are doing great," while a singer is inhaling can be interpreted like a listener is impatient and does not think the singer is doing well on their own. However, when the singer is in the throes of an outpouring the same phrase can seem completely different. Then, it is like adding fuel to the fire. It always feels good to get a pat on the shoulder, to be accepted and cheered on when you are fully engaged in action.

It is a possibility to glide tonally with the singer, so he/she feels "we are together" and the others in the group accept, hear, feel, enjoy and get inspired and healed by the emotionally-charged expression. Enthusiastic shouts of encouragement are important during the singing, otherwise the thought "I wonder what the others are thinking?" might just creep in and stop the process. "Am I being embarrassing?" "No – we are with you and are truly enjoying your release."

The girl screamed and screamed while flinging her slender body about. An empathetic participant handed the girl a tissue for the tears that followed after the screams. The tissue was angrily crumpled up, hurled to the ground and trampled on in an almost euphoric dance. The girl began to smile, and so did the rest of us. This was a body beginning to discover the woman within – a body that had been frozen in a state of "I don't want to be here."

After two minutes of screaming, the woman's true voice broke through, as if coming directly from heaven.

In the pauses between the singer's breathing, I did what I normally do – repeat the images that appeared during her expression of the Note from Heaven:

"Fishing boat on a rough sea with a pink, ragged sky. The fishermen have caught a beautiful dolphin in their net. The dolphin fights its way loose from the Filipino fishermen and slides back into the sea. Shaking of the fear, it dives down and meets a male dolphin. They briefly rub each other's noses, before the female dolphin swims up to the surface of the sea again. The dolphin moves so violently in the water that the fishing boat is washed away by the tidal wave caused by the anger. The dolphin stands up on its tail fin still singing powerfully. The male dolphin waits in the distance."

In the end, the singer burned the tissue that she had trampled on. This was done ceremonially in my teacup. She poured the ashes down the toilet. After three follow-up one-day courses, this woman was finally able to get on with her life. The last I heard she had begun painting and was planning an exhibition, and she had also enrolled for a university course.

There are no rules or recommendations regarding the number of sessions. This particular woman felt she needed additional courses – each time with an interval of approximately one or two months to digest the cellular changes from the previous course. It is up to the individual to decide how many courses they need and how long the time period between them should be. There have been cases where participants have come again, but could clearly sense that they had already outlived their trauma. Such a realization is a golden full stop. It's over and they are moving on in life.

Example 2: Wishing for more than you can handle

Another time I had to create a wall was when treating a journalist, whose interest in regressive cell-singing appeared to be more professional than personal. The episode added much to my experience, which is why I mention it here.

The session showed that *when a singer intellectually works out their ultimate wish it will be met head on.* If the person is not able to handle the ultimate, a mirror image is created that can be extremely provocative when the singer is confronted by it.

When I asked for the first volunteer at the start of the session, the journalist put herself forward without hesitation.

Her wish was for unconditional love – both to receive it and to be able to give it – and her primary feeling was that she was not good enough. Very unusually, she did not have any code words. Never accept to start a session without code words! The images started to come and at first nothing seemed amiss.

Steep, dark cliffs surrounding water. Dark sky, grey clouds. *The singer started to grunt and hiss demonically.* A black, oblong, narrow wooden boat. A woman dressed in black with a baby, a man dressed in a dark cowl propels the boat with a long pole. Hopeless feeling. Is it death? *The singer did not answer, but continued with the deep hissing tones. There was no ground in the tones, they went in circles and felt unpleasant, in that they seemed to affirm themselves in the darkness. After a while, the atmosphere became really heavy.* "Sing the child up into the light; we need an opening up to heaven." The boat glides drearily on. *The singer's sound expression was the same.*

The child is up on the cliff and the boat has gone. *No change in the singer's vocal expression.* The little, naked child is lying on the cold, hard cliff. It will die if no one takes care of it. *The singer continued grunting and by now the energy in the group had completely dropped. I felt heavy and noticed that I was being drained of energy. It was as if the singer was opposing every opportunity for release out of an inconsolable self-loathing.*

Now a stork is coming. It stands waiting beside the child with a nappy in its beak.

The singing continued in the same dark, demonic groove. "The stork says that it will fly off again if you don't help it get the child up into the light."

With that, the singer cracked: "I need more time, and by the way, the child is not going up into the light at all. It's going to stay on the cliff!"

"Then the child will die."

"Yeah, well let it die!" she yelled. "Therapists don't do that. You are not a good therapist!"

I let her know that I needed to be loyal to the energy I channel.

"You're no channel. Do you think you're so pure that you can be a channel?"

At that moment, I created an imaginary wall and invited the singer to shout at me. The journalist did not let herself be drawn in. All of my urgings for her to shout out her anger at me were demolished by her own self-view: "Don't you dare think you're somebody special!" (In other words: I don't want any help, I am not worth anything, I don't deserve it.)

Obstinately, she continued with her grumbling. I closed my eyes and prayed for a way out.

"The stork suggests flying you and the baby over to a strong, warm-hearted peasant woman, who is sitting on a newly harvested field on a pile of hay. Will you go along with that?"

The singer nodded slowly and began to sing. The voice was softer now, but still without the slightest contact to the Note from Heaven.

"The peasant woman is bringing you up to her breast and rocking you. You grow warm and feel safe and good."

The singer obviously wanted to call the shots. It was difficult to guide her through breathing. She strongly resisted every bit of advice, as if I were the enemy.

"A huge, golden sunflower appears in the distance. You are being offered the chance of being lifted up into the sunflower's golden center by the peasant woman. Here you can receive the light of heaven. Do you want that?"

"'No.' *The reply came without a moment's hesitation.* "But I would like to pick the sunflower and take it with me." *The singer now sang with a self-conscious softness and I got the impression that her attention was focused on the others' opinion of her.*

As she had now been singing twice as long as her allotted time, I rounded off.

The rest of the day she smiled politely and kept her distance. In the following days, I received quite a number of aggressive e-mails from her; however, they did become softer towards the end of the week: "I sing now with the cows out in the field and that feels good."

Wishes can be so contrived that they miss the target. You can have your greatest wish granted and yet be unable to accept it...

General Problems

When a singer does not hear the story

In some cases, the singer can get so caught up in the Note from Heaven that they "disappear" into their own world. When this happens, I choose to tell the story anyway, as it influences the subconscious mind. I follow the same principle when a singer sings so powerfully that they can't hear what I am saying.

After a long and colorful story, where the voice seems to have sung the story forwards, singers sometimes complain that they didn't catch what I said. I point out that the story is secondary to the release that has occurred. If they have been so "gone" that they didn't hear the story, this is usually an excellent sign – it suggests that they have been on a higher plane and have been released there. It is my impression that the story gets the voice going and gives the singer a private space in which to feel free. While all the rest of us are engaged in the "plot", the singer can float around in the healing energy. However, I do retell the story if that's what they want, as the echo of the story offers security, a link to the world so that they can easily find their way home again.

When a singer does not recognize a miracle

Jesus said: "I am the light that is above them all. I am the All. The All comes forth from me and the All reaches towards me. Cleave the wood, I am there; lift up the stone, and you shall find me there."
Gospel of Thomas, log. 77

A miracle is within reach for everybody, just as the Oneness level is a part of all life. But we have to recognize the wonder in order to experience it. So, *if you ask for a miracle to happen, you must, at the same time, ask to be open enough to receive it.*

The stronger a singer's trust in the higher powers, the more miraculous the manifestations, and the greater the gratitude and surrendering.

When a miracle causes healing or the improvement of imbalances, the effect will only manifest itself permanently if the singer simultaneously expands their consciousness.

It happens that the healed person will not accept the physical proof of a healing as a miracle nor will they feel gratitude in their heart. Singers sometimes deny everything immediately after a miraculous healing: "Well, I wasn't that sick anyway. It probably would have gone away by itself."

Alternatively, a client may give the therapist all the credit: "Thank you, Githa, for having healed me." Such gratitude is natural, but testifies to their inability to open up to the essence of the miracle.

It is not out of humility that I refuse their gratitude: it's just that it wasn't my doing! I opened myself up so the energy could flow through me. My trust in the higher power gave the energy the opportunity to work. The power of the Note from Heaven is much greater than that of one person.

The healing is free, but my time is certainly not!
Calle Montsegur (*The Seer* by Lars Muhl)

So, there is no guarantee that a singer will realize that a miracle has occurred, even if the listener and the other course participants have, without any doubt, experienced it to be so.

"The cure" and the process of the disease have a higher meaning that perishes if they are not also bound up with a strengthening of the client's trust in the divine. The miracle turns a minus into a plus, as the vertical line represents fervent trust. Without connection between the shadow and the light, the plus power vanishes.[65]

A person, for whom the miraculous stardust gets lost, is bound to the material plane and is then also subject to the laws that apply there. If someone has been physically cured through a miracle, but has been unable to embrace the miracle within their consciousness, it is very likely that the disease will soon reappear.

So if the participant does not recognize that a miracle has occurred, it won't be long before the soul is undernourished once more and cries for help using physical pain as its medium.

Our consciousness is kept supple and elastic through daily singing and surrender to the Note from Heaven. When the fruit falls from its branch with a soft thud, we can lay the table for a feast.

Example

An elderly woman had signed up for regressive cell-singing, because a clairvoyant had recommended she work with her voice.

For seven years she had suffered from a long list of asthma-related illnesses. These had started immediately after her only son had died in a car accident. Since asthma affects breathing, and with that the whole intake of energy, the reason for her illness seemed clear: the death of her son had given her a tremendous shock with ensuing stiffening that weakened her desire to live/breathe.

The woman sang herself into her illness and a miracle happened:

A captain, wearing blue sailor's clothes and a cap, is on his little yacht enjoying the sun and the spray from the sea. He feels free and happy. *At this point, the singer's voice opens and her breathing becomes deep. After a while the asthma disappears. The Note from Heaven breaks through on long breaths with its infinitely light and beautiful overtones. Everyone in the room listens in rapt silence.*

The sailor wants to help and work together with the singer. The woman is deeply touched and her whole demeanor is changed. Her face is radiant.

When the singer had recovered, she told us that her son had been a ship's captain and had worn a cap and the blue uniform described in the story. The pain in her body had gone and her breathing had become normal. I felt there was probably more that needed releasing, but that had to wait until this release had had time to be integrated into the body's energy system.

The woman had released so much energy that the air in the whole room quivered.

When she contacted me a couple of weeks later, it was to cancel our appointment: her new clairvoyant had told her it was not good for her to sing.

Trauma Due To Being Ignored

I have given you examples of singers releasing past traumas that stemmed from active abuse, but in fact one of the hardest kinds of trauma to release is that which comes from having been ignored. The following story is an illustration of the harm that can be done by suffering prolonged indifference.

Experiment with rice

When my eldest son started school, his vocabulary developed explosively. To put it plainly, swear words and vulgar terms flew through the air without his understanding the meaning and effect of these words on the people around him. These were words whose vibration has been distorted by deformed, suppressed feelings. They affect our bodies negatively, because they carry negative vibrations that can ignite repressed, as yet unlit emotional bonfires.

Innocence isn't affected by these words, which is why children have fun playing around with them until the day they run into someone who takes exception. Then it becomes even more fun. In the end, the child gets into trouble for it. Then the penny drops! Dangerous, forbidden, interesting. Their innocence is gradually degraded.

Around that time I gave presentations on Sound Healing at two conferences where the main speaker was Masaru Emoto,[66] a Japanese scientist and author renowned for his research into how the molecular structure of water reacts to a wide range of vibrational influences. His photos of frozen water crystals at minus five degrees centigrade clearly show that water is not only influenced by music, but by specific pieces of music. In fact, all forms of vibration influence the structure of water, and that includes feelings, thoughts and words.

In his book *Messages from Water*, Emoto describes an experiment with rice. My son and I decided to try the experiment out for ourselves. I must admit, it is one thing to read about something and quite another to experience it for yourself. So, dear reader, by all means give it a go.

We took three identical sterilized jam jars with lids and with the same, clean, spoon put 20 grams of freshly cooked brown rice into each glass. After the rice had cooled down, we put the lids on and put a white label on each.

On the label of the first jar, we wrote the worst swear words my son could imagine: "Fuck you, idiot!"

On the next jar, we wrote the most loving words he could imagine: "Love, gratitude".

We didn't write anything on the last jar.

After that the three jars stood on the same shelf in the refrigerator for four months. For the first two months we spoke to the jars we had written on at least once a day. We ignored the third jar.

Later, we expressed our feelings to the rice more sporadically. Every time my son had learned new swear words, he went and said them to the "Fuck you" rice. He also remembered the "love" rice and would loudly and solemnly sing to it: "Love and gratitude," "I love you."

Soon the rice in the three jars began to look and smell significantly different from each other.

The ignored rice started turning black after about ten days. Its smell was weak and not at all aggressive. It seemed to have given up, as if it were saying: "There is no need for me. I am withdrawing."

A little later, the negatively charged "fuck you" rice turned brown-yellow and greasy. But whereas the ignored rice withdrew and seemed to shrink, the brown-yellow rice expanded, as if it were fighting back and saying: "Do what you want, I will survive." Over time, the smell in the jar slowly turned from pungent and sharp to fermented. It was so strong that it made your eyes water. The color gradually changed from brown-yellow to turquoise.

The love-charged rice was gradually covered with a white, mold-like layer. The smell was sickly sweet with hints of vanilla, not pungent or sharp.

My son was so enthralled by the experiment that he asked if he could take the rice with him to school. There just happened to be a parents' meeting, so I chose to inform the parents about it so there wouldn't be any misunderstandings regarding rotten rice, bacteria, crazy healers and that kind of thing.

The parents showed only moderate interest in the rice, but I was allowed to show the rice to the children in the class and a couple of them dared to lift off the lids and sniff the contents. "Well that is incredible!" They looked at me with wonder.

The children were so interested that we had to keep bringing the rice back in to show them whenever it showed any further changes in appearance or smell.

Examples of being ignored

The biggest challenge for a therapist is in those unfortunate cases where a child has been isolated, ignored and treated with indifference. A grown-up's presence and loving touch are vital for an infant and their absence, at worst, will cause a child's death – withdrawing into itself, just as the ignored rice shrank and turned black.

Of course, the ignored souls who turn up to a course have received enough care to survive. They have survived like molluscs that have their own safe world under their shells where they can hide and, now and then, stick the tips of their antennae out into the world.

There are many different causes and background stories here. A classic example is the mother who suffers from guilt because she is not able to open her heart to her infant child. The child's presence hurts the mother, because it reminds her about her own lack of love. Therefore the child from birth experiences itself as a burden for its mother,[67] although everything on the surface may seem perfect. If the father also is absent or unfeeling the traumatization becomes complete. Often the course participant has not realized how "bad" their situation is. An ignored person punches into thin air. Their trauma comes from an absence rather than the presence of anything actively harmful that they can react to. "I was given food, clothes, driven to school... My parents were good to me. They never hit me." Fortunately, the organism protects itself by accepting the state of things. You can't lament feelings you don't know exist.

As an adult, the ignored person senses they are stunted emotionally when compared to the people around them. They find it difficult to be aware of emotional reactions in their body.

Some children may also be affected by an experience of physical isolation in the hospital when diagnosed with a serious infectious disease. For example, before widespread vaccination children with cerebrospinal meningitis were isolated in hospital, treated by nurses wearing masks and received their food through a hatch. It was normal to ask parents to visit only once a week, at most.

When a small child receives that sort of treatment, they

become seriously traumatized. In several of the examples I have encountered, the isolation lasted for months.

Treating people who have been ignored

The treatment in regressive cell-singing for course participants with symptoms of having been ignored is very individual and, as always, relies on the listener's intuition developed by working with the Note from Heaven. There may be the merest hint of something that, with sensitivity, can be drawn out using the right word, sound or intonation. Or sometimes the image of a cherished childhood toy can awaken long-suppressed feelings.

Let us say that an infant was never stimulated by the feeling "red".[68] The color still exists in adulthood as a possibility, but is imperceptible on the palette of feelings, because the emotional strings in the child that have never been stimulated will atrophy and lose the ability to resonate, just as a leg in a plaster cast loses its muscle tone. So the encounter with "red" doesn't awaken any resonance, because its tone is not to be found in the ignored person's fundamental existential patterns.

The question is whether you can soften an atrophied emotional string. In my experience you can, but only with the same kind of repeated training you would use to recondition an atrophied muscle. In most cases I would combine sound scanning[69] with regressive cell-singing, reflexology and/or massage. With sound scanning, the ignored person receives a gentle stimulation of the passive cells (similar to ultrasound therapy, for example); and with regressive cell-singing, the breathing is activated, and gradually unfolded as the ignored person's feelings are brought back to life. In this way the situation is worked on from two angles that are mutually stimulating. Combining the vocal sound therapy with reflexology and/or massage will support the body to integrate the new feelings in the body.

The ignored person's soul is led back to its original essence in the Oneness level – that is, to a state where the emotional string that was not stimulated by the feeling "red" is intact.

Singing the Note from Heaven daily would further support this process.

Another supplementary method is vocal regression (see page 244), where the singer goes back to a time, early in their infancy, in the embryo or in a past life, when they were able to access their whole palette of feelings. When you can contact your emotions, you can sing the feelings free.

Physical touch

When a singer who was ignored as a child regresses to the infant stage, manually touching him or her lightly while humming for them can help them open up to resonance.

As a female listener, it can feel natural to take on the mothering role, but only if it happens spontaneously. It is easiest to do this with one's own gender (if you are heterosexual). When communicating with an infant, words become secondary to touch and sounds.

When the little child is whimpering and reaching out for mummy or daddy a trained ear can register it in the singer's voice. In the cases where it feels right I ask, "Do you have a need to be held?" If the answer is yes, I start by putting my hand gently on the forehead, or wherever it happens to feel best. If the participant leans their head on me, the next step is to sit on the floor behind them, so they can be rocked while "mummy" is close by, and wants to hear *everything* the little one has to say. While the child is singing you can choose, as the listener, to sing along if the sound feels more healing that way.

The inner child in the client experiences being heard and understood on a wordless level. A client once explained after a séance that she felt we were as one. The breathing, the sound, everything.

When the "child" feels safe the body will, in some cases, make involuntary movements, as if it is trying to wind itself into place again (see the Paula Technique, below). Here I follow along and support them as well as I can. When the head lifts and turns around, I have a hand ready the whole time to support, so the neck can rest on a "care cushion" at any time.

At the end of a regressive singing process, the singer is sound-healed. Close contact between the listener's stomach and the singer's back, where the singer is sitting on the floor with the listener embracing from behind, is an especially rewarding Sound Healing position for "babies".

In that way energy coming directly from the *hara* chakra resonates over a large area and leads to an experience of melting and becoming whole in the energy, which is extraordinarily healing. Before the séance finishes, it is, as always, important to bring the singer back up to the adult level, where they should be able to sing the Note from Heaven on their own.

In the days following a release, feelings start vibrating in the body and can feel quite overwhelming and frightening for a formerly silent and ignored inner child. The reaction is a positive sign that life has returned to previously atrophied emotional strings. It is now time to master your inner harp. Embrace the tones instead of running away from them.

Paula Technique – Interrelationship Between the Sphincter Muscles

Paula Garbourg (1907-2004) was a German-Jewish classical ballet dancer and professional opera singer. In Israel I became acquainted with her book *The Secret of the Ring Muscles: Healing Yourself Through Sphincter Exercises* through a student who had been trained in the Paula technique. In brief, the Paula technique is based on the mutual strengths of the body's many sphincter muscles and the fact that they are connected to each other. Sphincters are ring-shaped muscles that control the opening and closing of bodily passages, orifices, feet and hands (in P.

Garbourg's method).

In her youth, Paula lost her voice for a long period of time and discovered, during dance training, that she could activate her voice by stepping up on her toes. She continued the movements and retrained her voice in that way.

This led to a wish to understand the muscular connection and she found out that the activation of a strong sphincter muscle can influence and strengthen a weaker sphincter muscle. A baby trains sphincter muscles the whole day. The hands, the feet, the mouth open and close in reflexive movements and these simultaneously stimulate the voice, the digestion; they get the entire body going.

In Paula Garbourg's book there are numerous examples of the healing of autism, intellectual disability, asthma, migraine, rheumatism, impotence, incontinence, etc.

During regressive cell-singing, a participant's body can start making involuntary movements. Some participants shyly suppress the body's impulses, while others attract attention to the phenomenon. In these situations, I encourage them to let the body do what it wants, no matter how awkward or embarrassing it may feel. The soft palate contains a sphincter muscle. The Note from Heaven can only break through when that muscle is stretched like a dome up in the rear part of the oral cavity. The use of the soft palate's sphincter muscle activates and strengthens the sphincter muscles in the entire body. A pulsating network of imperceptible movements is set in motion.

The interrelationship between the sphincter muscles causes the involuntary movements that occur in some singers. So, there is no reason to panic if a client's body begins to make strange movements. Everything is all right. You can safely let the singer continue their process with the strange facial expressions and body movements, which can be stopped at any moment when and if the singer takes over control of him or herself.

The listener's confidence in everything being all right gives the singer room to feel free.

Pulse and rhythm

If a singer is too inhibited to allow the involuntary movements to happen, then rhythm or a simple pulse beat can do wonders. Dancing becomes a natural extension of the voice's expression. The body joins in.

On my CD *Rising* there is a recording of fetus sounds, where you can hear the pulsating sounds of the umbilical cord vibrating and the beating of the mother's heart. We have all heard and felt the rhythm of these sounds 24 hours a day, from when we were a four-month-old embryo in the womb until we were born. So incorporating a pulse-like rhythm into the session can make it easier for some people to let go. Four-part rhythms give grounding, while three-part rhythms are calming and open up for contact with the heart.

In the warm-up session of a course, I like to work with low tones, rhythm and the body. Grounding is a prerequisite for complete surrender. With the roots well anchored in the earth, the organism is able to carry its crown, even endure strong storms, without breaking the smallest twig.

Release Through Changing the Story

Religious effort is not to be free of sin, but to be equal to God.
Plotinus

Fear squeezes the life energy out of the nerves to such a degree that it lowers the level of vitality in the entire body.
Yogananda

Readiness for release

Fearful, shameful, disempowering, terrible, painful traumas become attached to the body, not only as bound-up energy in the cells, but also as rigid existential patterns.

These can be characterized by anger and judgment of "the sinners" – those whom the person blames for his or her state. When blame is in focus, the body is nourished with negatively charged energy, which is a delicious treat for the pain body. Therefore, guilt and shame function like a thorn in the flesh.

We can heal and treat through eternity and this may even soothe the pain, but we must remove the thorn if the infection is to be eradicated. This can be achieved through forgiveness and/or changing the stories and the events that a client has attached to their identity.

Out with all the negative-acting stories and in with some new, refreshing pictures and feelings that build up healthy energy structures.

In the timeless state that opens up when working with the Note from Heaven, everything is possible because past present and future merge into oneness. Just by thinking that freedom is possible you start the healing process. In addition, the Note from Heaven can lift you to enter the gate of heaven.[2] Thus the singer can turn the feeling of disempowerment into a plus power. The question is, are you ready to leave your pain body? Do you really wish to leave your negative habits of complaining?

When the need to backbite and complain comes with its attractive, bittersweet taste, stop for a moment and think carefully before you continue. As long as the pain body has power over you, then your organism will not be able to integrate new, positive energy structures.

The human being is surrounded by potential positive energy. If we are open to its possibility, we will be able to receive it. Fear contracts and closes off. Devotion relaxes and opens up.

In the Aramaic language, which was spoken in the time of Jesus, sin is synonymous with making a mistake: "To miss the target. To be absent in the moment."

Considerations

"Can you change something that you know has happened?" is one of the questions I am most commonly asked.

Yes – you can change the energy around the event by emptying its content. You will still remember the event, but you will have restructured it into a harmless memory; an old, empty cardboard box in the attic.

You have moved on. But how will you deal with your newfound freedom if you have been chained for most of your life? Do not be too hard on yourself.

Remember that, even though the world now lies at your feet, you can still choose to remain living in your dog kennel. Before, you didn't have any choice, but now you do. The freedom to take responsibility for your own life is fundamental to a happy body.

Lars Muhl once wrote to me: *"Just be you, wish for everything you want and you will get it. Everything is love."*

It sounds so wonderful, and I have experienced the truth of those words myself. But how challenging they are – because if I don't know who I am, how can I then wish for what I want? What if I make the wrong wish and it backfires!

The fear of wishing for what is best for yourself is an aspect of the fear of changing an identity that has been formed by expectations from your surroundings. An adapted "I" that, like an outer skin, holds a liquid interior together.

What should I choose, consideration of others or consideration of myself?

Can the true self be happy if it considers itself at the expense of others?

A human being with a balanced, positive, surplus energy projects light and joy onto their surroundings.

A human being that is burnt-out and negative for a long period of time drains their surroundings.

The Buddha pursued always to seek balance, which led him to enlightenment.

The lifeline is the divine plan. There is only one path that is yours. Maybe you are walking it, maybe you have gone astray. Search for the path and when you have found it, serve it.

Jesus said: "He who seeks shall find, and to him who knocks the door shall be opened."
Gospel of Thomas, log. 94

By playing with the thought that *all my dreams can come true*, a seed of trust is planted in the universal mind. A heartfelt wish is, in fact, a desire for a miracle. The purpose of the miracle is not the miracle itself, but to strengthen trust in God. "Knowing" that my true "I" is a living miracle in this universe will teach me to listen carefully for signs of the divine.

By searching for the higher meaning in all aspects of life, your focus keeps you grounded, but at the same time leaves space for the higher energies to be present. In that way you take responsibility for your higher Self.

Be prepared that the signs from the higher energies manifest in many surprising ways and can be quite amusing! When we change a story or event in regressive cell-singing, we invoke the divine. Your wish calls on the higher energies to lead you. You cannot go wrong in this process, because anything that might be seen as a mistake will actually expand your consciousness.

Energy is extinguished without free space to maneuver in, just as a fire is extinguished without oxygen.

Changing the first layer of a multilayered trauma

A two-year-old boy with cerebrospinal meningitis was isolated in hospital and his mother was only allowed to visit him once a week. This went on for two months. As an adult, the man suffered from an extreme need for sex. When his partner was not in the mood – for example, because she was breastfeeding their baby during the night – the man felt unloved and letdown.

For him, sex was love.

Whenever the man felt rejected, he reacted like a forsaken two-year-old calling for his mother. The male sexual urge is located in the root chakra, which is also the source of the survival instinct. This suggested to me that the trauma of this singer was probably connected to a fear of being unwanted and abandoned.

His primary feeling was: "I get abandoned because I am not good enough." His code words: "You've been letdown," "You feel powerless," "You're not lovable" and "Only when you have sex can you be yourself."

As soon as the singer released the excess emotional pressure, the Note from Heaven broke purifyingly through. In that state, the man came to a psychological and physical realization of the emotional state induced by the two-year-old boy's experience. The story was already starting to change at this point.

The boy experienced being heard and loved unconditionally as he became filled up by the light and energy of the state of consciousness the Note from Heaven led him into.

Experiencing this state once was not enough, because the child's sense of being let down became thoroughly embedded during the two-month period of isolation. The singer and listener had to be prepared to uncover several layers in this trauma. The cleansing could only be completed if the singer sang the Note from Heaven every day to care for his wounded inner child. On a practical level, his energy was diverted from sex to the Note from Heaven, which improved the relationship with his partner.

Changing the story

The listener asks the singer if he or she is willing to change their story. In order to change the story, not only must the singer consent but he or she must establish an emotional contact to the trauma. Normally the singer and the listener change the story together. This is because, as discussed, it is difficult for the singer to keep a clear head when strong emotions are raging. The listener elicits the singer's wishes by suggesting new ways for the story to pan out.

In the case of the man suffering from a trauma induced by being isolated in hospital as a child, I suggested removing the whole experience of his illness. But this was too big a change of identity for him, so we needed to find a compromise. The reworking that emerged was that the boy was taken care of at home by his mother and the illness was a bad case of flu instead of meningitis. The mother was reading him fairy tales, singing to him, serving him his favorite meals (here we can go into great detail, because the food is very important to a small child), washing his face with a cool cloth, stroking and kissing him.

During the reconstruction of their story, singers usually become overwhelmed by strong feelings. They might chuckle happily or weep with joy.

When certain details in the story seem to nourish a singer, it is good to dwell on these parts for a while and always let singers take the story forward themselves when, and if, they get hold of a main thread. They may get in touch with new facets of their unfulfilled needs.

The listener can add to the story and make it even better, although only ever with the singer's consent. Returning to the example: "Daddy comes home with a present. What would you like? A teddy bear?" – "No, a red car" – "... and mummy and daddy sit close together and hold you."

"Your siblings are on holiday and your mummy has taken time off work, so there is a lot of extra energy and time for your parents to be present with you. Daddy is a loyal and kind husband."

The listener asked how the singer felt inside when mummy and daddy said that they loved him. The singer's reaction here spoke a clear message. Was there something special that he has always wished his parents would do?

"I want my parents to love each other!" Now his voice was, at last, thick with emotion. There was some deeper issue here.

During the whole reformulation process the singer sings. The sound immediately and unfailingly indicates when a release is occurring. The depth of the transformation is dependent on the brain-wave level the singer has reached. If they are in the alpha-stage, i.e. completely relaxed, the information can easily be led further down to the theta and delta brain-wave length, corresponding to the infant's mind and the grown-up's subconscious mind. If the singer's conscious mind is still active, then his brain waves will be at beta 1 or beta 2 and the transformation won't penetrate so deeply into the subconscious mind.[70]

In this particular case, the child was not released from his betrayal trauma during the first session. There were numerous layers to work on. A little corner had been lifted, but cleaning up under the carpet needed to continue if the trauma was to be released. It took several sessions before a release occurred and the singer had the will to take the path of self-development. This man's whole identity was based on his sexuality. He had left a trail of failed relationships, children here and there, infidelity, letting others down. He was troubled by a strong sense of guilt, but this was coupled with a devil-may-care attitude that hid the pain of a two-year-old boy who had lost his grip on life; he alternated between bragging and feeling sorry for himself.

Forgiveness

Storytelling often throws up situations involving forgiveness. When a singer meets another person in the story, the listener can choose to enquire if that person is familiar. If the singer is in doubt about the other person's identity the listener can describe the person's appearance in more detail.

I remember a case where a woman calmly said, "That is my

mother."

"She is asking you to forgive her."

"Well – no, I'm not ready for that."

I was annoyed by the answer, because I had a feeling that release was just around the corner. But as the listener, I had to accept and respect the singer's attitude as "right". If she wasn't ready, then she wasn't ready. You can't flap another person's wings for them. The mother continued to ask for forgiveness throughout the whole story, but the singer was totally closed towards her and was quite irritated in the end. The Note from Heaven did not manifest itself.

Afterwards, the participant told me that she had had therapy for years to get her mother out of her system. That is why it irritated her that she had now turned up again. The singer thought that she had finished with her mother. A couple of weeks later she wrote to me that she regretted not accepting the chance to forgive and was now ready to do so. This shows how regressive cell-singing can set in motion a process of forgiveness even if a singer resists it at first.

If the person (or people) who seeks out the singer in the story is still alive, then the forgiveness and release still occurs on the soul level. It will happen in much the same way as when the story is changed. The energy structure is opened and balanced. When the singer subsequently meets the person they have forgiven, both parties will clearly sense a change, even without the other person having any knowledge of what has happened. The singer's changed consciousness now carries a different energy that opens up new ways of relating to the other person.

In storytelling I have experienced several variations of the forgiveness process. Unlike the woman in the above example, the singer is usually ready to forgive. However, before forgiveness takes place the person who has shown up may want to explain themselves, and they start a dialogue with the singer. If it is difficult for the singer to forgive, and there are still differences between the two, the listener can invite the singer to ask for a helping tool (see the following section).

When the forgiveness is complete, the listener might suggest an embrace, if it hasn't already happened naturally. If the singer is unwilling to take this step, this indicates that his or her heart chakra is still closed and the forgiveness process is not yet complete.

Personal tools

Another way to effect change through storytelling is to provide the singer with a virtual helping tool. The singer closes the eyes and asks for a tool to, for example, protect herself with, so that she can feel safe in daily life. If the singer doesn't see any tool, the listener can share what he or she can see and then often the singer suddenly sees something. "No, it's not a hat; it's a cloak that I can protect myself with."

Example 1

A Native American (the singer's "character" in the story) is standing in front of the tribe that has killed his entire beloved family while he was out hunting. He can't forgive them. The listener suggests that the Native American asks for a forgiveness tool.

"Close your eyes. The first thing you see is your tool. Don't reject the tool if it seems strange or out of place. There is always a meaning."

The Native American gets a drinking straw. He blows into the straw and one by one the members of his family appear in front of him. In their spiritual state, they forgive the enemy tribe, which now bows before them. The family members reach out to the Native American and ask him to join them in forgiving the tribe. It pains them that he is suffering. They assure him that they are fine where they are and that he must walk his path on earth until it is his time.

I ask the singer if the Native American needs singing support from the group. The female singer nods. The singer now finally gets in touch with her grief, which is released through cry-toning.

After the session, the singer could make contact with the Native American and his deceased family at any time by blowing into her imaginary straw. The tool opened the door to past lives, and enabled her to contact the deceased, as well as other states of consciousness.

Example 2

A singer with mental problems was given a beetle, which she saw as a scarab, the sacred Egyptian symbol that was carved in turquoises and used as a protective amulet. The scarab was given as a key to the state of consciousness she had been in during work with the Note from Heaven – a meditative state she normally had difficulty finding on her own. Following the session, the singer would be able to find that state at any time, using the scarab as a starting point.

Example 3

In one of the fastest and most convincing releases I have experienced in regressive cell-singing, the tool that was given was not an object but a high-pitched vocal sound. A female executive had become so worn out by stress that she had been close to being admitted to a psychiatric hospital. She had been on sick leave for several months.

When she arrived at the course, it was hard for me to believe that she was ill. "Appearances are deceptive," she said. Before the course, she had told me that a number of years ago she had lost one of her twin sons in a cot [crib] death. Now, many years later, she had become overwhelmed by a grief that had totally knocked her for six. The woman was not accustomed to using her voice and was anxious about being able to sing in tune.

She was the first in the group to put herself forward as a singer and her voice went right up into the high notes after only a few seconds. The woman's crisp tones were as clear as a bell and fairly rang out of her mouth.

"He's there, isn't he?" I asked. "Yes." The tears were running down her cheeks and she smiled blissfully. She sang and sang and sang. At the end I suggested that she ask for a tool to keep in touch with her son, and the answer came promptly: "I want the high tones." At the end of the one-day course, we tried the tool out. The clear bell tones were still there.

After the course, the woman was back at work. A few weeks later we exchanged e-mails. "I can get in touch with my son whenever I want to. The tones are still there and I have regained my strength."

When the Singer Sees Images

Inspiration without grounding leads to apathetic or hyperactive image sequences. When the singer sees images, it requires skill from the listener to sense if these images will lead to release or if they are unconscious diversions that will knock the process off course. The listener's navigation signs usually give the answer. If the sound or images don't arouse any sensations in my heart, I interrupt the singer and set them straight.

Not everyone sees images. Many have access to them, but do not take them seriously, dismissing them as nothing but flights of fancy. In cases where a singer hasn't been able to see anything before, and suddenly receives images, the listener should proceed with caution. A new dimension has opened up to the singer, and the mere fact of being able to see images is like stepping into exciting and unexplored territory. What people see differs. Some get colors and sense impressions and experience different, subtle light phenomena. Others suddenly cut into the listener's storytelling and say: "No, it's like this and this."

Here the listener can rely only on their hearing and intuition. Does the singer seem excited and authentic? Does the voice sound open? In which case, do the means (the images) justify the ends (the Note from Heaven)?

It is the listener's responsibility to see through the ego's diversions.

Example 1: A successful distraction maneuver

A well-educated woman was in the process of singing herself into contact with the Note from Heaven. She had a hard time getting in touch with her feelings. In the story she was singing, I could see a house with yellow walls. It was in a mountainous area in South America. A volcano was smoldering in the background. The singer got stuck at the yellow walls. Apparently she didn't want to go into the house. Her expression stiffened.

I asked if she could see something. Yes, she could. "I'm walking by the edge of a lake. There are ducks and reeds, the trees are beautiful..." As the listener I should have stopped her, but unfortunately, I decided to respect her authority.

She continued describing her ramble as if she was actually going for a walk down by the local lake. Her voice was monotonous, both when singing and talking. The description of the walk was really boring me.

"Maybe we should try to find that yellow house."

"No, it feels right." The woman was determined to walk round the lake. I didn't have the heart to stop her, and that was my next mistake.

She had been talking continuously ever since I asked if she could see anything, and in that way, had avoided the Note from Heaven. I spotted that too late. It would now be an impossible power game to force her back to the yellow house from her beloved lake.

By the time she had walked all around the lake and was about to go round again, which she swore was absolutely necessary,

I was forced to admit to her, the other course participants and myself that her images had deceived me.

I should have kept to the yellow walls and endeavored to move forward from that point, because I sensed an impending crisis in the story, and that the woman would do anything not to confront it. Before then, I had believed that all appearing images were important and carried a message. They certainly do, but the question is, what purpose do they serve?

In almost all cases, the ego will try to protect the singer from confrontations with any emotions based on fear. This is a natural instinct. If a listener lets a singer's ego have its way, he or she might as well throw in the towel and bring the session to a halt. With some people, the astral images float to and fro as if they were on an LSD trip, so when singers see images during their own singing, the listener must be fully alert.

Absorption in the Note from Heaven connects us to an all-encompassing, intelligent, mythological power that expresses itself through images, among other media. I refer to this power as the Akashic field, or the universal mind.

When a listener listens to a singer's voice, he or she is aiming to surrender to a consciousness that communicates with this universal mind. I rely totally on what I sense when listening. I don't have any choice but to trust the images and impressions that turn up, because "I am not there", when I step to one side.

The field between the singer and listener is like a magnet. If either the singer or the listener is held back by their ego, their pole will weaken the information coming in.

Example 2: Images without a main thread

There was one female singer who saw lots of images. They intertwined with my story, and what started as a wrecked ship at the bottom of the ocean now became a large tanker, which the woman boarded. The whole crew had died of the plague, it stank, and suddenly creatures with abscesses and black spots rose up from the ocean, and parrots, and... I tried to figure out the meaning and felt nauseous from my attempt to gather the threads. Images from the astral plane were pouring out of the woman's subconscious mind.

The singer's sound was vague and reflected her inner state.

With a great effort I got the story and the ship back on course. The woman had to walk the plank, jump into the water and receive the grounding from her tonal power that she needed.

Mindful of similar cases I had come across previously, I interrupted her and told her the truth as I experienced it. This, for me, is always the fairest way to treat a delicate subject: "It feels to me as if your images are leading us astray. Try to sing yourself into your primary feeling and let me see what images turn up."

This is when it is particularly useful to have the singer's code words, wish and primary feeling ready on a piece of paper. They are invaluable in helping to keep the participant on track. As far as possible, I try to retain the original story and let it develop further with the images that appear.

When a singer suffers from a large inferiority complex, it can, paradoxically, show itself in delusions of grandeur.[71] Talents have to be displayed somehow or other, and they can, for example, burst out in exaggerated images. The listener needs to use his or her ears. If the breakthrough to the Note from Heaven fails to come or the séance feels heavy and tiring, it is the listener's responsibility to change course as quickly as possible by taking over the helm.

Regression

My personal experience with regression

After the first ten years of work, and deep involvement with surrendering to the Note from Heaven, I noticed that long, coherent, film-like stories full of exciting and dramatic events would pass by my inner eye when I was in a relaxed state.

The first time it happened, I thought my destiny was to become a writer of novels. The inspiration for the stories simply came to me, without demanding any sort of effort on my part. In the days that followed, however, my body began to react and I was emotionally shaken and deeply involved in the story. These after-effects wore off after about a week.

I went on to experiment with enquiring about past lives and each time I immediately got a new story.

It is difficult to generate an effective release by practicing regression on your own. The ego will fight desperately to protect you from fear and stop you from going to the roots of a traumatic experience. This is only truly possible together with a therapist.

As I had singing pupils that might possibly open up to past lives while working with the Note from Heaven, I felt I needed to become trained in regression, so I registered with André Corell's education in regression therapy in Copenhagen.[72] Among other things, we learned basic techniques on how to lead a client in and out of a regression, how to zoom in on a trauma and then release it.

My experience, derived both from my work with clients and my training, is that it can be very heavy, even burdensome, to keep diving down into the dark areas of the subconscious. The moment of death – the terror – the experience can easily tip over into the kind of sensationalism that you might find in a tabloid news story. The pain body grabs some tasty morsels along the way.

The most far-reaching regressions I have ever experienced involved being healed between two lives. I especially remember one regression where, after only a few minutes of lying down, my body hummed in a weightless state and was warm with a tingling energy. I felt blissful, as if I were in heaven! Soft hands surrounded my body and healed it with the utmost gentleness and love.

My fellow student, who was supposed to be practicing on me, tried to get me out of the state. I asked to remain where I was. Fortunately, André came by and said: "She is being healed on a higher plane. Give her five minutes, before you continue practicing."

The experience remained with me, and now new methods in the field of regression therapy focus on precisely this type of approach in healing – which can you also can experience during Grail Meditation see page 464.[73]

Clients who are heavily laden with guilt can have a hard time surrendering to the Note from Heaven. We have grown up with guilt and taboos that steer our instincts and urges in the direction of hell rather than heaven. Many of us, therefore, believe we have to suffer before we can be uplifted. But it doesn't have to be like that.

In regressive cell-singing, I experience more and more cases where the stories become transformed into myths full of symbols, and that it is these that release the course participants. The myths can easily cover over tragic events in past lives.

In traditional regressions, it is the client who tells the story with the support of a listening therapist who asks leading questions. In regressive cell-singing, the listener does the seeing, sensing and telling, so that the singer is free to sing him or herself into a state of being that is pure listening. Thus, the chance of the transformation being ushered down to the subconscious mind during the session is much greater.

The inner pictures the listener sees and/or senses are reflections of the singer's sound. If the singing goes round in circles, then the images do as well. The story and sound merge together.

Experience has shown me that the pictures are usually correct. Time and again I have been surprised at their accuracy. For me, it is always a game. I have no idea where the story is heading. When all the pieces of the puzzle finally fall into place, I am amazed at how much humor and wisdom can be channeled through my brain. I present the storytelling as a "singing game", where the message of the pictures is secondary to the vocal release through the Note from Heaven.

Regression to heaven

Here is an example of a woman who was expecting to undergo a painful regression, but ascended to heaven instead.

In just a few breaths, the singer sang herself directly up to heaven. She described an incredibly beautiful, paradise-like garden, where she was floating around, feeling light and whole. "I just feel so good, so completely blissful," she said in wonder. The process took just a few minutes, but then her intellect asked: "Can it really be so very simple? I was convinced that I had to get down into something bad in order to release my problems."

After that, the woman asked to go down and experience a past life related to her problem. The energy became heavy, the air dry. A desert, a Muslim woman dressed in black. Drought, deep sorrow, no water, dying children. The singer looked round, and we agreed. "No thanks, it's not necessary."

We could all feel the change in the energy level and returning to the pain in the incarnation seemed superfluous. The singer's voice still carried gilded veils from heaven – why let it gather dust in the baking sun, death and deprivation? The singer could clearly feel that her trauma had already been released.

Paradoxical Myth

In my International Education for Vocal Sound Healing a male singer and composer was entering regressive cell-singing. His wish was to dissolve the root cause of his feeling of powerlessness. His voice manifests a flagpole in the midst of nowhere, a deserted place with no vegetation, dried out carrions spread around in the sand. The singer has travelled a long distance to reach his destination and bring his own colorful pennant. As he drags the pennant up the flagpole it is a big moment for him. But he is then overwhelmed by a feeling of emptiness and drags it down again. After returning home, he gives his small daughter the pennant, which is then used as a cover for her doll. He is with his wife and family. Also this feels empty. The musician needs to accept that his life is a paradox. The word "paradox" allows the Note from Heaven to manifest. The musician needs to bring his family with him on his journey, even it would be faster to travel without them. Why? Because in the presence of his family the ground around the flagpole turns into a green and fruitful oasis the moment he drags his colorful pennant up the pole.

After this ten minute demonstration session, the singer slept for two hours and a physical pain under his left rib vanished.

Women in orgasmic ceremonies

There are many different themes in regressions. One of the most intriguing ones is when ordinary, conventional women experience being courtesans or temple priestesses, serving the gods through their erotic devotion. Beautiful women radiating an uninhibited erotic life force have always presented a huge threat to the efforts of the religions to suppress human sexual urges.

Example

A woman decorated with flowers and precious jewels is sitting on an elephant on a beautifully decorated howdah.[74]

Her womanly qualities are scantily covered by a net of golden opals. Her breasts lie sensually under the rose mala, she is plump and delicious. There is a heavy layer of black kohl makeup around her eyes. Small diamonds on her nose. Tika[75] on her forehead. Long, loose black hair with elaborately woven pearls and flowers.

She can be seen bobbing above the heads of the masses. Women and men raise their hands up in the air and praise her.

The way this living goddess writhes with soft rolling movements causes the air to almost stand still. She is a manifestation of innocence combined with liberated erotic instinct.

The procession enters the temple and proceeds along the central avenue towards the shrine's altar, where the young woman will be united with a chosen priest. The foreplay has begun. The whole crowd is participating.

The woman is true to her gender, her sexuality, without any hint of reservation. She radiates total confidence in her own purity in the holy grail of reproduction and this is passed on as inspiration to the people.

The singer, a woman in her fifties, had as a primary wish: "I want to completely acknowledge myself as I am." Although she had reached a stage in her life where her sexuality was on the back burner, she was totally into the story and I was glad there were no men present in this group. The sound was sensual and powerful at the same time. We were all carried away by the singing and the story.

A special regression

At a one-day course in regressive cell-singing with a group of five, two of the women were friends. While one of them was singing into her problem, she shot back into a regression, to Venice in the year 1365, where a wealthy woman was dying in childbirth. The child survived. The mother's sense of guilt and powerlessness at having left her first child to fend for itself was overwhelming. The Note from Heaven came through strongly in the process of release.

During the birth, the singer's friend suddenly started getting intense spasms in her heart. She writhed back and forth, gasping for air and was unable to explain what was happening. When her face went dark red, my first thought was to call an ambulance. Fortunately, one of the course participants was trained in first aid and, before I could get all the way out of the door to the phone, the woman with the heart pain was able to stammer: "No, don't go, I am the child!"

We changed the story to a happy one in which mother and child were united, and the woman's pain eased. The two women cried and hugged each other repeatedly.

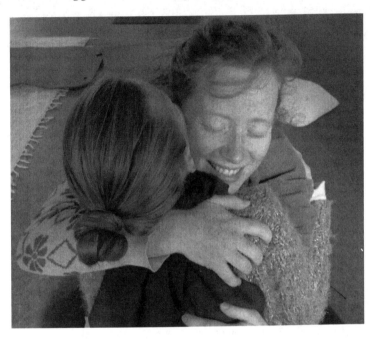

Boundaries

People who lack boundaries

The primary feeling: "I am not good enough" is one of the most common themes on courses in regressive cell-singing. Therefore it is relevant that listeners explore the core of this feeling, which I see as being based in having an unbalanced relationship with regard to boundaries. In what follows, two variations of the same theme are described.

Those children, who have had to strive particularly hard to meet the conditions of their parents' or close relatives' conditional love have, like rubber bands, had their boundaries stretched to breaking point. Although neglected children are especially prone to this problem, it is also true to varying degrees for those with a "normal" upbringing.

In an environment without reasonable boundaries, there is no mirror in which to reflect and thus love one's self.

Some children are raised with the feeling that life consists of an endless list of deeds they need to carry out to earn love. Little pats on the head in passing, a nod, a smile, the giving of sweets and so on come to function as rewards in a power game. It is a sad, but unfortunately quite common pressure cooker in which to preserve our most outstanding fruit and it is often the first-born or children who have taken on great responsibility at too early an age who are most affected. The fear of not being able to do things well enough leads to over-responsibility, which becomes a substitute for setting boundaries for what the self, as a person, agrees to.

"I have done my duty; therefore you are not allowed to hurt me."

"I have done my duty; therefore I deserve love."

How do you feel about the sentences above and the two following sentences?

"I won't put up with you hurting me."

"I am lovable."

We increase our self-respect when we stand up for ourselves unconditionally. If we experience ourselves as lovable, we don't need to have arguments. Conditional love trains children to achieve in order to feel good enough, and gives them the understanding, that they are not complete in their essence.

In that way, their whole basic foundation is being defined outside the self. They fumble around, caught in the unhealthy pattern, hungry for approval from others, as if that is the only possible peg on which they can hang their identity.

People who have overly controlled boundaries

In contrast, people who do not have many demands or expectations placed on them or who have been overprotected may lose their self-confidence and, to a greater or lesser degree, their natural feeling of responsibility for themselves. Often the people who have this problem are only children or the youngest in a family.

As I see it, the basis of the problematic of unemployment lies in the amputation of our self-confidence. *We don't need you!* An individual can lose their basic sense of self-worth to such a degree that they become handicapped for the rest of their life. Even trying to live up to being good enough and experiencing ourselves as efficient can be such an overwhelming step to take. We can become sick with fear in the soul, causing a self-perpetuating circle of paralysis. "No one needs me, I am nobody, I can't do anything, I don't belong."[76]

This can lead us towards irresponsibility as we push our all too painful emotions aside and put a protective membrane over an increasingly infected boil. "I will only do something if I feel like it."

Instead of feeling satisfaction at rising to a challenge, we are pulled down by fear of risk. What if mum and dad aren't around to lend a hand in case I can't do it? We lose interest, because: *What if I am not good enough?* This pattern can lead even highly intelligent adults to throw out their arms and say: "I don't feel like it."

"I am helpless, therefore you can't permit yourself to hurt me."

"I am helpless, therefore I deserve love."

How do you feel about the sentences above and the two following sentences?

"I won't put up with you hurting me."

"I am lovable."

The overly responsible and the overly irresponsible fit

together hand in glove, but this is not a perfect relationship as they enable each other to indulge the extremes of their characters. The false self-confidence of the irresponsible one hits rock bottom through overdependence on the responsible one, who becomes exhausted by the excessive demands of his or her mate.

The overly responsible person admires the irresponsible person's ability to set boundaries without the slightest hesitation, even in small, insignificant situations. This false respect – a substitute for the real thing, which they will never deserve – validates the irresponsible person's behavior and compounds their loss of self-confidence. Boundary setting effectively covers up the hollow echo of the individual's painful secret: I am not good enough.

Of course, the overly responsible person doesn't see this.

Conversely, the irresponsible person will be attracted to the overly responsible in the belief that the other person has the self-confidence that they lack. In reality, they both lack self-confidence, but one reacts outwardly and the other inwardly – two variations of the same theme. I come across these themes again and again in regressive cell-singing. They come in countless different guises, but they can all be traced back to the same negative primary root. "I am not good enough. I am not worth anything. I am unlovable."

When a person's foundation collapses

When a person makes big decisions in their life, their foundation can be shaken to the core. This can be so painful that the person comes into contact with the fundamental essence of their existence.

The fear of hurting loved ones, of being mistaken, of being hurt by other people's opinions – we can come up with plenty of reasons to hold on to the old patterns.

Your body will always tell you if your soul is not happy

and well. Through illness or physical pain or psychological imbalances, it rebels in a way that demands a reaction. If you ignore this call it will, in the long term, result in serious illness that is rooted in the soul's wish to leave the Earth.

When facing a major crisis like the impending end of a long-term relationship, people often lose their zest for life. They can wish themselves far away, be deeply depressed and escape into sleep. It can seem easier to die than to take that terrible step. In so many cases the organism speaks its own language in the form of the sudden appearance of a serious disease – the "step" is taken for the person.

"Do you want to live or die?" "I want to live, my feelings have the right to exist despite the consequences they will have on my surroundings." Ought you to say that?

Only your heart can answer that question. When the fruit is ripe, it falls. One can feel lost in disempowerment.

It is possible to liberate your breathing and emotions on your own with regressive cell-singing when in a crisis. Go for a drive and practice cry-toning when everything becomes overwhelming. If you don't have a car available, put your head in a pillow and go all out. Be prepared to do it daily, as the emotions during a crisis will continue to pop up, until the pattern that triggered them has been changed.

I have had course participants who knew that the structure of their marriage was the cause of their cancer.

One participant with terminal cancer, who for most of her married life had not been able to communicate, either verbally or sexually, with her husband, wished to stay with him till the end of her life. She was fully aware that she would pay with her life. For many years she had kept herself alive keeping the cancer on hold by singing the Note from Heaven, not knowing what to do. Two months after making her decision to stay with her husband, she died.

Should a person sacrifice him or herself? Is it a good thing to be silent about your own pain?

A crisis can be the catalyst leading to a quantum leap in life. Just like when you encounter the Note from Heaven, you have to jump without a safety net.

Are you ready? Dare you jump? Do you want it and does it feel right? In my experience, if a person is truly ready to take full responsibility for their life, and, therefore, to accept the consequences of making the leap, they receive wings that carry them through even the most painful feelings. There are no shortcuts to the wisdom of a broken heart. Remember that even if you take the jump, the world still remains. There is the sun, moon, trees and bird song.

To dare is to lose one's footing for a while. Not to dare is to lose one's self.
Søren Kierkegaard

Release of Guilt

Since guilt gets its nourishment from the repressions lurking in the subconscious mind, the feeling of guilt dies when the root is dug up and brought into the light.

Guilt is one of the most destructive emotions of all. It gnaws away relentlessly within and can also be perpetuated by external situations. For example, a mother might feel guilty when she looks at her child. This causes her pain, so she distances herself from her child. The more she distances herself, the guiltier she feels, the greater the pain, and so on.

The mother doesn't know the reason for her sense of guilt. It has possessed her like a chronic disease.

The child becomes traumatized and inherits the mother's sense of guilt. Unconsciously, the child knows that it is inflicting pain on the mother, but it does not know why and it certainly feels guilty! The snowball rolls on, growing bigger and bigger from generation to generation.

Fortunately for all those carrying guilt, an acknowledged guilt can be removed, and what a catharsis the release brings about!

The following example shows how it can be done.

On a course, one woman had the courage to be honest about her relationship with her young children: "I have two children. I love my baby girl with all my heart, but there is distance between me and my three-year-old son. I don't know why it is so difficult for me to hold him close. Problems have now started in kindergarten. When I look at my son I feel guilty, because I know he needs my love, but I cannot give it to him. Something is in the way. It makes me feel miserable."

The woman sang herself back to a past life in the Mongolian steppes:

A woman with Mongolian features was cutting grass with a little circular knife and putting the grass in a big basket. Her six-month-old son was lying sleeping near the edge of the road, bundled in woven fabric.

Suddenly a group Tartar horsemen came thundering by. They looked mean and had bloody weapons. In a flurry, one of the warriors speared the woman's baby boy, laughing coarsely all the while. The woman had thrown herself down into the long grass, so they wouldn't see her. The Tartar rode on with the boy on the tip of his lance, before slinging him roughly out over the steppe.

The woman rushed over to her son as soon as the men were out of sight. The baby was dead. She was overcome with guilt at being alive, at having thrown herself down into the grass instead of protecting her son. She reproached herself for having laid him so close to the road. If only she had done this or that. The memory gnawed at the woman for the rest of her life.

We changed the story to a happy one, so the boy and mother remained unharmed (the Tartars rode the other way). The singer practiced cry-toning during the whole séance and the Note from Heaven came through powerfully.

A few days after the course, the woman sent me a joyous e-mail. The distance and sense of guilt had gone. Now she could hug her son, and love him with all her heart. Things were also going much better with him in kindergarten.

This example is not unique. A sense of guilt towards one of your children is always possible to remove, because a mother's love is one of the strongest instincts that exists. So, dear, guilt-ridden mothers, step forward and throw off your cloaks.

Release through contact with wise light beings
Jeshua, yes you are – reflecting the highest degree of love and compassion in me.
Githa Ben-David

Some people feel particularly connected to a certain prophet, archangel, saint or other sacred figure.

Because of the deep meaning these archetypes have for people of different religions, their energies can manifest themselves during regressive cell-singing. The effect is especially strong when the listener doesn't know anything about the singer's special connection to the Virgin Mary in advance, for example, and then this figure becomes part of the story. The magic moment creates an opening. An opening for the belief that anything can happen – and then it happens!

Sometimes I see a figure wearing robes of glory, but I am not able to identify them, due to a lack of mythological or religious knowledge. If I have the slightest doubt, I describe the figure's appearance and the singer often then recognizes the figure.

In other cases, the singer may explicitly wish to get in touch with a certain high energy form that they have faith in. The wish is formulated and we see what happens.

A third way is for the singer to ask to be meditatively guided to a spiritual level where they can ask and receive answers to their questions.[77] The singer may formulate their wish during the process, or it may occur spontaneously.

Gratitude ritual

At the end of a session, meditation or of a course, everyone participates in a short ritual of gratitude to round off the release that has taken place. This is a ceremony for a conscious exit from the Oneness level. By placing your hands on your heart, you close the veil and return to the world of duality. Through the gesture of gratitude you confirm the healing that has occurred to be manifested in duality.

When a person gives thanks for a healing, they acknowledge the miracle and create space for the consciousness to expand. One can say that the course participant takes the miracle home with them in the pocket of their heart.

Healing lies in strengthening our faith. Not necessarily faith in a particular understanding of God, but rather a general faith in the existence of higher energies which our antennae can pick up and communicate with whenever we need to.

Example

Close your eyes and put your hands on your chest. Give thanks for the love and light that you have received today.

Many course participants are moved, because the heart chakra opens when the release is affirmed. If a participant has difficulty in being moved, then either the heart has not opened up enough or the participant has transferred the credit for any release to the listener.

"Behold, my masters and mistresses and, above all, the emperor! We never know what the real nightingale will bring forth, but with the artificial bird all is certain beforehand!" And the nightingale sang so beautifully that it brought tears to the emperor's eyes. The

tears rolled down his cheeks and the nightingale sang even more beautifully. This went straight to the emperor's heart. He was so happy that he declared the nightingale should have his golden slipper to wear round its neck, but the nightingale merely thanked him. It had already received reward enough. "I have seen tears in the eyes of the emperor, and that is the richest treasure for me. God knows I have indeed been richly rewarded!"

Hans Christian Andersen (*The Nightingale*)

Physical Reactions

During regressive cell-singing

Spittle, slime, coughing, irritation of the throat and spasm-like movements are normal (see page 154). The listener cannot be squeamish. Be ready with a spittoon and be prepared to urge the singer to spit out their slime. If the hoarseness continues, then you need to find a "hole" in the voice in a higher or lower region – a place where it is "clear" so the voice can ring through.

If a singer's need to cough and spit comes after contacting the Note from Heaven, it is a healthy, cleansing reaction due to an activation of muscles and feelings that have hitherto been suppressed.

When the singer is united with the Note from Heaven, he or she often will have involuntary eye movements under their closed eyelids like those that occur during REM sleep.

Some participants need to get up and use their whole body during singing – arms outstretched, head back, eyes closed.

Stretching out the arms with the palms of the hands open and turned upwards while leaning the head slightly back strengthens the surrender to the Note from Heaven. Most singers do this gesture instinctively.

The right side represents the outwardly moving, dynamic, giving, masculine power.

The left side is the inwardly moving, spiritual, receiving,

feminine power.[78]

Some course participants can feel a fine electric energy only on the one side. If a person has difficulty feeling "good enough", then they will often feel they have no right to receive anything. This will lead to their left side being more or less closed. A person who has experienced shock will often have a weakened right side. Their ability to actively respond is reduced. In the case of a child having been ignored, the whole body can be closed down. Those who have been ignored or who have experienced shock will typically say, "I can't feel myself/my feelings/my body."

In such cases it is important to bring the "dead" part of the body to life. The vibrations of singing can resonate and work only in areas of the body where the cells are energetically open and therefore resonant. The sound can move through the opening and gradually reach the part of the body that cannot be felt if the listener and singer will focus on this part. The sound follows the focus. The body will open only when and if it is ready. Here the right code word can open the gates of heaven.

The muscles can ache and hurt when the body wakes up from its slumber through regressive cell-singing.

A hand that has fallen asleep always hurts when you begin to move it. Illness and pain are the body's request for attention.

Pain teaches us to listen to our body. Only when our organism has received what it is calling out for, will we have peace. Regressive cell-singing is about expressing, and thereby understanding, the body's call.

After regressive cell-singing

Many singers feel charged with energy for days after making contact with the Note from Heaven. Sometimes this energetic opening process continues for months afterwards. In such cases there has really been a breakthrough and the participant can apparently cope with remaining open. This means the energy will continue to work in the person, and a gradual development of intuition will occur. The singer will also experience more synchronistic happenings than can be put down to mere coincidence.

It is normal to feel tired after regressive cell-singing, even totally exhausted in some cases. A woman participating in a one-day course once slept for a whole day and night afterwards. When I have week courses I purposely make a long break in the afternoon, in order to support the body to integrate the heightened energy level in the body. If we continue working all day long, people get exhausted. It is recommended to move, relax, detox in the breaks. Listen for your body's need.

When the body has been strained by illness it is in particular need of peace and quiet to assimilate the new energy structure. The process of releasing cells that were bound usually continues for a week to ten days after the séance.

Symptoms resembling influenza can appear at the start of the purification process. If this does happen, the symptoms will develop immediately after or during the course and recede within two days. For support of the healing process you can drink purified water and do fasting combined with compresses with castor oil on the liver.[79]

In rare cases where very intense feelings have surfaced, and not all feelings have been released during the singing process, people have experienced vomiting. A woman was fine at the end of the course, but then felt nauseous in the car on the way home and threw up periodically during the journey. The vomiting continued through the night and then passed. She felt very relieved afterwards. Her theme was incest.

In another case, a male Arabic immigrant vomited during the vocal release of an overwhelming fear brought on by the thought of a hearing the next day involving rights of access to his son. The father's emotions had been so effectively released that the next day he managed to stay calm and in control during the hearing.

Some people react with physical pains or general soreness. The pains signify that the body is starting to acknowledge suppressed emotions. The pain is closely followed by mood swings – a part of every purification process.

Waves oxidize brackish water.

Yawning

Yawning during singing the Note from Heaven is a good sign because it is a natural physical reaction to the body's letting go of tensions. A true yawn can only happen when the body instinctively takes a deep breath. The mere thought of yawning makes you yawn. I'm sitting here writing and yawning away.

The body yawns when it releases. You can almost picture steam spewing out of a little hole on the top of the head.

During one course where we yawned and yawned, a female participant let us in on a memory that had plagued her for years:

"Someone close to me was being buried. The priest was delivering a speech and earth was being thrown down onto the coffin in the grave. I was yawning almost constantly and weeping at the same time. It was impossible for me to hold back my reaction, despite the fact that I must have appeared rather arrogant and I felt so embarrassed about it."

The soft palate in the oral cavity lifts up every time you express a genuine feeling. The yawning sets a physical reaction in motion from the lower abdomen up to the crown of the head. The jaw – the joint in the body with the highest number of nerve reactions[80] – is extended and a stretching occurs in the oral cavity. It feels almost like a parachute opening out. Try stretching out your arm and bend the wrist coquettishly downwards and stretch out the pinkie like a ballet dancer.

The movement supports the stretching of the soft palate, the domed roof of the oral cavity. The stretch affects pituitary, hypothalamus and pineal glands. Yawn – the eyes start watering.

Surrender. The hormone system is activated.

The only vowel that completely stretches out the dome of the oral cavity is "Aaar". This vowel has led me and numerous course participants and readers to the Note from Heaven.

Giving birth supported by the Note from Heaven

During my second pregnancy, I was assigned a community midwife named Annie Brehmer. She presented herself as an odd type who could get women to deliver easily by moaning and singing on "Aaar".

We both experienced goosebumps of pleasure at this first meeting. I have never before or since heard of a midwife who asks those giving birth to sing. Nor could she believe she was dealing with a pregnant woman who had written a whole book on singing "Aaar". What's more, it turned out that she lived only 200 meters away from me, so we were able to collaborate closely, among other things on a composition called *Womb* (a recording of fetal sounds in the womb) on my CD *Rising*.[81]

Annie's many years' experience and a wide range of holistic studies had taught her that the mouth corresponds to the vagina, so that when you open the mouth and sing "Aaar", the vagina also opens – the muscles work in partnership.[82]

Annie offered to assist me in a singing delivery at the hospital. I felt so very lucky, because I realized it meant our first-born child, then almost seven years old, could be present at the birth. He was used to the Note from Heaven and would understand my way of using it much better than if I was screaming in pain.

The time came, but when my waters had broken and the labor pains were strong, it felt much more natural to go into a deep meditation than to sing. The pains brought me into a state of elation as I stood leaning over a beanbag absorbed in my own inner world.

None of us were aware of how quickly everything was going. Annie filled the bath with water. Once in the bath the second-stage labor pains started and then I felt the urge to sing.

The Note from Heaven became so powerful that at one point there were four curious midwives watching in amazement. When I stopped the singing because Annie wanted to check down between my legs, the pain reappeared with such a shocking intensity that I instinctively kicked out at her. "My God, the head is just about to come out."

With two more pushes accompanied by the Note from Heaven, a new soul had come into the world. Our newborn son immediately clung tightly to my breast. The birth had taken one and a quarter hours from the breaking of the waters. Our elder son, now a big brother, had been present the whole time. My first experience of giving birth had been long, hard and traumatic, so it was enormously releasing to deliver my second child so easily with the Note from Heaven on my lips.

Giving birth is an initiation. So, mothers-to-be, please do not take any unnecessary painkillers. This is such a sacred moment and can expand your whole being. Do not let fear take the lead. Sing your child out with the help of the Note from Heaven.

Gender and Sexuality

The gateway between Oneness and duality

In the moment of surrender to the Note from Heaven, a letting go occurs that is much like the release of an orgasm. You can no longer resist, you have no choice but to let yourself surrender to the flow of the current in the body's river.

When we stifle a yawn, we stop our mouth from opening and thereby protect ourselves physically and psychologically from momentary exposure. I believe that the erotic surrendering unreservedly to another being is the physical reflection of the yearning for the spiritual experience of Oneness in the heart.

What arouses us most is to overstep the bounds of what is permitted and set foot in the forbidden land. This land is actually a holy land, but as long as we keep it in the shadows we cannot experience it in all its light and glory.

When guilt is linked to our sexuality, it reduces the likelihood of an orgasmic awakening of spirituality.

In Walter Schubart's fantastic book *Religion and Eroticism* (1941), the words glow under the professor's pen. It gives me a pleasant jolt of surprise that he defines female sexuality as the "joy of creation":

> *In the joy of creation, it is not coarse feelings of lust that are made divine, but eroticism's uninhibited, bubbling source of all life; the origin of the universe, shrouded in mystery. The joy of creation is a religious feeling. Creation's beauty and fertility overwhelm the human being and force it into a state of worship. The joy of creation leads religious thinking towards speculation about the world's creation, not the world's purpose. It raises the question of where from, not where to.*

To a remarkable degree, Schubart's definition of female eroticism reminds me of the power that is generated while singing the Note from Heaven. It is almost identical to the feelings aroused in my chest during surrender. The experience of the bubbling, whirling energy shower, which wraps up my organism, awakens a deep, overwhelming gratitude for this divine wonder.

The oral cavity has aspects of both female and male genitalia. It has a uvula (corresponding to the clitoris), a hard palate in front (the vulva), a throat (the vagina); the soft palate and the oral cavity can extend and stretch upwards like the uterus. The tongue corresponds to the penis. Try in a private moment to open your mouth and stick out your tongue: I open myself; let myself be filled, while simultaneously giving everything I have. I unite the masculine and feminine principle.

The tension between man and woman, the tension between matter and spirit: polarity.

In the experience of the Note from Heaven, the Singer is not one or two in that moment. He is both.

Jesus saw children who were being suckled. He said to his disciples: "These children who are being suckled are like those who enter the Kingdom." They said to him: "Shall we then, being children, enter the Kingdom?" Jesus said to them: "When you make the two One, and you make the inner even as the outer, and the outer even as the inner, and the above even as the below so that you will make the male and the female into a single One, in order that the male is not made male nor the female made female... then shall you enter the Kingdom."
Gospel of Thomas, log. 22

The power of the feminine
What will the consequences be for your life if you become your self?

For women in particular, fear of getting in touch with one's own spiritual power is a common problem in regressive cell-singing. This fear is well founded. The conventional male reaction to meeting a woman who is clearly in touch with her spiritual potential is to position himself for a cock fight: can I possess her/outdo her? This instinct is natural. The primeval sexual power is built around a man's ability to possess a woman. He must be strong for her to want him. This ensures the quality of the offspring.

A woman unconsciously tests a man's boundaries, because she needs to be able to float in his vessel. If she senses that she can trust him to carry her in all her completeness, she will be able to surrender; which means totally yielding to the man's penetrating power (equivalent to surrendering to the Note from Heaven, which is also a question of trust).

The very moment one partner in a relationship changes,

the other must adjust. Since women are instinctively created to surrender and, for that reason, are emotionally more fluid than men, they are also more likely to surrender to spirituality. Therefore it is an archetypal challenge for a man the moment faith in a higher power takes his wife by the hand. Does he see it as a blessing, or does he see the higher power as a rival, threatening his sturdy castle, in which wife and offspring are kept in a safe strongbox?

If he is able to see her spiritual process as a gift, he will not only win her, but strengthen their love relationship as well. The man shows with his openheartedness that he is not afraid to be tried by the higher powers. His castle, his strength is unshakable. She can feel completely safe in the knowledge he will go to the ends of the Earth for her. But he acts on his own terms, and she acts on hers.

This is where all partners should wake up: conservative dominance and rigid family patterns are no longer acceptable today. When a man/woman clearly works against their partner's aspirations to raise their consciousness, they dig the grave of their marriage. It is as if the partner turns off the light in the relationship, saying, "You must not shine, darling. Stay with me in the darkness."

Men and women can easily raise their consciousness together. Real men are intuitive.

Business leaders recognize the need for intuition to help them make the right decisions in their fast-paced, pressurized working environment. Interest in the Akashic field is growing; scientists talk about the zero-point field, a similar all-knowing layer of consciousness.

Man, keep the feminine energy in your vessel.
Woman, surrender safely in the vessel's encircling power.
A vessel without fluid is empty. Fluid without a vessel is wasted.

It wasn't until I was 40 that I realized bubbling with energy and inspiration is a positive thing. There is no reason to hold back my buoyant energy. My power is a gift, a gift that rises above the constraints of marriage. Make or break. No one can take this power from you and it is there for both you and your partner, if he is able to resonate with it. The feminine power is just as important for the man as for the woman. Like a yearning for the all, it is now knocking on your door, stronger than ever before. It is a question of life and death, Nature's aspiring to reestablish balance on Earth. If you are looking for a partner, you will get one that fits who you are right now. So why not be yourself? Does your most optimal sound resonate within you? I'm telling you, everything is possible. Love is unlimited.

Open your arms so that you can contain as much light as possible. Receive everything that is given to you. The more you shine, the better you can serve Oneness. Pure energy flows like water, catches like fire, spreads like love. It must be passed on. If you push it away, you lose it. If you hold on to it, it will be taken from you.

Fear is the yoke that switches off all light.

Woman, pluck your emotional strings. The world needs information in the form of sound. The sound behind the words, the unconscious, the mother ocean – all are of feminine lineage. The woman is of the all. She is closely connected to the universe through the process of pregnancy. The world mother, the pregnant stomach. An egg, a globe, a fertile planet with oceans and lands. Mystery is a natural thing for a woman, because she feels it within herself and is influenced without asking any questions. She knows. Life and death are intertwined with pregnancy. Facial features change, become softer and more open. You are humankind's oracle. Lead the masculine power to the Oneness level and let it fortify its seed there.

Man, speak your mind and lead the woman back to the Earth. Plant your seed in the name of unity. Let the woman vibrate under your wings and know that she loves you more each time you pour her flowing essence into your vessel and gently cool it with your patient breath.

If you put a lid on the vessel, you will lose her. Let her ebb and flow freely within her cycle. Like a moon orbiting and reflecting you, the sun. The stable, unwavering power.

Footnotes:
1. Read about detox in Help (Gilalai 2021) by Githa Ben-David.
2. See page 464 Grail Meditation.

Part III

Resonance with Domino Effect

What is Resonance with Domino Effect (RDE)?

In Resonance with Domino Effect (RDE) the liberated prince or princess overwhelms the troll and leads their fellow prisoners out into the light of freedom. Not only are the prisoners liberated, they too liberate others with their song of freedom. Some participators will not be ready to leave the troll's fortress, as they may feel as if they are still chained to the pain body. Even when the chains have been cast aside and the troll is dead a few prefer to imagine he is still alive, so that they can justify staying in the safe and familiar darkness.

In my International Education, demonstrations and workshops each person usually takes their turn to sing themselves free. Whoever in process should be given special attention and not be disturbed by anyone else's spontaneous need for emotional expression.

However, it is a fact that the tonal expression of an emotional release from a person with a particular trauma will activate resonance in fellow human beings who carry a similar emotional trauma. When a tuning fork tuned to 440 Hz is activated with a club, it will resonate with all other tuning forks present in the same room at a frequency of 440 Hz without any physical stimulation.

When I demonstrated Sound Healing at a large Power of Sound event with 450 participants, a young woman from the audience volunteered to sing herself free up on stage. I started the introductory interview and inquired into her primary feeling as she opened her mouth and screamed so it went straight through you. The crowded hall shook.

The important thing with screaming is to listen beyond the expression in to the energy. This woman really aired out her innermost chambers. As earlier mentioned, it is the listener's duty to help the singer to reach the Note from Heaven. By vocally emphasizing the scream's basic note, I led her with me. Soon her voice stood like a shimmering column in the air, compelling and full of light. After two minutes' expression of the Note from Heaven the woman had finished. We had hardly exchanged a word.

The séance made a deep impression on everyone. Many were wholeheartedly enthusiastic, but I also got responses from people who admitted they had been shaken to their very foundation. The scream had frightened them and the experience had caused stifled sobs, nausea and discomfort. One had even needed to leave the hall.

I wondered how to prevent this kind of emotional domino effect from happening, and finally decided to try an experiment.

When doing an introductory course at a Holistic Festival, I conducted an experiment with a group of 65 people who had just opened up to the Note from Heaven by offering them the opportunity to experience collective regressive cell-singing. This experiment developed into RDE. After a woman had sung herself free of a past life trauma, a number of the course participants had lumps in their throats and said the woman's singing had touched something within them. Like a horse that has been given its freedom, she had happily whinnied outside the stable, while her fellow course participants were still tethered inside. Of course, they became restless. "We also want to get out and run around!"

I asked those course participants who had been touched to sit in the center of the group. There were eight people. Each person was assigned two or three helpers who were instructed in how to support their release. One by one they purified their emotions and more people from the group were touched – it went on and on.

Principles of RDE singing

1. When working on a collective level, the identity of the person being released is of secondary importance.

The goal of RDE is the release of bound-up energy through contact with the Note from Heaven by using regressive cell-singing.

We are all part of the Oneness level. Therefore, when one person sings down the light, everyone receives it. The course leader has to see the group as one energy field – one being, metaphorically speaking, where the pores of the skin are open to varying degrees.

2. In RDE singing, participants can spontaneously sing themselves free when an unresolved emotion knocks on their door.

The law of resonance applies to every expression of feeling. Emotions are archetypal, and certain emotions resonate with certain vibrations. Most of us carry the same set of differently tuned tuning forks within us, which pick up these archetypal, universal emotions. This is how we can understand each other's feelings. We are on the same wavelength.

Anyone carrying the same unresolved emotion as the singer will be affected by the sound produced during a release and will clearly feel an emotional reaction starting in their own body. This emotional chain reaction is at the heart of RDE.

When the body resonates with a fellow human being's feelings, it reacts before the intellect has time to intervene.

The feeling of isolation created by a huge taboo of a problem is dissolved in that wonderful moment when we realize that we are not alone. There is sympathy and total understanding from those who carry the same emotional burden. During the release of RDE singing a flame is lit that awakens true compassion.

3. RDE requires a ratio of one-three listeners per singer.

It is impossible to know in advance how many people in a group will resonate with the same unresolved archetypal emotion. In a group of 30 participants, a singer will, on average, affect one or two fellow participants in the first round. These will then affect between two and four more and so on, until the emotion is discharged from the group. When, on occasion, many are affected at the same time, it is important, as the leader, to keep your composure and take it as it comes.

Singers who have gone into mutual resonance are assembled in the middle of the circle where the rest of the group is located.

For participants who feel powerless by passively watching RDE, it can be rewarding to get involved as a helper in the process. The needs of the resonating singers are explored before anyone begins to support them. Although it is normal to feel safer with some helpers than with others, there are seldom major problems because those who have a burning urge to offer care are usually inspired by a feeling they recognize from their relationships in their own lives.

The listener should be supporting the neck and hold a hand lightly on the "resonating singer's" forehead, while listening to their sound. There can easily be several supporters at the same time. For an example a second listener might do grounding work by healing/holding the singer's legs and feet. A third listener might hold a hand lightly on the singer's stomach, while supporting deep breathing. The singer gets as much attention as they need. By the end of the session, the singer should be able to sing alone. Laughter rolling around in the spaces between the tones is a signal that release has occurred. It can take from two to six minutes. If the process goes on longer than this it may indicate that the emotion has been discharged, closed down or that the singer has gone into melodramatic performance/ hamster in the wheel.

4. Keep an eye out for "shy resonants".

Shy resonants are people who resonate with the same emotion as the resonating singers, but are too shy to put themselves forward for release. During RDE, it is important that the leader keeps a watchful eye on the flock, because there may be shy souls sitting wringing their hands, battling with roused emotions. They can be too proud (particularly in the case of men) or too shy to draw attention to themselves.

Shy resonants usually only need to be offered a helping hand, then the release occurs quite naturally. "Come on, dear, it looks to me as if you have been affected; your voice can fill the whole room if you want to. We want to hear your power. Let us hear you sing down the light to all of us." Sentences like these, when expressed honestly, can have an opening and particularly powerful effect on participants who were ignored as children or whose parents didn't have the energy to give them the attention they needed.

RDE is especially good for shy resonants, because they are in a situation where they can wait for others to make the first move before stepping forward. Some people hold back because they are tied down by a deep rooted shame – a shame that has isolated them with an inner primary feeling of fear of being discovered. They have had no choice but to hide themselves and their all too heavy emotion. When this emotion is openly acknowledged in a fellow course participant's sound, it activates a wish to pull free of the mire. This might never have happened if I had been sitting alone with them as a client with an uninterrupted focus on "No I can't do it".

For some participants the prospect is too frightening: To open up they would have to cast the chains binding them to their identification with the pain body. However, the experience can easily prick a hole in the membrane of a negatively functioning life pattern, and suddenly one day the person is ready to let go. A negative emotional reaction from a course participant can be a sign that a positive process has been set in motion.

5. Dealing with images.

It can be difficult to listen in to an individual singer's sound expression in Resonance with Domino Effect. For an example the sound might come from four singers simultaneously and resemble an infernal fire of energy in its bursting-out phase. Here the main thing is to lead the singers one by one to the Note from Heaven. The principle is the same as for regressive cell-singing. However, if images appear, it can be difficult to use them constructively when the sound is coming from several people at once. You can't distinguish who the message is for. But, if you sense the message is for the group, then the images can help focus the energies.

On one course there was a group of resonating singers whose common theme was Native Americans. They acted like a little tribe and the images I received gathered them in a euphoric song and dance that drew in the rest of the course participants. In such a situation there is no question of "willing" something to happen. It happens and feels quite natural. When what you are arises spontaneously from within, it is genuine. Afterwards you can remember it had something to do with Native Americans, but since it all took place in the moment, the memory has vanished. You only remember that it was a good feeling: a sweaty face, a plant and the sun outside. A feeling has been acted out.

6. Melodramatic performing.

In RDE, anything can happen. The method attracts melodramatic performers, who unconsciously see it as their chance to get attention.

Even in a large group the leader must be able to spot melodramatic performers and neutralize them as quickly as possible, because the others who have just opened up cannot tolerate the presence of such heavy energy for very long.

A melodramatic performance with a stuck expression can be recognized by a competitive edge to the singing. Usually the melodramatic performer will sing or scream so loudly that none of the others can be heard. The expressed sound does not touch the heart.

Melodramatic performance is an archetypal reaction learned in childhood. The person underneath is innocent and calling for help. It is easy to get irritated because an individual acting in this mode takes center stage with no regard for anyone else. The whole group atmosphere can become negative if the person is allowed to drain them of energy and that is why the leader of RDE singing must be experienced.

7. The element of surprise.

When I, as course leader, sense the slightest trace of melodramatic performance/hamster in the wheel, I immediately hand the release of any remaining resonating singers over to helpers and concentrate fully on activating the true feeling behind the melodramatic performance. Here an element of surprise is helpful. For example playing a cheerful melodious phrase on the piano or a guitar: The melodramatic performer will stop for a moment to hear what is going on. In that short moment I will improvise what I really want to say and what the person couldn't hear: "You are so precious. You are perfect as you are. We love your voice, we want to hear the genuine you. We want to see you – to feel your light. You are loved, you are so wonderful, how nicely you are letting go. Wow, how beautifully you're singing now…"

Energy-drainers are used to being met with resistance. Their surprise at being valued can transform the energy. The person may be touched and burst into tears and then the true emotion can be released through cry-toning.

If the listener is able to quickly recognize a stuck expression and be precise in the treatment, very few will even notice the character of the outburst. The harm will be minimized, the energy raised, the singer released and happy, and the séance will continue without interruption.

Group singing for dissolving melodramatic performance

The group's singing can also be used to dissipate melodramatic performance. The leading listener needs to use their intuition here. The melodramatic performer can be surrounded and sung to. Give him or her love. Focus on their expression and mimic it, in order to resonate with and understand the expressed emotion. Soon the melodramatic performance will be drowned out by the echoing of his or her own expression. This leads very naturally to the person stopping short in amazement and listening. In daily life, the same thing can be done with small children.

It is actually fun to copy someone else's expression. The participants can use this mirror as a shield against the heavy, draining energy. Soon all the heavy vibrations are lightened again by the releasing effect of laughter.

All for one...

Make it clear from the start – as soon as people apply for the course – that the strength of RDE is that anything can happen and that one person's release is everyone's release. In this way you effectively avoid people resenting each other, because they feel this one or that one received more time or attention than they did.

Practical organization

Although RDE is inherently unpredictable, courses tend to follow a certain structure.

1. Body and voice warm-ups, grounding and breathing exercises.

2. Singing on the Note from Heaven for half an hour. If anyone reacts emotionally they are led into regressive cell-singing, and if others resonate with them, RDE is allowed to develop naturally.

3. During a course there can be three to five rounds with different emotional themes, integrated with relaxation and surrendering to the Note from Heaven. If no one becomes overwhelmed by trauma while singing the Note from Heaven, I release a volunteer and then resonating singers start to pop up.

4. The course is rounded off by sound healing. I either heal the whole group myself, or we split up and take turns to heal each other with intuitive healing.

For a course you need: Tissues, drinking water, spittoon, mattresses, pillows and blankets.

After a trauma release most people feel like they have been born into a whole new peaceful universe. Most released singers like to relax by lying like a baby who has settled down happily on a mattress while they still feel part of the assembled company.

For some adults, especially shy resonants, it can be difficult to accept being cared for. Out of sheer politeness they will refuse the offer. If the listener persists, the shy person will succumb with a sigh of relief.

Example from a course of RDE singing

The Note from Heaven flowed through the course participants one by one. There was an infernal noise in the room. Each singer had their own tone, sharp and powerful as a siren. I disappeared into the sound and pure joy flowed through me as I was whirled into a spiral of energy. A common note appeared gradually. As a young woman with breast cancer leaned her head back, closed her eyes and spread out her arms and surrendered to the Note from Heaven, an older man who also had cancer broke down in tears. He had participated in other courses but had always kept a trace of self-control. The man's cry-toning was unusually energetic, drawing the whole group into it.

He and the young woman formed a symbiosis in a bonfire of prayer. The two of them showed a mature realization: "Everything in me vibrates in the presence of Oneness. I am vibration – I am light – I am the Note from Heaven."

Book III

Sound Healing: With the Note from Heaven

*The voice has all the magnetism that musical instruments lack;
for voice is nature's ideal instrument, upon which all other
instruments of the world are modeled.*

Hazrat Inayat Khan

*Once you have worked with the voice and have cultivated it,
deepened and widened it, you may leave it for months and years;
the voice may take a different shape and appearance, but at the same
time, what you have once developed remains with you somewhere.
It is just like a deposit kept in a bank. You have forgotten it perhaps;
yet it is there.*

Githa Ben-David

The only true wisdom is in knowing that you know nothing.

Socrates

Introduction

In recent times, the discoveries of science and physics have come so close to the understandings of spirituality and metaphysics that, combined, they illuminate what before was hidden in darkness. Like two shining stars, each field of knowledge sheds light on half of life's mysterious unknowns, and together, they reveal to us completely new dimensions, which broaden the consciousness of mankind.

What is important for me in this illumination of knowledge is not so much who is holding the lamp, but rather, what the light of that lamp reveals to us.

If you, dear reader, become surprised, astonished or even provoked by some of the sources I use in Book III, bear in mind that these are included because the information they contain is beneficial for illuminating the reason why the vocal expression of resonance has such a tremendous effect on the body.

According to quantum physics and religious scriptures, vibration is the foundation of all life. Thus sound is an expression of energy that man, within audible frequencies, can detect and the human voice is able to transmit.

In the description of sound, there is a limited and an unlimited perspective:

1. The well-tempered tuning where the notes of the piano in the 17th century were tuned as equal as possible. This tuning dictates the rules of today for "being in tune".

2. The natural tuning/the music of the Spheres, which is representing the free and unlimited natural sound corresponding with the Fibonacci sequence/the Golden Ratio.

When you play a wind instrument you automatically learn to adjust the tones in order to tune to the piano. The natural overtones, which are the true expression of the pipe of for example a saxophone, are suppressed by the player in certain keys because they will sound false compared to the inflexible sound source of the piano. The reason for this is the Pythagorean comma, which is corresponding to "The Golden Ratio" which naturally corresponds to the infinite spiral movement of fractals – DNA – Cells – Life. The music of the spheres reconnect us with creation, because it *is* creation.

Ancient music styles like Indian, Chinese, Mongolian, Tibetan, African music are "enharmonic" music which is developed in harmony with the free natural sound.

Johann Sebastian Bach and the composers after him based their music on modulation which means moving around from key to key in well-tempered tuning.

The question is, does the reason for the Western world's medical scientist's rigid denial of natural medicine, energy, nutrition, healing, miracles, etcetera, have its origin from our musical tradition? There is no Pythagorean comma, no place for a prayer in conventional medicine.

The natural sound is linked to the creating principle. Why? Because we are all shaped from frequencies.

The moment you *listen* attentively for your sound, you tune in to a state of presence. In this state, the true character of the voice opens and connects the singer to his/her full energetic potential. This potential is a projection of the golden electrical matrix of who we truly were when we entered this incarnation and who we still are in the higher dimension of the Oneness level.

Like the first overtone in the fractal line of overtones is close to an octave, where an A will be an A1, each living being has a complete energetic matrix. When we die we reunite with our matrix. The enlightened state is a state where you reunite with your energetic matrix while being on Earth. Jesus was united with his matrix, that is why people with faith were healed by touching him. Their cells got a glimpse of their own complete energetic matrix and were instantly healed.

The foundation of Sound Healing with the Note from Heaven

is to express the sounds that resonate with the receiver's energy body and retune it into the original energetic matrix.

The Sound Healer's search for resonance, I have called: Vocal Sound Scanning. When a Sound Healer's voice resonates with a recipient's energetic matrix you will be able to hear it easily. The sound expands and becomes rich in overtones – almost luminous. When I demonstrate this phenomenon, people almost always get an "a-ha" experience, either as a spectator, or as a recipient noticing how the sound resonates and tingles in their body.

Those who learn to sound scan get yet another "a-ha" experience, often already after a single one-day course.

At first it can seem strange to sound scan each other, but once you have experienced how pleasant it feels and the depth of impact it has, you can experience difficulty in stopping again.

In Book III: *Sound Healing: With the Note from Heaven* the reader is instructed how to deliberately scan a receiver's organism for resonance through the use of their voice – and how this can activate a healing process in another being's cells.

It is my hope and wish that my personal story – told here for the very first time – will encourage a fuller understanding of the key position, that can be attributed to the human voice.

Sound Healing: With The Note from Heaven is intended for anyone with an interest in learning an extraordinarily powerful healing method – a method proven to have an effect in areas where conventional treatment methods fall short. No prior knowledge of music or special vocal skills are necessary to practice Sound Healing. The primary talents required are an open heart and devotion.

Healing is by nature a union of love, empathy, compassion and gratitude practiced with humbleness.

If your heart is alive and warm, then you are "good enough".

If your heart is beyond reach, then sound can reestablish contact.

Part 1:

My Path Into the Universe of Sound Healing

Meeting with The Note from Heaven

The study of classical, North Indian khyal singing led me as a 25-year-old to the Note from Heaven – an experience of resonant sound, which opens the mind to a state of consciousness that has a profound healing effect on the organism.

My in-depth work with the Note from Heaven resulted in a process of deep, personal transformation which I, brought up as an atheist, was completely unprepared for. The Note from Heaven came out of the blue, and I had no other choice than to follow it, even if it worked against my career as a professional saxophone player, songwriter and composer.

It was only when I became pregnant at the age of 35 that the Note from Heaven began to give my life true direction.

Our firstborn son was born with an unknown chromosome translocation that almost cost him his life. At that time, my husband and I lived in Israel and supported ourselves playing music. Our son's tough start in life changed all of that. We moved back to Denmark, so that we could have time for his daily treatments. He was born without kneecaps, and with arms that couldn't be stretched out. Uncertainty reigned concerning his future. Would he ever be able to walk normally? Would he be able to keep up in school? Would he be able to function in daily life? Back in Denmark, in those fragile years after his birth, I wrote my first book, *The Note From Heaven*, while taking care of our wonderful and loving son. Later it turned out that song would play a decisive role not only in his treatment, but especially in how he treated his surroundings.

It is amazing how frustrated you can be when caught up in the moment, and by contrast how in hindsight it is possible to see that same situation as both brilliant and preordained. And so it was in this case. Therefore, dear reader, if you are currently experiencing a crisis in your life, take heart!

Dr. Karl

When our son was two years old, his muscles were too weak and his joints too soft for him to be able to function normally. For example, he was unable to raise himself if he fell. At night he slept with splints on his arms and legs – the latter to correct his all-too soft, outward-facing ankles. Specialists at the National Hospital warned us that he might never be able to walk normally, and even if he could, that cycling, running and other similar activities would simply be out of the question. When my husband by chance looked in on an event at the local library, he saw how a woman with an incurable ailment got healed with Sound Healing given through an English medium called Graham Bishop.

After the healing session, the spirit Dr. Karl spoke through the body of Graham. Dr. Karl was at the same time wise, compassionate, precise and scientifically very well founded. My husband and I decided to book a "sitting" with Graham after some research about him. Neither of us had any previous experience with a medium or the like, but because our son's prognosis was by all accounts doubtful, we felt we had nothing to lose and everything to gain.

When the day for the sitting arrived in February, a snowstorm raged the likes of which are seldom seen, even in Denmark. Winds howled and mounds of snow covered the roads. Schools across the entire country were closed, and radio announcers advised against any travelling unless it was absolutely necessary. We drove for several hours in order to reach the meeting in Copenhagen, equipped with a shovel, blankets and tea.

Because of the snowstorm, Graham, his wife Mie, my husband, our son and I were the only ones present at the sitting. For that reason, there was extra time for our session, giving all three of us the opportunity to communicate with Dr. Karl. To our amazement, after Graham had gasped several times, his appearance changed to that of an older man, and Dr. Karl's crisp yet husky voice chuckled in a friendly manner: "We are ready for your requests."

In response to our question regarding our son's missing kneecaps, Dr. Karl replied, "The doctors say many things, but they don't know everything. Your boy's kneecaps are located in his thighs. Continue to ask the specialist to look for your son's kneecaps. One day he will find them."

It was reassuring that someone could make such a confident statement – finally, a positive message! Later in the séance Dr. Karl told us that children coming into this world with a handicap are always given a gift as compensation.

"Have you not noticed how much love your son spreads to those around him? Have you seen how he cares for and heals any new person that enters your living room?"

"We see so often disappointed parents of children with Down's syndrome, for example. They only see the problems and never realize that their child has been born with all the love they themselves have so desperately been seeking all their lives."

After answering our questions, Dr. Karl (Graham cannot sing) carried out Sound Healing on our son for about an hour.

Our son lay still and was sung to by Dr. Karl, who for most of the time emitted a sound, much like a tractor, that reverberated out through Graham's nose. The sound reminded me unmistakably of one that regularly occurred when I did Sound Healings. It's a sound that I had experienced as quite disturbing, because of its hoarse, guttural noise, almost demonic and far from what would normally be considered musically pleasing. However, our son clearly loved it.

"Gut, gut" said Dr. Karl, with his German-English accent, and then continued making his grunting sounds. From time to time, he summoned other spirits and higher-pitched female voices could be heard coming through Graham. We were politely informed by Dr. Karl that other members of a spirit group of about 700 members came to lend a hand when necessary.

Dr. Karl came to the conclusion that our son had a digestive problem because he lacked certain enzymes for breaking down proteins. The spirits wanted to try to solve the problem, but apparently it would hurt for a short moment. A gentle lullaby from a light tenor voice calmed all of us before the procedure, which consisted of a combination of sound, and energetic palpation of our son's stomach. He cried briefly, and then it was over.

We were then instructed to give our son a specific medicinal cure every day: A mixture of mashed avocado, freshly squeezed pink grapefruit juice, garlic and a pinch of salt. If necessary, we could sweeten the remedy with "currant juice". None of us understood this last ingredient, and neither Graham who is English, nor the German Dr. Karl could speak Danish.[83]

"Wait a moment, while we ask one of our Danish members." The spirits apparently conversed. Dr. Karl politely thanked the "helper" and said in broken Danish: "Solbaaersaft" (currant juice in Danish).

Spiritual knockout

I don't know what I'm doing. We are constantly driven by invisible forces – we are quite simply actors on the stage of life. We think we are the ones pulling the strings, controlling what happens, when in actual fact it is we who are the puppets. Don't complain, weep or pray, rather, open your intuitive eye and become aware of the light in you and around you – it is always there.
Emmanuel Sørensen, Sunyata (*A Danish Mystic's Life and Words of Wisdom*)

Just two days prior to the meeting with Dr. Karl, I had sent the manuscript of my first book, *The Note From Heaven*, to the publisher – and for the third time. Every time I sent it, they wanted this or that changed. I had written the book to get the Note from Heaven out of my system, so that I could move on. I could not see what practical use there was for the Note from Heaven in this world. Was the publisher's concern to adapt the book to make it more marketable a sign that I should give it all up?

My private life suffered under the strain, and we dreaded what our son's future might be. We had cut short our musical careers in Israel and declined an offer for a recording contract, something we had desired for many years. We were back in Denmark with our new career as parents, and prepared to do anything for our fantastic, but different child.

Graham Bishop knew nothing about me or my writing before the session.

Below is a transcript of some of my questions and Dr. Karl's answers, copied from the audio recording of the sitting.

How can I serve the whole?

"We are here to follow each opportunity to serve what is brought before us with the fullness of all our enthusiasm and effort."

"In your case, we bring you, at this time, an understanding of certain aspects of tonal creation and combination."

"We bring thoughts to your mind that are not totally in accordance with normal musical practice. We do this in order to extend mankind's understanding of the utilization of sound – to show that sound and vibration have the potential to heal. And this is what we are teaching you now. Other things will come at a later point."

"As we have said, the important thing is merely to follow the opportunity that comes to you, and not to have limitations within your own mind. Some of this inspiration that is brought into your mind does not comply with the accepted rules, regulations and normal patterns of activity within the musical spectrum, but it should not be cast aside. Simply follow the inspiration that is being presented. It is there for a purpose."

I felt faint at Dr. Karl's words. During the writing of my book, the thought had struck me, "Where do all of these ideas come from? Is it possible they come from somewhere else?" But I had quickly pushed these questions aside, because in my family and circle of friends, it was taboo to believe that you were in contact with the spirit world. But even so, I had noticed how the gentle flow of ideas, which I had my hands full with just sorting through, were always followed by a warm and pleasant tingling sensation in my scalp. In fact, I always felt great when in that fascinating, writing state.

Dr. Karl spoke as if putting thoughts into my head were the most natural thing in the world.

"So, is it not me who has written my book?"

"Of course it is not you, my dear."

"Shall I write in my book that the information comes from you?"

"That is up to you. It is more important that the information is brought forth. You see, once we are divided from the physical form, we no longer need for things to be attributed to us. We merely wish to impart the understanding. We care not whether you state that it comes from us or whether you take the credit yourself."

"Is it so that the type of sound I have described is dependent on being open to you, the spirits?"

"As we said, it is a healing vibration. By increasing the understanding of this vibration, we intend to decrease the barrier between your world and ours over the coming years. This is all a part of the healing process. So, my dear, continue the good work and always hold this within your heart: No matter how much these ideas appear to deviate from normal musical thought, there is a reason why they are being brought forth. Some may consider it to be musically deficient, but of course what we inspire you with has in reality very little to do with music and more to do with the vibrational energy that it can create. So we hope this answers your question on that subject. Is there something else you would like to ask?"

"Should I sing jazz or is it more important that I work with Sound Healing?"

(I had the opportunity to sing with the well-known jazz pianist Horace Parlan and bass player Jimmi Roger Pedersen, but frustratingly enough felt no desire to practice.)

"Well, my dear, let us say that one has to create perspectives. Of course, we would essentially agree with you, that what is being brought forth from us to you in this time is of significant importance. However, one also has to have an earthly life connection too. One needs to create a symbiosis of the work involving those from our realm and normal earthly activities. Therefore we would say to you that it is not detrimental to the work we are bringing forth for you to also work with other aspects of musical expression – though of course one has to have balance. Remember, that which is being brought to you **is** important."

"We have found a channel through which we can deliver our message, and we are using it. But we do not wish you to dedicate your entire life to the message, that we bring forth through this channel. You also need to have your own aspects of expression. So of course it is not for us to say whether you should sing jazz – that is your choice. But perhaps our words have helped you to understand, that we do not intend or wish that you should dedicate all of your available time to the undertaking, that we are bringing in to your mind, otherwise you may become disassociated with the reality of your earthly world, and that is not what we wish."

"You have found already that the reality of the world can seem a little strange when you first come back after having spent an extended period of time with us. And of course, if you were to spend more and more time, you would find the reality of the world becoming even stranger. That would be detrimental, because it is important for you to be able to share with the material world that which is being brought to you. Therefore you need to have your feet upon the ground in the earthly aspect also. Otherwise, people will merely dismiss you as a crackpot."

"What about healing? Is that something I should do?"

(I had had a hard time taking myself seriously in the role of a healer, as my identity was so tightly interwoven with being a musician and composer.)

"My dear, have you not heard our words? When opportunity and inspiration come into your mind you should grasp them. In other words, the answer is yes!"

"I just wondered, am I good enough?"

"Oh, my dear! This is always a problem with you foolish humans – the question of 'Am I good enough?' Let us ask you one question: Do you go into the process of healing with love and compassion for those who come before you? Then what more is necessary? Hmm, you see all that can be asked of anyone is to bring forth the intention of love and compassion. So, providing you have the full focus of love and compassion, then whatever you bring forth is good enough. The healing doesn't have to be at the same level as another could do it, but that is irrelevant."

"You would not be given the inspiration, my dear, if you were not capable. This is such a foolish human problem. We sometimes wish we could take human brains and wash them in a washing machine."

"When you heal others, is there a risk of taking on their problems?"

"Well, my dear, the answer is rather complex: Yes and no is the answer. Essentially, my dear, what you have to do is... just a moment." (Dr. Karl consults the rest of the spirit group.)

"You must learn to separate compassion from pity. You see,

when you pity another being, that is where you can take on part of their problem as your own. It is not the compassion but the pity that is the problem. But, it is not that you take it on permanently. However, when you have pity, there is an opening within your own energy field to accept some of the other person's energy. And so these problems occur. One should never go into the process of healing with pity in one's mind. If that is there, then one should take a few moments to eliminate the aspect of pity before you commence the healing process. It is compassion and love. If pity is present then you run the risk of causing yourself some difficulty for a short time, but it will pass. Usually after one or two days."

Transformation

The séance continued with more private questions.

When we returned home, my son and I were completely out of it. I remember us sitting, almost lying down, on a mattress more or less like zombies. The air was thick and appeared to move slowly. It took several days to fully integrate this first personal meeting with Dr. Karl into our bodies. In just a couple of hours my entire perspective of reality had been turned 180 degrees: My role was no longer purely a question of "me" and my ego. The straightforward wisdom, precision and love Dr. Karl had shown convinced me that no one is alone here on this Earth. If we dare to open ourselves, inspiration can sing through us. And this inspiration is not one's own – it is universal.

The chronic inner doubt of "Am I good enough?" had been a leak in my system that had tied my power with a fear of unfolding myself in life. The Note from Heaven had transformed that fear to a burning need to serve the whole. The reunion with "my sound" led me to an experience of resonating with the whole universe. "Am I good enough?" I understood now why this question was not relevant at all. You are a part of a cosmic vibration, which is a holy sound. You are nothing and everything just like all of creation is. Serve the best you can. Finally I understood everything. There is no death, just different levels of creation. Higher or lower frequencies. When we die, we shift to a denser vibration, and therefore must leave our earthly body. A level that is invisible for the physical body, but with which we can communicate through the cultivation of listening.

It felt as if I had been set free, everything fell into place and I understood at once the frustration of the previous years. In reality, I had been fighting against my own unity with the whole. I realized that the best way to serve my purpose on Earth would be to surrender to the Note from Heaven and to let the other side work through me as long as I could be of any help.

Dr. Karl's words hold water

In the six weeks that followed, we gave our boy his avocado medicine, and noticed that his vitality and lust for life began to increase. About half a year after the meeting with Dr. Karl, a specialist at the National Hospital by the name of Steen Bach Christensen found our son's kneecaps, which had slid into place.

He walked normally and could even jog, which surprised everyone. By the time he was five years old he could ride a bike normally. He had some smaller difficulties intellectually when he started in school, and our son seemed to drift away into his own world. He loved to copy Mr. Bean and put on such a convincing "Mr. Bean" impression for the school psychologist, that he was sent to a special school for children that had more or less come to a halt in their development.

We moved to another county that had a state school with room for the individual. Today, our oldest son functions normally. As a kid he sang almost constantly. The power of his voice has always felt life-giving. I can't get enough – it has a special quality that I myself cannot produce. You can feel the innermost chambers of the heart resonate when his voice unfolds.

Working with the other side

My approach to further work in the spiritual field was underlined by the thought that the group of spirits[84] had used me without my knowledge, and that they just could continue doing so. The experience had changed my life, but my surroundings remained the same. I couldn't share all of these new experiences with anyone. The fear of awakening the ego through a public proclamation of my collaboration with the other side was paralyzing. I would lose everything – every last piece of respect from normal people, from my circle of musician friends and colleagues, and from my family who already saw me as an outsider.

So I hid it within me. But from then on I saw my son's connection clearly – the higher meaning, that he is perfect exactly as he is. When he slips into a daydream, when all children and adults daydream, they are in a state where time and space disappears – a place where intuition subconsciously communicates with other planes. The conscious use of that intuition and the service such awareness implies is only possible once the ego has matured.

An advanced use of intuition corresponds to an increase in the electrical currents flowing through the body. Therefore the prerequisite for the development of the body's electrical network is grounding, and in this way, each and every earthbound person, regardless of their background, has the capacity to develop their spiritual abilities.

For me, the current ideas on holism are about waking up the parts of our brain that are connected with the heart. The stronger connection the brain has to the heart, the more holistic the way of thinking.

Society's basic skepticism for the alternative world is part of this process and a prerequisite for the weeding out of large, self-promoting "guru-flowers". We all have to deal with our shadows and thereby with the weakness within ourselves where the ego sneaks up on stage and wishes to bathe in glamour and sequins. So, long live the skeptical! The spiritual connection becomes lost in static, when the ego tunes in to its own program. Minute changes in frequencies can make a world of difference.

So these, and the following words about spiritual connection, are first and foremost a balancing act.

Ego fitness. A flexible ego understands that it needs to take a back seat when the music is playing through the flute – an instrument whose most important function is to be hollow and resonant. The less present the ego, the better. It is a most liberating feeling when the wind is at your back. All fear disappears.

Follow with your utmost enthusiasm that which is given to you.

Opening

The meeting with Dr. Karl forced me to choose a new direction. I had been at a standstill on the banks of the river of life at a place where that river split into two. I chose the left branch of the river – whose current turned out to be far stronger than the river I had previously been floating down.

My publishing company accepted the third submission of *The Note from Heaven*. The editor, Flemming Bindslev, was an amazing gift to me. In his own way, he gave me an education that forced me to think in modern concepts. What use is it to be ahead of one's time if the message you are trying to portray doesn't get through? I am extremely grateful to him for his hard work removing every single superfluous word – he was indeed a gift from above!

The book release was approaching, and the publishing company Borgen was on the lookout for someone who could write a foreword to my book. Several of the people I had suggested, including the author Lars Muhl, who had supported me throughout the final part of the writing process, did not suit them. The company suggested one of my former teachers at the

Academy of Music, Peter Bastian. However, he didn't know much about singing and healing.

I therefore, on the spur of the moment, e-mailed Graham Bishop in August of 2001 and asked if Dr. Karl would write a foreword to my new book, as he obviously knew me inside and out. At the same time I was eager to receive verification that the spirits really were still present. The following day I received an e-mail from Graham:

Hi Githa,

I have passed your request to Karl and this is his response:

Within the realms of humankind there is more and more understanding being brought forth to those who are willing to open their minds to the flow. Once you have gained the understanding that your whole existence is based upon a vibrational structure, then it becomes obvious that vibrations can affect your structures both positively and negatively. Sound, light, magnetism, all have powerful potential within the process of creating harmony and reducing disease. Herein lie the first steps for simply using the abilities of the human voice to affect the disrupting vibrations which create disharmony within the energy flow of the physical structure. Its use is not restricted to humankind. It can be used for the benefit of all living things. This is just a beginning. There will be much more over the coming years. Those of you who open your minds in freedom and clarity, with absence of ego, will receive guidance for that which you are capable of bringing forth into the earthly realm. Take that which is given here and start a journey towards the simplicity of tonal healing.

Dr. Karl

And these are the words and feelings that came into my thoughts (Graham Bishop):

Spirits have for many years spoken of the power of sound, stressing the importance of the undertones that are created by the physical voice. They have frequently created sounds from my voice system that I cannot make myself. These tones have affected many people greatly in many ways. It has long been known that music has an effect upon all forms of life. This book takes this age-old knowledge and puts it into a simple form that can be built upon and extended by the reader. Why not start the flow within yourself and see where it takes you...

Graham Bishop

I was thrilled having read the e-mail. *"They are out there – I am not alone."*

Ecstatic, I called my publisher, Borgen. The mood there, however, was not as enthusiastic. At that point in time, Graham Bishop was well-known through the Danish television program *The Power of the Spirits*. If *The Note from Heaven* should be considered reliable and reach a wide Danish "normal" audience, it better be without a foreword by Dr. Karl and Graham.

A physical initiation

People responded positively to my Sound Healing, but clients weren't exactly queuing up to see me, and I only took a symbolic fee. So I continued with my life, but began, more and more, to dare to believe in giving Sound Healing. With trembling hands I started teaching an evening class in song and healing, this after having given my first lecture on *The Note from Heaven* at a library.

Cancer sufferers began to seek me out, sang themselves free and received Sound Healing. One particular client who overcame cancer with a combination of holistic treatment, song and Sound Healing, invited me to a one-day workshop with Andrew Cohen, a renowned spiritual teacher.

The hall was full of around 200 people. Several of the men wore suits.

Andrew Cohen entered the stage enthusiastically, in a shiny

blue and black silk waistcoat, white shirt, pressed trousers and tie. His moustache bounced merrily over an infectious, short, nasal laugh supported by a powerful push from the diaphragm: "Ha!" He began by meditating for half an hour.

I felt bad. My whole body ached. People sitting close by glared irritably as I fidgeted and sat uneasily, feeling anything but spiritual, thinking that the next half hour would be a nightmare.

Suddenly I noticed the presence of a soft, fluttering, energetic movement above my head. There is no doubt in my mind that someone made a decision: "Now!"

A force struck down through the middle of the crown of my head and everything became instantly black.

– I woke as I fell against the back of the man sitting in front of me. He looked strangely at me while I excused and straightened myself up. I woke, as it seemed to me, merely a moment later, with one of the suited ushers helping me up from the floor. Subsequently my chair had fallen over backwards and apparently I had too. How embarrassing – and strange! It felt as if I was gone for just a split second.

The meditation continued unaffected. I was feeling better now and was finally able to slip into a meditative state. When Andrew Cohen cleared his throat and told the group that the meditation was over, he said directly to me, "Are you okay?" At first I thought he was speaking to the man beside me as my blackout was over so quickly that Andrew Cohen might not have noticed it.

In the interval, my client explained to me that I had been lying on the floor for three minutes and said something like, "Don't worry. I am okay. Everything is fine."

I wondered, who had really said that? It wasn't me at least. I was out like a light!

Strangely enough I felt completely comfortable with and in fact relieved by what had happened.

My body was relaxed, happy and peaceful. Intuitively I knew that "they" had performed a necessary procedure on me – but why in a public place like this? Perhaps because it needed to happen in a place where someone could help me up – a place with high energy? If it had happened at home my husband would have called for an ambulance. But not here. Everything felt perfect, and I had a clear sensation of the energy that had made the decision there and then for me. It was a good energy, despite the fact that it had struck me down.

During a round of questions, Andrew Cohen mentioned that this wasn't the first time that someone had lost consciousness during one of his meditations, although it didn't happen often.

A change of identity

I signed up for a course as a regression therapist because I had begun to experience previous lives when I lay down and relaxed.[85]

The course took place over six weekends in Copenhagen, and was led by the Swiss-Danish André Corell.[86]

If the work with the Note from Heaven had been able to release psychological blockages within myself, it would surely be possible for others to experience the same. It was necessary for me to be able to cope with a regression, in case it should spontaneously occur in one of my students during singing lessons or during Sound Healing. The course began shortly after my book and practice CD *The Note from Heaven* was finally released.

On the release date 02.20.2002, I became sick. Following this date I coughed for three months, and neither doctors nor specialists could explain why. They found no infections and diagnosed it to be a virus that couldn't be treated. I, normally, suffered very seldom from colds.

In any case, I sniffled my way through the weekend courses with André.

During the final weekend, one of the course participants was suffering from such a powerful migraine that she was on the verge of going home. In the break I offered her a short Sound Healing session, in my usual apologetic manner. It was still a struggle for me to take on the identity of a healer in a public arena. The Sound Healing seemed not to have any visible effect on the migraine, so my insecurity was confirmed.

The woman arrived at the course the following day and told me that she now was able to hear again in her previously deaf ear. She believed that this must have been due to my Sound Healing. Apparently, her neighbors had had a party the night before. Normally she would simply have turned her deaf ear towards the sound – however, that trick no longer worked!

In the lunch break I gave her another Sound Healing session for ten minutes, during which her hearing improved further. The woman's regained hearing gave me the confidence I needed to finally call myself a Sound Healer. By that transformation, my cold promptly disappeared. The healing occurred a couple of months after the blackout at Andrew Cohen's course. Again, it needed to happen in public.

In the afternoon we were to take an examination in regression therapy. The participants that hadn't yet worked together would work on each other. The girl I was paired up with was very different from me, and we didn't get along well. First, she brought me back to a former life. I didn't feel released afterwards and was irritated by her controlling way of treating me. When it was my turn to release her, she was obviously not comfortable with me either. She was stuck in her body and I didn't succeed in leading her into a previous life. Following my success with Sound Healing from earlier in the day, I felt brave enough to follow a sudden impulse, "Shall I sing on you?"

"I would hate that... but you should," she replied.

So as not to disrupt the others who were in middle of their examinations in the nearby rooms, I sang undertones from her toes all the way up to her stomach. During the process, I asked her the questions we had been told to ask during the course, but received no answer – she was in another world.

André Corell came in to watch our séance. My partner still didn't respond to my questions. It was probably not the smartest thing to do to use Sound Healing as this wasn't requested as part of the examination. André left the room without a word and I began to feel nervous. My partner hadn't answered me for a full fifteen minutes. Her hands were warm and her pulse okay. I sat down on a chair and contemplated the situation. She awoke in the same moment that André reentered the room. What a relief! I was about to embrace her when she looked sternly at me and said, "When you began making sounds I wanted to scream, but was pulled away into darkness before I was able. It felt like I was anesthetized!" She didn't say much more, but it had obviously been a rather violent experience for her.

I called her later to find out if the Sound Healing had had any effect on her. I also asked her to write down her experiences. She remembered nothing of the actual event, except for the feeling of being completely "out of it". However, three out of four allergies were now gone. Her oversensitivity had occurred due to a traumatic operation as a 12-year-old while under general anesthetic.

The two healing sessions I did during the final weekend course in regression therapy were the start of a definite change of identity for me. What had I done? Nothing more than singing and listening for resonance, as usual. Whatever the spirits might achieve through me was up to them!

And with this I became a servant. The responsibility for the outcome of the healing was no longer mine. The only thing that mattered now was to listen for resonance in a state of compassion and love.

An attempt to cure tinnitus

But, nevertheless, I had a worried feeling about using undertones after experiencing that the client had lost consciousness for fifteen minutes. I wondered if subtones were simply too powerful? Some medical arguments were needed.

I therefore contacted Audun Myskja, a Norwegian medical Professor and researcher in musical medicine, whose highly recommended book *Den Musiske Medisin*[87] I had previously read.

Audun replied, stating that sub-harmonic tones in Sound Healing were not dangerous, and calmed me by saying that he had also used undertones without his clients ever losing consciousness. If a client had needed to enter a full narcosis in order to become healed, I should accept it. Audun became most enthusiastic when we spoke about using Sound Healing to cure tinnitus, as that was a subject of great interest for him as a scientist. He wrote, "Try to sing at tinnitus and tell me what happens!"

A week later a craftsman responded to an advertisement I had put up in the kindergarten about free Sound Healing for tinnitus sufferers. I was clear regarding the fact that I had no experience in the field. The 38-year-old man had suffered with tinnitus since he was 17 years old. It occurred when he worked with an angle grinder without hearing protection. An audiologist had diagnosed him as having second degree tinnitus. The sound of the tinnitus was powerful and always present. The man had managed to learn how to cope so that he could sleep at night.

After the vocal Sound Healing session his tinnitus became worse. He agreed to call me in the coming days and let me know if his tinnitus had returned to normal levels. Meanwhile I blamed myself for presuming that I would be able to heal him. I lost all desire to Sound Heal again. Dr. Karl and The White Brotherhood had promised to help me, but now I stood alone knowing that I had injured a fellow human being.

Two days passed without any word from the client, so with a shaking hand, I called him. He sounded happy. "I had actually completely forgotten to call you because my tinnitus has gone now!" A month later he rang me and said, "Can you help me again? You know, I'm used to working without hearing protection, and I used the angle grinder again. The tinnitus is back. But I'm sure you can fix that in a jiffy!"

Measuring brain waves during singing and Sound Healing

When Audun Myskja found out that I had cured a tinnitus case, he was prepared to fly to Denmark to observe my Sound Healing method. I contacted the psychologist and researcher Professor Erik Hoffman[88] and made an agreement with him that we, in connection with Audun's visit, should meet and carry out brain-wave measurements during Sound Healing, with the intention of possibly starting a research project with Audun in the future. Before the meeting with Dr. Karl, I had searched for scientific explanations of the state of consciousness that the Note from Heaven brought me into. Because of this, I had contacted Erik Hoffman. He is a retired professor of psychology and has developed his own brain mapping system that shows the brain's wavelengths corresponding to gamma, beta, alpha, theta and delta waves. These measured states of consciousness are displayed on a color scale that shows frequencies from extreme alertness to a comatose state.

The measurements made while I was singing showed no significant deviation from a normal brain-wave map. But when Erik later examined the graphical representations of the movements of my eyeballs, he couldn't explain the phenomena: My eyes demonstrated the same rapid eye movement patterns which normally only occur during REM sleep. Today I know this is a normal phenomenon for any person surrendering to the

Note from Heaven.

I met Audun Myskja at Kastrup Airport in Copenhagen and was struck by his direct and focused energy – a combination of cool distance and completely uncensored openness at the same time. The atmosphere was already intense even before we arrived at the Cymbion Science Center to meet Hoffman. I especially remember one of Audun's statements, in his singing Norwegian accent, "On fire!" In some way we were family. Sound had ignited us. He had just like me a burning passion for the power of sound, just as more and more people nowadays are becoming impassioned by its amazing effects.

So when Audun and I strolled into the room where Erik Hoffman was sitting ready with coffee, biscuits and electrodes, he asked with an astonished expression, "Have you two met previously?"

We began. Erik was obviously feeling a little out of things in the beginning, and sat down, fiddling with his coffee cup, looking a little distant while Audun lay on the dining table with electrodes on his head receiving Sound Healing.

It didn't take long, however, for his gaze to be fixed on his computer screen.

Audun's brain waves moved systematically from beta to alpha to theta to delta and then back through the spectrum. His brain waves continued to change in this way throughout the entire Sound Healing session.

Following the session, Erik Hoffman made it clear that it would not be possible to draw any formal scientific conclusions without a minimum of 30 test subjects. "However! It seems that there is a clear movement between consciousness and unconsciousness during the Sound Healing." Erik continued, "It is possible that information is fetched from a subconscious to a conscious level, where it is then processed."

Erik's assumptions were in keeping with the reactions that I had seen and continue to see today during Sound Healing: Many clients slip away into another state, snore occasionally and then gradually return back to a state of normal consciousness again. Certain clients fall into a deep slumber during the entire séance, others lie awake, but most glide to and fro between conscious and unconscious states.

Now it was Audun's turn to observe the method, and Erik Hoffman was eager to try Sound Healing. Audun sat calmly in a corner. Erik's brain waves were not measured.

After the Sound Healing, Audun admitted that he had seen the Holy Spirit. Based on his vision he believed it was the forces that sang through me that were so powerful, and not my method itself. The scientist in him was disappointed, but the mystic was overjoyed. Being both a scientist and possessing clairvoyant abilities, Audun as a prize-winning professor and researcher was plagued by an inner conflict.

We will return to Audun later on.

Part 2:

The Effects of Sound Healing

The whole physical mechanism – the muscles, the blood circulation, the nerves – are all moved by the power of vibration. As there is resonance for every sound, so the human body is a living resonator for sound.

Hazrat Inayat Khan

Lectures and Sound Healing Demonstrations

I began to give a fair number of lectures following the release of my book *The Note from Heaven*, and was often asked, "Do you teach courses as well?" My answer was always, "No, I don't. I can't teach a course in something I don't truly understand."

I carried on giving lectures over an extended period of time, and treated more and more clients. This book could give an account of the illnesses and conditions Sound Healing has and has not cured, but, to tell the truth, I cannot remember all of the cases as there are several hundred. I will mention the ones that I recall when the inspiration strikes me. Here follow two cases from Sound Healing demonstrations made in lectures.

The concert pianist's curse (tinnitus and hearing loss)

A retired concert pianist approached me and requested treatment for tinnitus. She had awoken after an operation for cancer, hearing one by one all of the piano pieces she had ever performed from her repertoire throughout the course of her career – much to her amazement!

The pianist asked the nurse on duty how they had known about her repertoire. "Repertoire? We don't play music here," replied the nurse. The pianist was puzzled. The music continued. When all of the pieces of music she had played throughout her life had finished playing in her head, they began to play again two at a time, then three, and so on until all of the pieces played simultaneously in an infernal noise which tortured the woman night and day. The doctors wanted to admit her to a psychiatric ward. She refused, as she was far from mentally ill, but took sleeping pills in large doses because it was impossible for her to get any respite from the din.

315

And now the woman had contacted me. Her hearing had become so bad that she could no longer hear the birds sing, and the noise had turned into tinnitus.

The woman was probably not the easiest person to spend time with. She was a spinster and bitter, but her story was fascinating to me – a fellow classically-trained musician.

As the woman was unable to travel, I invited her to a lecture I was giving in Copenhagen near her residence. I asked her to arrive during the intermission, as she was hypersensitive to the slightest noise. I would then demonstrate Sound Healing on her in front of the audience.

A small, fragile, well-dressed woman stepped out of a taxi precisely when we had agreed to meet. I escorted her to a packed lecture room at the Mental Research Association's premises. If I had known how sick she was I would have never agreed to the meeting. The woman was extremely frail. Once she lay down on the treatment couch, the audience huddled around to observe the séance.

I prayed that there must be some higher purpose to all of this. In these critical situations, I am thankful from the bottom of my heart that it is not I, but the spirit world, which is responsible for everything that transpires.

What would I do if she should sit bolt upright screaming when I began to produce a sound? We'd just have to take it from there. The woman seemed extremely sensitive in every cell of her body. She hadn't slept a wink for the past four nights.

I began with an opening ceremony, tucked her in gently under the blanket and hummed softly for her. The woman lay still with her eyes closed. I then Sound Healed her entire body relatively quickly in about ten minutes.

As I was finishing and hummed directly over her, I was accompanied by the sound of her snoring. The audience looked somewhat amused. There was rather a lot at stake. She hadn't been able to sleep, and now there she was, asleep! What now?

We let her sleep and retreated to the other end of the room where I answered questions from the audience.

The woman was still asleep when we had finished. I managed to awaken her by nudging her body. The pianist blinked and wandered dazedly out of the door, following me into my car.

I tried calling her the following day, but nobody answered. This of course made me somewhat nervous. She finally called me back later that evening and told that she had been out walking all day. The pianist was particularly happy as she had regained her hearing and could now hear the birds singing once again.

A week later the same pianist called me, although this time she was in a bad mood. She complained that she was able to hear her tinnitus much more strongly now that her hearing had returned.

Because the woman didn't feel well enough to visit me, we had no further treatment sessions.

The Psychologists' Association (tinnitus)

The organizer of the lecture in the Association for Psychological Research recommended me to the Psychologists' Association. It was a more intellectual audience this time, but a surprisingly open one. One of the psychologists volunteered himself for the final demonstration of Sound Healing. "I have tinnitus which I'd like to get rid of."

The man lay down on the treatment couch, and the atmosphere in the room was filled with the question as to whether he could be cured or not. This was essentially just a demonstration, but his clear definition of what he wanted raised people's expectations.

I scanned him as usual and found the sounds that resonated. The notes affect not only the person in the demonstration, but the audience as well. When I was finished it felt as if I was playing the lottery: What if his tinnitus had become worse? And what if it took two days to have an effect, like the first tinnitus I treated? What if nothing at all had happened? Again it was a relief to leave everything in the hands of the spiritual helpers.

The man gradually returned to consciousness. He sat up and shook his head in disbelief, "Well I'll be darned, it's gone!"

It was as if the entire building breathed a sigh of relief. I could have fallen to my knees and thanked the higher powers, but contented myself with placing my hands over my heart and feeling my body singing with gratitude. Soon after, everyone was eager to buy my books and the money fairly flew about!

Measurements with an audiometer

It is a mammoth task to immerse oneself in a method which is scientifically unexplored, and which can affect any aspect of life because every living thing in reality is sound.

The results are all we have to go on. Sound does have an effect, and it has its own life. But what sort of life? It can feel like being blown out to sea on a little raft. Where is one to begin in relation to treating illnesses?

After having consulted with Audun Myskja, I decided to concentrate on healing hearing problems, especially deafness and tinnitus which I had already had good results with.

In an attempt to approach the subject from a scientific point of view, I borrowed an old audiometer, created questionnaires, wrote journals and carried out audiograms before and after each Sound Healing session. The hearing tests took a long time to carry out, which had a detrimental effect on the Recipient's experience of the session. If their hearing improved, they thanked me for the treatment and went on with their lives. However, personally, I didn't find myself particularly suited to the role of an audiologist.

The measurements and readings from the hearing tests left me with an emptiness that I myself had created by attempting to be "scientific". How could I unite a scientific approach with my belief that the greatest healing effect in the séance would be if the client could strengthen their own bond with the higher powers? And how should I explain to the clients that it was possible for them to reach a contact with previously unknown states of consciousness which can have a healing effect on the entire organism?

None of this was exactly in harmony with hearing tests and journal writing.

Sacré Cœur

Sound can awaken a feeling of deep affection and gratitude which allows the heart to open, the chest to be engulfed in warmth, followed by involuntary yawning. This kind of physically-felt heart opening can be compared to an orgasm. Sacré Cœur – the engorged, bleeding or blooming, but always burning heart – is a state, which can be awakened by a resonating sound.

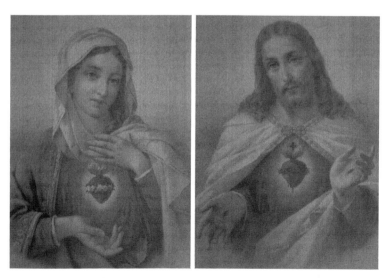

Jesus and Mary Magdalena, each depicted with a glowing heart. (Origin: Southern France)

When the effect of a sound healing is measured, intellectual analysis takes place, and therefore the left hemisphere of the brain, that deals with logical thinking, achievement and control, is activated. Scientific, left hemisphere-based thought hinders affection and gratitude – emotions which are based in the right hemisphere of the brain, and which allow access to the heart.

It is a fact that no apparent opening of the heart occurred in the clients whose hearing was measured with the audiometer. However, clients whose hearing wasn't measured almost always experienced an opening of the heart.

The Sound Healer can also be affected by measurements and tests, becoming focused on the results. Was I Sound Healing well enough? Wow, *I* can cure deafness – something no one else can cure! The moment *"I"* comes into the picture, the Sound Healer loses power, and the effect of the healing is diminished instantaneously.

In Niels Bohr's Principle of Complementarity in quantum physics, the state of "being" and "observing" cannot coexist even if they are part of the same reality. When you observe, the "being" state is excluded. In the "being" state it is impossible to observe.

I had learnt a good lesson. As a Sound Healer you must learn to balance on the tightrope of humility, not over an abyss, but just high enough so that you land with a bump if you fall. And I fell.

Not my will, but thine, be done.
Luke 22:42

The hearing tests did seem to have some effect, but I didn't experience the same level of healing of tinnitus and deafness that I did in the treatments where the tests were not made. The tests did show, however, that partial deafness was positively affected in approximately 60 percent of clients after their first Sound Healing session.

Albert Einstein and Niels Bohr had long and involved discussions about quantum physics. One of these discussions was about this exact topic: How much a research situation affects that which is being examined. Bohr concluded that experiment and reality would always affect each other.

The Primary Cilium

Each of our trillions of cells are coated with different kinds of sensitive cilium – sensory hairs. One kind is the primary cilium, which is required for the ability of retinal cells to detect light, and is critically involved in an array of other cell communication processes.

> *Much of this cell communication machinery occurs at the primary cilium, partly because this organ extends out from the cell body where it can access environmental signals. Thus, the primary cilium serves as a sort of molecular antenna, receiving and transmitting signals for the cell.*
> **Nicholette Zeliadt** on June 29, 2010, *Scientific American*

If the primary cilium's ability to detect electrical signals is dependent on a client's confidence in a cure and/or a therapist, then that confidence has a lot to say in a Sound Healing session.

Imagine that we with our subconscious mind can affect our primary cilium antennas to open and close. This seems reasonable and could be linked to an open/closed attitude of a client.

Conducive conditions for Sound Healing

Every person is an instrument in the orchestra that is the whole universe; and every voice is the music that comes from one of its instruments, each instrument being made distinct and particular, so that no other voice can take the place of that particular voice. If then, with the instrument that God has made and the music that God intended to be played in the world, one does not allow that music to be played and develops a voice that is not one's own, this

is naturally a great loss to oneself and to others.
Hazrat Inayat Khan

The Recipient's Soul wishes to be cured.

The Recipient has faith in the treatment.

The surroundings are supportive and safe.

The Recipient's body is receptive to Sound Healing.

The Recipient is being illuminated by the resonance of the Note from Heaven.

A week-long Sound Healing course in beautiful and natural surroundings with fresh healing rock water and healthy food.

When the hospital system has difficulty making a diagnosis.

When all other hope fails. For example, when a doctor provokes a patient by saying, "You will never be able to hear again," or, "You have two months left to live." This sort of news can in some cases awaken a person's self-belief mechanism, and light a fire in them: "I refuse to believe it! I'm going to prove the expert is wrong."

When the Sound Healer is able to maintain a balance between humility and enough authority and confidence to radiate to the client: "Now you are with me, and I am acting as an intermediary between you and your higher powers!"

Non-conducive conditions for Sound Healing

When the Recipient's soul doesn't wish to be cured and/or wants to end its life on Earth.

When a person is bound to the pain body[89] on a deeper level. In these situations, I combine Sound Healing with regressive cell-singing.[90]

When the Recipient is skeptical or wants to prove that Sound Healing doesn't work.

When a Recipient subconsciously uses the illness to receive care or attention, or maybe even causes their illness for the same subconscious reason.

When the Recipient attends treatment to make their relatives or a friend happy.

Sound Healing of tinnitus

Tinnitus is in my experience linked to the vagus nerve. The vagus nerve is connected to the stomach, and all internal organs. It divides at the breastbone, continues at each side of the neck up to the jaw into the ears and sends signals to the pineal gland and reptile brain. When the main cause of tinnitus is known, the chance to eliminate it with Vocal Sound Scanning is about 70 percent. This is especially true when tinnitus is caused by a loud sound, because we then know that the root of the trauma is placed around the ears.

Stress-related tinnitus is more complex to cure, because the Sound Healer has to scan the entire body in order to locate the imbalance causing the tinnitus. On top of that, the cause of stress is usually created from impulses outside the body, and these impulses need to be eliminated before a lasting cure of tinnitus can occur. For example if the stress is caused by a tense atmosphere at work or at home or by an environment with strong radiation, the tinnitus can return shortly after a cure during a vocal sound scanning. The same applies especially if there is radiation in the bedroom. You can compare it to saving a drowning man and then placing him in a rubber boat with a hole in it.

Sound Healing of hearing problems

Voices with flair for sound healing hearing conditions can have a positive impact on – and/or – cure hearing loss after ear draining procedures and cases of middle ear infections in about 70 percent of the cases. However, there are of course no guarantees.

When the small cilia in the ear have been flattened, there is a chance that a resonant sound can raise/repair them.

One of the common signs that healing is taking place with the Note from Heaven is that the Recipient feels warmth in the ear canal, and that the sound bounces from one ear to the other. This is also felt by the Sound Healer, who in this way can feel the effect of the Sound Healing. It can quite simply itch in the middle ear.

Artificial implants in the ear/body obviously can't resonate with the Note from Heaven, because they are comprised of inert material. As a Sound Healer you must be careful as it can be difficult to find resonance when a foreign object prevents vibration in the living cells.

Sound Healing of cancer

When treating cancer with the Note from Heaven, it is the Recipient who is in charge and therefore has responsibility for his/her own progress.

If Sound Healing is the right form of treatment for a specific case, the Recipient will become enkindled by the sound. If the cancer is aggressive, the Recipient must continue his/her own treatment with daily song. Practical experience has shown that half an hour to one hour daily singing on the Note from Heaven seems to stop further development of cancer. In one case the PSI numbers fell drastically and became normal after only ten days of singing.

In another case a woman given up because of terminal leukemia was Sound Healed and opened her voice beautifully to the Note from Heaven. She sang daily for one hour. After one week she got the answer from a blood test taken the day after our first Sound Healing. Her immune system reacted fine, and the blood level was close to normal. The woman had asked me to call upon Jesus to Heal her. The healing was extraordinarily strong, so strong that the water ran out of my eyes. The same thing has happened before for example with a man that had cancer in the lungs. He got healed instantly. Jesus – higher beings can only be present when the receiver is asking them for healing.

Many cancer sufferers are conscientious, have a strong sense of duty, are brave, selfless and have a hard time relinquishing control.

Therefore, the Listener must sense whether a process of sound healing should be started by regressive cell-singing or solely by opening the voice of the Singer to the Note from Heaven. The experience of the state of Oneness ignites the life forces of the immune system. But if the Singer is too sick to sing, you start by Sound Healing them or by teaching them "Hung Song" (see link to film).

It is important to sing with the Recipient's family and to give them Sound Healing too. In this way, they will be able to feel and physically understand the effect of the sound. It is of crucial importance that the family supports the treatment. Doubt weakens faith more than anything else. Sound Healing of family members can also have a preventative effect because the Recipient's close ones often suffer just as much as the cancer patient. When a relative's sickness has passed, it is not uncommon for other members of the family to fall seriously ill due to exhaustion.

If I myself got cancer and had faith in that a certain treatment could cure me, I would follow my intuition, because if you are not true to yourself, then you lose everything. In case my family would try to persuade me to choose a traditional chemo treatment, I would isolate myself in Nature in order to be able to feel my organism and to take a decision without distortion of other people's emotions. The best for you is the best for your family. The reason you got the cancer is that you have taken everybody other than yourself into account. The cancer is a challenge: Now the time has come to return to who you truly are.

Cancer cells sound different than healthy cells

All matter is made up of vibration. Every type of cell has its own signature note. In this way, liver cells can recognize each other via their common special frequency.[91]

Seen from this perspective, the cause of cancer could be attributed to a change of signature note in a group of cells.

The healthy cells can no longer resonate with the changed cells, and therefore reject them as foreign matter. "You are not a liver cell. Find somewhere else to live." In cases where the immune system is too stressed to eliminate these "foreign" cells, the fugitives seek a new abode and in time build an entirely new organ in the form of a tumor.

Back in 2006, researchers at University of Missouri, Columbia showed that the spread of skin cancer cells through the blood system can be revealed literally by amplifying their sound (the vibrational frequency of melanin) using a special laser technique. This amazing technique highlights the sound of skin cancer cells/melanoma and can help oncologists discover early signs of metastases. The detector can reveal down to a precision of ten cells, and track them before they establish themselves in other organs.

In 1933 the brilliant scientist Royal Raymond Rife healed 16 out of 16 terminal cancer cases in three months by using electronic sound treatment with the "Rife Machine". None of the participants experienced relapses or any side effects.

"Rife learned that **different species of life have their own electromagnetic 'signature', or pattern of oscillation (frequency)** based on its individual genetic chemical blueprint. It's different for all. Dr. Rife discovered that viruses, bacteria, and parasites are particularly sensitive to their own specific 'bio frequencies' and could be destroyed by intensifying those frequencies until chemical changes occur within the pathogen and it would devitalize and die. Sometimes they could see them literally explode... like an intense musical note that can shatter a wine glass."[92]

In my book *Help* there is a chapter about the work of Royal Raymond Rife.

Sound Healing of stress

A prolonged exhalation is the key to release stress. Singing long notes therefore is a quick method of resolving stress, especially if the Recipient is aware that he/she needs to change the conditions that have created the stress in the first place.

It can be difficult for a stressed person to "take a deep breath" on command because the diaphragm usually is locked due to tension. However, the instruction, "Listen to your stomach. Which sounds are hiding within?" tends to allow the breathing to open up. This is because the body calls for attention and loves when you listen to it, rather than give it orders.

A playful attitude creates space for oppressed emotions. Without play, control takes over. A natural counter-reaction takes place in every cell when it is forced to do something.

If the Singer's solar plexus is still tensed up, the Listener can sound heal the area with undertones until the tension in the solar plexus is dissolved and results in a detached lump of emotions that will be released as a deep cry. When the cry breaks through, the Listener encourages the Singer to do cry singing on long notes, which will activate the parasympathetic nervous system and release noradrenaline, oxytocin and result in a deep relaxation.[93]

Pain Relief with Sound Healing

Sound Healing and especially undertones are excellent for pain relief, as they induce the body to produce endorphins which have pharmacological effects. This applies when treating others, but also for the person that is singing. As an example I have experienced singing for hours with a sore throat, without noticing any pain.

Endorphins can apparently have a marked increase on

the effects of some medicines as for example methadone.[94] Therefore, be aware to be careful when treating a Recipient that has taken high doses of medicine.

Happy pills (serotonin re-uptake inhibitors like Prozac) and other medicines that affect the nervous system reduce the sensitivity of a person, because some of the body's own chemical processes are put on standby. The connection to the higher forms of consciousness is restricted and the effect of Sound Healing is reduced. The cells can resonate, but they are lethargic.

In general, pain is soothed during singing and receiving of Sound Healing. People with serious ailments can arrive for a course in severe pain, and, shortly after, during the singing, they sit smiling, accepting and seemingly pain free.

During the birth of my second son I sang the Note from Heaven and experienced the pain being soothed to such a degree that I did not notice that his head was on the way out. So I have personally no doubt that singing long notes releases painkilling endorphins.

Karen Guldager, a woman who had lived with breast cancer for more than ten years, had in the beginning of her illness joined a week course in the Note from Heaven, where her tumor diminished one centimeter during the week. Many years later I heard from her girlfriend, that the cancer all of a sudden had spread to Karen's liver and bones too and that she had died in her home denying any hospital treatment.

As Karen was allergic to painkillers of any kind, she had sung undertones for hours and throughout the death process.

The body's chemistry during singing and Sound Healing

When we sing the Note from Heaven, the level of the feel-good hormone oxytocin in the blood rises – the same hormone which is released when a woman breastfeeds her baby; during loving physical contact; during orgasm – all in all a hormone which increases the feeling of compassion, togetherness and belonging.

Therefore any teamwork can benefit from singing the Note from Heaven. For example before a challenging rugby fight.[95] Like the individual body's cell communication is intensified, a team's common spirit can be strengthened and the members' intuition linked together in Oneness with the result that the communication level is increased.

Listening to and performing music has a marked influence on immunoglobulin A – a chemical that helps to fight viral infections. Melatonin, norephedrine and ephedrine are also produced in copious amounts and each one helps us to regulate sleep, fight depression and to be more alert. Finally, music has a marked effect on our serotonin levels, which are directly connected to mood.
Daniel Levitin

Endorphins are the body's natural chemical medicine (it produces 20 different types) which have a broad range of amazing effects, such as reducing pain and age, strengthening the immune system, and allowing creativity to flourish.

Studies have shown that body temperature rises 0.2-0.3 degrees Celsius when singing. Heat is a sign of an accumulation of energy, an activation of the immune system. I have observed that daily singing rejuvenates seriously ill people as it ignites their life force.[96]

Music releases endorphins in the blood and changes the mood. Change in mood is directly proportional to endorphin. The bad or depressed mood of a patient changes when they are given external endorphin injections. Endorphin also protects us from stress, hypertension, depression and heart attacks.[97]

An acquaintance was admitted to a mental hospital. She believed she was Elvis Presley. Something had snapped inside her after a long period of sleep deprivation and constipation. With the aid of powerful sleeping pills she was able to sleep at most a couple of hours per night. At the end of visiting hours I was alone with the woman, and gave her a Sound Healing session with undertones, during which she immediately fell into a deep sleep.

There was a knock at the door at the end of the session. A male nurse came to give my acquaintance her sleeping pills. He was astonished to see that the woman was already asleep.

Part 3:
Spiritual Science and Traditional Science

Einstein, H.C. Ørsted, and Dr. Karl

I am of the opinion that all the finer speculations in the realm of science spring from a deep religious feeling, and that without such feeling they would not be fruitful.
Albert Einstein

Music is more than mere vibration and sound waves that can be measured in Hertz. It is a bridge to the subconscious – a concept that is of great significance for the scientist.
H.C. Ørsted

Music connects precise, empirically visual, acoustic signals with our entire perception of reality. When you hear a string quartet by Schubert, it is the feelings and emotions that the music awakens that are of most interest to us. Finding a principle for these feelings preoccupied Ørsted. After all, they transform our lives. In this way the boundaries of natural science are challenged, and it becomes truly interesting because science begins to move into the field of aesthetics.
Dan Charly Christensen, about H.C. Ørsted

Hans Christian Ørsted (the father of electromagnetism) saw art and science as two dimensions of the same thing, both of which are governed by underlying, invisible laws.

Sound and Science

We come forth and assist even those scientists who do not believe in our existence. For instance, you might be interested to know that the discovery of penicillin was not an accident. It was a very specific and arranged process because the gentleman concerned was not willing to accept our (Spirits') existence. Therefore, we brought it forth in a manner in which he was able to accept.
Dr. Karl

During the studies of the healing properties of the human voice, my focus has been on obtaining scientific confirmation of the healing effect of sound. For example, many deaf people would be able to achieve a partial or even full recovery of their hearing with relatively few sound treatments if we had a scientifically-based investigation of which particular hearing problems are positively affected by sound.

The fact that no ear specialist has yet shown any interest in the many cures of tinnitus and deafness must be due to the fact that Sound Healing is still ahead of its time. The same must be the case when I've met resistance to the method in other fields. For example, I had regular meetings with The Danish Cancer Society (Kræftens Bekæmpelse) over a period of six months trying to get Sound Healing research established. But when, in the end, I was limited, by the psychologist concerned, to using songs from a high-school songbook with the research group, I simply gave up. So much energy, and weeks of unpaid work creating research experiments, wasted.

Previously, senior doctor and cell expert Ulrik Dige and I had attempted to gain approval for an experiment through VIFAB, but this was denied on the basis that Ulrik himself had been a member of the approval committee.

The Danish Cancer Society also refused a very simple

research proposal as it was, in their view, *unethical*. The reply I received in 2003 was that, *"The Danish Cancer Society only works with traditional research methods."* It was our intention to Sound Heal cultivated cancer cells while they were being observed under a microscope.

My idea was inspired by the Frenchman Fabien Maman's experiment from 1981[98] in which, together with a biologist, he exposed cultivated hela cells to acoustic sound.

Song proved to be the sound source that had the strongest effect on the cancer cells, which exploded after 9-14 minutes.

Cell Type: Cancer - Hela
Instrument: Voice

I have realized that as long as our politicians are focusing on economic growth at any expense of the welfare of the citizens, then a "free" medicine such as song is uninteresting from a financial perspective. The scientists who have broken the code of cancer, like for example Royal Raymond Rife did, have paid a high price because it does not serve the economic system, that people get healthy. Why? Because medicine is big business.

In 2006 I established Association of Sound and Science with the hope to attract scientists and funds to do research into the healing power of sound. No one was interested, so in 2007 I decided to dissolve the only one year association by a last gathering: A session with the English medium, Graham Bishop with the hopeful purpose to get answers for some of our many questions relating to the healing effect of sound.

The following is an excerpt of Dr. Karl's[99] introduction transcribed from an audio recording of a sitting with the medium Graham Bishop arranged by Association for Sound and Science, February 2007.

Dr. Karl:

"It is unfortunate that in your world of science, they pooh-pooh our understanding and wisdom. Yet they do not apply their own rules of judgment to our work. If we now give you a range of tonal vibrations that were able to remove, let us say, 50% of all cases of migraine, and you go and make it public and encourage people to follow the tonal instructions, you would be ridiculed, for your medical people will say that it does not work on everyone, so it must be fake. We have observed this constantly. Yet, if they produce a little tablet that is effective in 30 cases out of a hundred, they will claim that that is a wonderful breakthrough of modern science. Now, one might ask, 'Why there is such an imbalance in existence?' It is because of the conceptual limitations within the minds of the majority.

The majority of humans must have something physical, or

it is not real. So, if we were to present you with a sugar tablet and play music at the same time, it would be the tablet that fixed you, not the music. And that is something that you need to bear in mind in taking your work forward. Do not attempt to force the concept too quickly on mankind, for you will hit a wall stronger than you can ever imagine."

Meeting with Spiritual Scientists

Graham Bishop and I had not been in touch since he and Dr. Karl wrote the foreword to *The Note from Heaven* six years earlier. During this time, Graham had become less active due to blood clots in his legs and lungs. However, I decided to contact Graham Bishop concerning a session with the Sound and Science group.

Due to his state of health, Graham's replies were discouraging. However, in the end, he invited us to meet him. The purpose of the meeting was to assess whether our energy was as it should be. If not, there was a chance that we would be putting his life in danger. It was necessary for six people to be present. So, the Sound and Science group met, together with Lars Muhl (then leader of the aid organization Hearts & Hands) and, after a meeting of around two hours, was approved. We were warned not to ask specific questions pertaining to illnesses. The questions would need to be general and non-specific. If we broke this rule, we risked the trance being immediately interrupted. In addition, we had to accept that Graham couldn't guarantee that Dr. Karl or other spirits would make contact with him in his current physical condition.

We met outside the town of Kalundborg on a rainy February afternoon in 2007. Graham's wife Mie joined us. Those present were: Graham Bishop, Rose Lübich, Thomas Christensen, Jette Lokvig, Githa Ben-David, Lars Muhl and Mie Bishop. We sat in a circle. The names here are given in the order that we sat, clockwise from Graham.

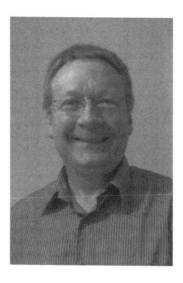

Graham Bishop, September 2008.

Graham gasped frenetically, and after a moment Dr. Karl was present, much to our relief. His wise and affectionate presence bade us welcome. It was an intense lecture full of enlightening information that lasted for two hours and 45 minutes. However, almost three years went by before I transcribed the séance word by word while I was snowed in by a howling snowstorm just after Christmas 2009.

Excerpts from the Sound and Science Session with Graham Bishop and Dr. Karl

General notes

It is recommended that the following information from Dr. Karl is to be treated with common sense, and that the reader should examine and test the advices for themselves. Dr. Karl is humorous and quick-witted. He is spokesman for a spirit group, The White Brotherhood, consisting of about 700 members, which he consults several times during the session.

For me, the recording of the session with Graham Bishop is a treasure trove. The spoken language of Dr. Karl is old-fashioned English with a German accent. He is very thorough in his explanations, and the importance of certain aspects is stressed time and again in different ways. I have chosen to distil these repetitions in order to clearly present the essence of Dr. Karl's message, but in so doing some of the benefit to be gained from the repetitions will be lost. Some of the points that are repeated several times are:

*The most effective healing will always occur by following one's intuition.

*It is not up to the Sound Healer to play God. It is generally the Recipient's Soul that decides if it wishes to receive the Sound Healing or not.

*A person's desire for ordinary control is alright, but unnecessary control has destructive effect.

*There is no rule without an exception.

*It is necessary for humanity to think holistically, rather than to focus on specific narrow points.

*Sound Healing has side effects, just as all other forms of treatment has. These side effects are minimized, however, when the Sound Healer is able to surrender themselves to intuition.

*A human being is limited without using his/her intuition.

*If you seriously wish to serve the spirit world and are open enough, you will be worked with, often for many years. You must be patient. The same action is repeated over and over again and you have no choice, because only the spirit world can see the bigger picture. If a given knowledge damages global unity, the process will be stopped.

Introductory lecture

Dr. Karl began with a 20-minute lecture about the other side's regard for wholeness. Here follows an excerpt:

"A grain of sand upon the beach can be compared to what

you know as your universe compared to the whole. We are observing all aspects. And that is something that man cannot do. So be aware. Those are the aspects from which our assistance comes.

The human being can be trained from the spiritual plane so that they may become excellent instruments.

The human brain, however, has not yet the cranial ability to contain for example knowledge about the specific tonal combinations that are able to cure specific illnesses."

Later Dr. Karl says:

"Essentially, those in our world have the capability to correct any error in the physical structure of a human being. And we mean any. Our only limitation is your own spirit."

I was asked the following hypothetical question directly: If my son were on his deathbed and I had been given the necessary knowledge to heal him, would I be able to stand by and let my son die, if that was what was meant to happen?

In a tough but loving way Dr. Karl tried to make the group understand that it would not be suitable for us to possess such knowledge, as it would cause an imbalance in humanity which would damage the wholeness.

Information must always be manifested at the right moment in global development. We humans are weakened by our egos yearning for power and control. We wish to play God, and therefore easily come to abuse our powers.

The majority of the following questions had been composed before the session by the Sound and Science group.

A voice's flair for healing specific illnesses

Githa: "Do the voices of different Sound Healers have specific gifts for healing certain illnesses?"

Dr. Karl: "Essentially, yes. That is of course attributable to the different selection of tones that are available from that particular human voice box. And it is not just the tones, it is the sub-tones, the super-tones, the undertones and overtones, call them what you wish. The combination of those tones that are available within the voice box will automatically determine that some Sound Healers will be more effective in certain aspects of illness than others. And this is absolutely a fact of existence that cannot be changed. You cannot alter the fact that your sound production is helpful to people in a specific area, where the other ladies here are effective for a different area. That is just the way things are."

"And the next question that is going through all of your minds is: Which aspect of illness is suited for my particular range of tonal vibration ability? We are not deaf, blind or stupid [laughter from the group]. And the answer is: We are not going to tell you. Why? Because you can easily work it out for yourselves."

"Observe those who have come before you for assistance, the types of problem that they have and the percentage of assistance that you have been able to give. You can easily begin to see a trend in the types of problems where you create the best results. You do not need us to tell you something so obvious."

Thomas: "But can that change?"

Dr. Karl: "It will change."

Thomas: "Has that something to do with the development that I am going through?"

Dr. Karl: "Absolutely, sir, absolutely. Essentially, although there is a relatively fixed vibrational range that can come forth through the vocal chords, it can be modified slightly by your own mental process – in other words, your mental or emotional states of being. Therefore, what you were most effective with three years ago may not now be the same. The voice may, apparently, have remained the same, but the whole vibrational flow within you can have changed. For some it changes more regularly than for others. And that has nothing to do with one being more spiritual than another. It is just an additional part of the development process of mankind."

"Each has a different pathway to follow. And for some, the rate of their vibrational structure will be completely different than in another. It does not mean that one is more advanced spiritually than the other, that must be borne in mind. It also adds to the reason why we do not tell you what aspect you are specialized in. Because, let us explain, we will then have destroyed your usefulness. If we said you were best with bones, would you then work with anything else? Unlikely. And what happens if in a year your vibrational system changes so that you are able to be of more use with digestive problems? You would have burned your boats and be focusing on the wrong thing, because you would not be able to be aware that it has changed."

Githa: "Then I wouldn't follow my intuition."

Dr. Karl: "Perhaps not and probably not if you were told by us. That is the danger. We can tell you that at the moment your greatest effect is upon the circulatory system. How do you say, the blood circulation, the heart and all of the aspects of the blood moving around the physical structure. But that is at the moment. And again, in a sense, please erase that from your mind."

Githa: "Right."

Dr. Karl: "It will change. It has been like this for the last 18 months. Prior to that, you had effect on people's digestive systems and prior to that, there was a great measurable effect on the emotional/mental plane. But, it will continue to change. What we are really trying to achieve through working with people such as yourself, is to widen your abilities. It is therefore necessary to go through certain periods where you will be presented with people who have similar conditions. You will find all of you that this occurs for you and will be surprised and think, 'How come that I meet so many people who have this kind of problem?' It's on purpose."

"For you to be trained you need to be exposed to these

aspects. Then we will bring different aspects. And we will leave those other aspects for a while. The end result is that you can be used for many different aspects, because you have a special openness to those particular frequency patterns which are required. So you need to understand this is a constantly changing ability. Though in essence, through the process of development, there will always be one aspect which will be stronger. So, as the Sound Healer goes through the different aspects of assisting with different conditions, inevitably each individual will have a specific area where they will be more effective. Do you understand our implication? If we show you how to help 30 different illnesses, you will have one, where you will be more effective. That cannot be avoided. But, the reason for undergoing these changes is partly because of changes in you, and partly because we are trying to broaden the range of help that you can offer."

Lars: "Does each human represent a specific tone?"

Dr. Karl: "Absolutely. Each person has a unique tonal vibration.[100] When the person is out of balance or sick, their tone is changed in some way. The basic tone is unchanged, but what does occur is that additional undertones and overtones are created. The actual identification of the unique tone will always remain the same. Indeed, that is how we recognize each other.

You are not recognized by us by your name, but by your tone. That is how we can find people so quickly.

All we have to do is to examine the tone. That tone exists in only one place. So we can find you immediately, whenever we want to. Imagine if we had to do that by name. Just in the small area that you call your country. We would have to tap people on the shoulder and ask, 'Are you the one I am looking for?' By utilizing unique tonal vibration, that is eliminated.

It's the tone that causes recognition within you when people get close, whether they have a body or not. You unconsciously become aware of that tone."

Lars: "Is it possible to know your own tone?"

Dr. Karl: "You cannot."

"The tone of an individual is far beyond any kind of measurement that you currently have. Therefore, you cannot know what tone you are. Your recognition is automatic. Under all circumstances, it is impossible and also not necessary for you to define that tone.

Realistically, while in your physical body, you will hardly ever use your ability for tonal vibrational recognition. It is not until you exit the physical body that the tonal uniqueness becomes of greater importance. So the answer is, *you cannot know your tone. It is not possible.* Hmm... However, what can be ascertained through a different method of conceptualization is, that *you will feel more comfortable with those who are of a similar tone to yourself, than those who are farther away*. It does not mean there is anything wrong with them or you, the notes just do not resonate so well together.

Thus, by this time, you should have realized that those in this room are of a similar frequency pattern to each other, otherwise the degree of compatibility would not exist. That is something else that is important to understand."

"We hope that this has brought some understanding to your thought."

Githa: "Is it the cells that resonate during Sound Healing?"

Dr. Karl: "My dear, let us point out to you. *You cannot hear the resonance of the human structure. What you are hearing is our guidance.* The resonance of the human structure is far beyond your capabilities to hear or any other human's capability. What happens is that there are those in our world who are working with you and they bring themselves down to a frequency level which is audible. Thus you can then follow the rhythm and procedure. You would not be capable of hearing the vibration of a human form. So the answer is twofold:

You are doing the right thing, but you are not doing what you thought you were doing."

How many treatments are necessary?

Githa: "We would like to know if sound treatment over a longer period will lead to healing even when nothing happens at the first treatment."

Dr. Karl: "The answer to that is simple, my dear: That is absolutely possible."

"Tell me, are you cured the first time you consult a physical therapist about a condition? Very often does the therapist not just listen to your words and then do nothing? And then sometime later you go back and the physical therapist does something. The time in between has still had an effect. The fact that the effect may not be obvious does not mean that it didn't work.

The same occurs with this. When you first present tonal vibrations to someone who is significantly out of balance in any particular organ of their physical structure, then initially there may be little or no response whatsoever. And one then repeats the process. All we would say to you is that if there is no response noticed of any kind, yes very well..." [Dr. Karl consults his group.]

"After six attempts to bring forth healing with no effect, then you are the wrong tonal vibration range for that assistance. Something will happen within a maximum of six times, if it is going to happen at all. So it may not happen on the first or the second time. If it has not happened by the sixth time then it is absolutely definite that you are the incorrect vibrational range to be of assistance to that person. But, of course, if something happens, then you keep going even if it takes much longer. We are not saying that everybody should be cured by six visits. We just felt the need to clarify that."

"It can take up to six attempts before the effect of Sound Healing shows."

Time between treatments

Githa: "Can you recommend a certain time between the treatments?"

Dr. Karl: "Well, it is variable. There are some who would benefit from several treatments within each 24-hour period. Though, in general, as a useful guideline, we would recommend that the majority of instances require at least four of your Earth days to assimilate the modifications the vibrational toning will have begun. And wherever possible, one should not have a period of greater than 21 of your Earth days between the tonal healings. Of course it does not mean that the process is useless if you have delays – merely that it will not be of the same degree of benefit."

"In general, there should be from four to maximum 21 days between Sound Healing sessions to keep an ongoing process."

Sound Healing and side effects

According to Dr. Karl, no method of treatment – Sound Healing included – is without side effects. If a liver condition is healed with a specific frequency used to strengthen the liver, this same frequency might somewhat reduce the quality of a man's sperm. *Side effects only last for a couple of days and are of no real harm.* The energies behind the intuition calculate the risks, and we therefore need to completely trust their assessments.

Dr. Karl explained, for example, that if someone were to sing the note "C" for more than five minutes at my, Githa's, digestive system, it would balance my digestion, but, in the longer term, would start a process in the brain which might lead to Alzheimer's 30 years later.

Sound Healing the same place on the body with the same constant note for more than three minutes is not recommended.

Dr. Karl speaks to those who feel unsure of their intuition: *To mechanically expose a fixed point on the body to an unrelenting sound over a long period of time is dangerous and unhealthy.* However, when we, in surrendering to the Note from Heaven, sing one note for an hour, the entire body is exposed to a sound that is created from within its own voice, and is kind of downloading an energy that is recharging the energy field. Despite this assurance, some of us were frightened when we heard Dr. Karl's information of side effects. Dr. Karl repeated the same answer several times to our questions as to how we could avoid hurting a client when Sound Healing – that is, if we dared Sound Heal at all, when there could be such dire consequences. We were given the following advice:

"Follow your intuition and everything will be fine."

Dr. Karl: "If you follow your intuition, you will be given the right notes."

"It is impossible to eliminate the fact that when you create the right note for the liver or kidneys or heart, that note will have elements of a detrimental effect on another part of the human form. But, it is all about balance. One must realize that it is a temporary side effect."

"For example, if we gave you a note that would help the function of the left ventricle, but would impede the digestive system by two percent, which problem would you prefer to have?"

"When we evaluate, we are always aware of what best serves a physical body in connection with healing. It is these considerations that we attempt to bring forward through your intuition when we guide you. You cannot eliminate this aspect. It is impossible, exactly as it would be in any other form of healing."

"With every form of what you call healing – whether it is

complementary, alternative therapy or medication – there are the same limitations. One is not more limited than another."

"For example, when a surgeon operates, and opens the physical body with the objective of curing a dysfunction, it will have a damaging effect on other parts of the body that are connected to the organ in question. But it has had an advantageous effect on that particular organ. Or at least, that is what is hoped for. That is also how it functions with Sound Healing. *There is not one single note that can be beneficial for the whole body.*"

Dr. Karl: "Very well. Are there further enquiries? Everyone seems to be very quiet. There is no need to be overawed by us. We have spoken to many, many thousands of people, and we are very nice and we have never eaten anyone." [The group relaxes with laughter.]

Githa: "Does gender polarity have any significance in Sound Healing?"

Dr. Karl: "My answer will sound a little evasive to you, because the question of whether a constructive resonance is created is dependent upon the individual man and woman's vibrational structure, not on whether they are male or female. That is the misconception of mankind. Mankind seems to consider that there is some enormous difference between the vibrational structure of the male body and the vibrational structure of the female."

"Well, between you [Githa] and the gentleman [Thomas] who asked the previous question, there is a large difference. Between you and the gentleman sitting next to you [Lars Muhl, who I later married] there is a very small difference. From an energy viewpoint you two are very equal. Thus, what is important is the combination of vibrational tone and energy frequency."

"On occasion, the utilization of two hundred voices would be vastly superior to one voice. On other occasions, the one voice would be best."

"When we observe mankind, we often hear both from their discussions and from their written material, that one needs to have a constant balance between the masculine and the feminine. We can tell you that energy-wise, some males have more essentially female energy than some females. We utilize that term for your benefit, not ours, because you term things male and female. *The point is compatibility.*

Hmm, that is the real point – if you are doing a healing together with another person, whether it be male or female. If you do not feel in complete harmony and compatibility with that person, then you should not undertake the healing process, hmm, because the lack of harmony and equality will interfere with the interfusion of the vibrating tones."

"Equality is more important than the sexual orientation of the other person."

Vocal, mechanical or electronic sound?

Githa: "It is important for us to know which type of sound is best for healing: Vocal, mechanical or electronic sound?"

Dr. Karl: "Which sound is the best? It is that which is correct in relation to a specific illness."

"Regarding the advantages and disadvantages of using the human voice, mechanical or electronic sound production, you must understand that the evaluation of what is best is dependent upon how exact or variable the vibrational tone needs to be."

"For example: It is impossible for mechanical or electronic machinery to express the variation of the human voice – just as it is impossible for the human voice to create the stability of a mechanical or electronic sound. So, it is a combination that will give the most benefits. In some cases, a stable tone production is required and in other cases, a variable tone production is necessary."

"So it is not as simple as saying that the voice is better

than electronic or mechanical machines and vice versa. All sound production can be advantageous when used in the right situation."

"Furthermore, it is necessary to understand that the setting of a sound is extremely important too. Let me give you an example: It is not about the human voice, but we will briefly talk about another sound area:

If we were to blindfold any one of you so you had no idea where you were, and we transported you out to the ocean and sat you down on the beach, your stress threshold would automatically be reduced. What would cause this? The sound of the rolling waves. But, not only the sound of the rolling waves. Again, we must expand our angle of understanding. When you sit on a beach, whether you are aware of them or not, there are millions of sounds: The wind moving every little grain of sand, the ocean moving clam shells and pebbles, the wind blowing through the leaves on the trees. It is a conglomeration – a composition – that creates the effect. If you take away one element, the effect will remain the same. But, if you take away one more element, then the whole effect disappears."

"This is important to understand. It is the same principle with medication. There are many, many aspects to compare. The human voice is able to create changes in vibrational intonation which at this time cannot be replaced with mechanical or electronic sound sources. Therefore, that which you are thinking to ask about later, and that we may choose to answer, these details will never be able to be represented by machines, as they can only be represented by the physical structure of the voice. Simply because of the limited technology that you humans use."

Difference in quality between live and recorded sound

"Let us give you an example: Huuuuuuuuuh" [a high, overtone-rich male voice].

"The vocal expression causes a reaction inside you. Not only because of the tonal vibration, but also, and especially, because of the energy that is being placed in the tonal vibration. This energy is impossible for your technology to reproduce.

Every sound production will be more effective live than it will be in any form of recording medium."

"This is because of the limited technical equipment that mankind controls at this moment in time. There are limitations in sharing recordings with others. When you create, what do you call it? Yes, one moment please." [Dr. Karl asks the other spirits for advice.] "When you produce a CD, the tonal register and the energy that can be transferred via these tones, and therefore shared with the listener, is limited. All you can do is to do your best."

Dr. Karl: "So, is it possible to produce one recorded tone that can be sold as a cure for migraines? *No.* Can you produce a recorded tone that can be sold as *a possible* assistance for some migraine sufferers? *Yes.* Do you see the difference? As an individual, you can produce an infinite spectrum of variable tones by following your intuition – whether you use your voice or electronic or mechanical assistance."

"The expression is dependent on your presence. And here it is important to understand the limitations of recording. When you publish recorded material it must be of a general nature – not specific. It sounds frightfully limiting, doesn't it? This is how it is. *The live situation is the circumstance where the strongest effect can be achieved, if it is being carried out correctly by ignoring the ego and following intuition.* Do you think we would worry about coming through in this way and straining *the instrument* (Graham Bishop), if we simply could download our thoughts into your brains? No. And it would be pointless to place them in written materials or recordings. Because it is this, our interaction, that is convincing. *It is the revealing of the energy that exists in the now, which is the prerequisite for the greatest benefits through the process.*"[101]

A reprimand for healers

"Many healers that we have observed, do not have the right focus in their minds. They are not here to play God. They do not decide who recovers and who does not. Actually, neither do we. If I carry out healing on you, who makes the decisions? You do. But, not your human mind, hmmm, your Soul. This you must understand. *Essentially, those from our world, like ourselves, are able to correct any type of physical problem in the physical structure of a living person. And we mean any problem.*"

"Our only limitation is your own Soul. And it is the same for a human that is carrying out a healing method on another human:

The individual Soul makes the final decision regarding what will happen or what will not happen."

"Hmm. This is the most important thing. If you should only remember one thing, from all of the time we have shared, it should be this:

If the Soul of a person that comes to you for healing does not want there to be any effect through your healing actions, there will be no effect – regardless of what the mouth of that person says. It is the decision of the Soul."

"In some cases, the human mind can have an influence, but in the great majority of cases, it is the Soul that makes the decision. The human mind can, for example, influence cases, where the Soul wishes success for the human, and the human mind says, 'No.' This happens. We need to make sure that you also understand this. The area that you have gone into is so complex – there are so many variables and possibilities – but you nevertheless seem to yearn for a step-by-step program to help with each and every problem. We are here for general assistance. Otherwise, it must come through your intuition in connection to specific events. We do not wish to be unsympathetic. We are simply trying to be brutally honest with you."

Sound, Light, Magnetism

Jette: "Can you give us a practical explanation of the connection between sound, light and magnetism?"

Dr. Karl: "First, we must explain why they are all part of the same process: Sound, light and magnetism are all different aspects of vibrational frequency. Some of the frequencies are visible to the eye, some can be detected by the ear. You have developed electronic equipment to measure magnetism, even though you are able to measure it within the ear also, because that is how you keep your balance.[102] Though, of course, you are not sensitive enough to be able to actually measure it with the ear. You cannot escape the fact that you are constantly exposed to the magnetic field. The very Earth upon which you live has a variable magnetic field across its entire surface. So you are constantly being affected by that."

"When sound, light and magnetism are combined correctly, the process of healing can be accelerated. Now, again you would require us to give you the precise requirements for each individual. But, let us give you some more general terms."

"For instance, if you create a tonal vibration which enters into this level of tone: 'Uuuuh' (a 'tenor spirit' sings the note Bb), then that tone would be aided by the additional function of creating an orange tint to the available light source. For the orange tint is a supportive vibration to that particular tone."

Githa: "Is that valid for everyone?"

Dr. Karl: "That is in general. There would be specific cases where it will not be of benefit, but those situations are impossible for us to define."

Githa: "Should we use a lamp to shine orange light on the person?"

Dr. Karl: "We are referring to the use of artificial light sources. In order to generate assistance, there are some small techniques that you can utilize. To be of greatest benefit, you would need an infinitely variable light source. In other words, the source of the orange nuance would need to be infinitely variable. Such a light source can be produced with the technology that mankind currently possesses."

"The way that we can help you to develop a clearer idea, regarding a vibrational light frequency that may enhance the vibrational audio frequency – whether that be from your voice or from a mechanical or electronic source – is this: *While subjecting yourself to tonal vibration and with a light source not directly before you, but a little above you, your own system will react, when the light resonates with your tonal expression.*"

"It is unfortunate, that we do not have colored lamps available so that we could demonstrate it to you. But from your own experiments, you will discover that some colors make you feel extremely irritable when you make certain tones. These are clearly outside the range of usefulness. That will give you a general ability, because obviously the exact effect on the individual that you are assisting will not be identical to your own. But, that is the nearest you can come to being able to work out the light frequency that goes with the sound frequency. With regard to magnetism, it is somewhat more complex to identify what would be helpful. There are no visible or audible means by which you can even begin to get a rough idea of what will go together. What we can say in general is, that in relation to what you wish to achieve, it is worth *isolating the magnetic energy while using light and sound.*"

"Therefore, what one should be trying to do is to create a neutral magnetic base below the person, who has come for treatment. The most effective way would be to have a treatment table that is constructed from five centimeter thick lead. That would create an entirely neutral magnetic field, though it might prove to be a little difficult to move. There are things which can be done to create a similar effect without utilizing such extreme measures. Obviously, a lead table would be inconceivable in most situations. Therefore, one must, as always, balance possible benefits against possible effects. Thus, to utilize 5 cm of solid lead would be impractical. We can substitute something else which will give us perhaps 80% of the effect. That is a reasonable compromise. Just as, when we create 80% healing in one organ, and one, two or three percent damage to another, it is a reasonable compromise. Now, what you can construct is – " [There is a pause while Dr. Karl asks the other members of the spirit group.]

"Very well: One of our colleagues informs us, that you must take a normal electrical flex, and place that in a figure of eight, twelve times under the bench upon which the Sound Healing client lies. Then, connect a fifteen watt source of energy to one end (a lamp, for example) and plug the other end into a power outlet at the wall and switch it on."

"What will occur is that the movement of the electricity, through the figure of eight cable causes a nullifying effect of the magnetic energy fields in the area, not entirely, but to a degree which will help. The use of magnetic energy is very complicated to control and utilize. Therefore, combining magnetism with sound or with light is out of the question. The best solution is to create a neutral magnetic field into which one can bring sound and/or light."

Crystals

"One can also use other aspects – for example, the use of crystalline structures also has a place in the healing process. Crystalline structures have a vibrational frequency. That is how they work. You know there are a lot of people who offer what they call crystal healing. It is the vibrational frequency of the crystal which is actually assisting, so if you generate precisely the same vibrational frequency as that crystal through electronic or mechanical means, you would produce the same effect. It is the vibrational structure which is important. Though, of course, one can ask if there is any point in creating a machine to simulate the vibrational structure of something which is easily available and of much less cost?"

"So, you need to understand when and where combinations are required. And that is one of the most difficult areas for us to give you rules for, because the danger is that if we give you generalizations, many people will try to interpret them as universal facts. For instance, it is absolute rubbish that rose quartz can help everybody with emotional problems. It can help some – it does help many. But, it does not help everyone. And these are the aspects which bring confusion and, to some degree, dismissal from the more accepted areas of human adjustment. The scientists can easily dismiss such a claim. Then, what happens is that, because they can so easily dismiss such a thing, the whole idea becomes dismissed as of no use."

Now suddenly the message from Dr. Karl was aimed directly at me.

Dr. Karl: "You need to be realistic about what you write, in order to remain within the boundaries of what can be publicly accepted. If you wish to take things beyond such acceptable boundaries, you must confine this to your own work. *If you claim 'this tone heals this illness,' you will be ridiculed. If you say this tone can in some cases benefit people who suffer from this illness, then you have a completely different level of credibility."*

Chromaticism

Githa: "Do chromatic, tonal progressions have a particular effect in Sound Healing?"

Dr. Karl: "For some it can have an effect. In fact, we have observed that a chromatic interval is only useful when it is conveyed through intuition rather than through any form of mathematical sequence.

Downward moving intervals can be just as useful as upward moving ones. Again, we meet the human aspect of judgment. Just as humans judge that white is better than black, they judge that upwards is better than downwards – for a high tone must be better than a low tone. Of course this is total rubbish, but it is the way the human mind seems to evaluate many things. Consider that. Because that is also an aspect which you, Githa, need to examine."

Part 4:

Being a Sound Healer

On saying "Yes" to being a Sound Healer

*The instrument (the Sound healer) has to follow our instruction.
That is part of the reason why we are able to do what we do through
the instrument.*
Dr. Karl

Inscription over the entrance to Carl Gustav Jung's house, and
above his tomb:

Called or uncalled, God is present.
The Oracle from Delphi

When you go into the process of becoming a Sound Healer, you
take on a responsibility. Uncertainty about what this entails
creates fear. When fear is present, it is the ego that takes on the
role of healer. Am I good enough? This doubt can either prevent
you from attempting healing or lead to over-educating yourself.
Regardless of how much education you have on your CV
[resume] as a healer, it will always be your ability to surrender
– your contact with your intuition – that counts.

If learned methods are practiced blindly on a client, you are
not taking responsibility for your actions.

Bring your playful self into the process. Let your intuition
smoothly intertwine with the techniques, just like sound colors
the meaning of words.

This corresponds to the Indian singing style that is described
in *The Note from Heaven*. A learned scale should never be sung
stiffly up and down. It must be given spirit in order to come
alive, inspired by the inspiration that spontaneously flow
through the performer.

The ego feels secure when it fully controls a situation.
It feels insecure in unknown territory. So the ego needs

to feel confident in cooperating with the intuition. In reality, spirituality is a natural force of vital importance, which is an integrated part of every human being. Inspiration is the knowledge we can access from the spiritual Internet. A net that is open to anyone with the courage to listen to him/herself.

Mum, we don't need to phone, we can just call each other inside the brain.
Ghil, five years old

We are constantly assisted by our intuition. Practically speaking, we don't need to be conscious about who or what it is that helps us, as long as the intuition works. It is, therefore often when we fall ill, and/or feel unhappy or desperate, that our consciousness of higher powers is awakened.

When you give Sound Healing, it is useful to be aware that there are higher powers working through you. This awareness makes it easier to set aside personal aspects that can block the flow of energy in a treatment session.

As I've already mentioned, I was not ready to say a wholehearted YES to being a Sound Healer until I had had the message spelt out for me by Dr. Karl. In fact, not even *that* was enough. To step into the healer's archetype is a process that takes time.

Dr. Karl says that *they must work on their instruments,* possibly because the instruments' ego must be convinced about the advantages of surrendering themselves.

In my opinion, common sense and skepticism are the basis on which to build a healthy foundation. If you trust too quickly at the outset you can lose your credibility and therefore your power, because power can only manifest where it finds itself in fertile ground, at the right time, and in the right environment. It is better to evaluate the power that you are working with once too often rather than once too little.

It was only when I experienced miraculous Sound Healing results, which I myself clearly did not feel responsible for, that a definitive and resounding "YES" manifested itself: The results were no longer my responsibility. Dr. Karl and The White Brotherhood had won my trust.

As a Sound Healer, my responsibility is solely to keep my flute open and unblocked, so that I can be serving as an instrument.
Githa Ben-David

We rise up by kneeling, we overcome by surrendering, and we win by giving up.
Alice Bailey

You cannot *decide* to say a wholehearted YES. *It happens*, when you are ready, when they are ready, when the time is right. If you offer yourself as a Sound Healer, or in fact anything else – as long as you have an uncompromising dedication and an open mind – the higher energies will help you to find your path here on Earth.

It is the degree of openness that determines the effect of Sound Healing.
Helle Hewau, psychiatrist, Sound Healer

Dr. Karl clearly pointed to me in one of his general statements on the recording made in 2007: *"The weakness of mankind is laziness."* He predicted that *"we"* will not listen to this recording for a very long time.[103]

But for me it is also a question of knowing when the right time has come, and I personally have had to be ready to accept all of this. Not to mention all of the suggestions for scientific experiments, which we were given.

On the necessity of cleaning your flute

Working with the Note from Heaven is an activity which, when correctly practiced, will keep your flute clean, so that higher energies can flow through you. The exact nature of these "higher energies" is up to each individual Sound Healer to define. The power operates through the Sound Healer's trust in a higher power, regardless of its name.

The definition of the concept "the Note from Heaven" is unmistakably linked to the physical experience of the energy of sound. When a singer sings flawlessly, with total focus and an absence of playfulness, motivated by the desire to prove his/ her worth through the performance, contact with the spiritual plane is lost.

A sound based on personal will, will always drain the audience rather than uplift them.

Nevertheless, we clap for the flawlessness and make ourselves judges by our applause. TV programs such as *The X Factor* and talent shows focus on energy. The judges often disagree with one another and the audience. But no one is in doubt when a genuine talent shines through, because the energy lifts everyone up.

The uplifting energies occur when we let go of our ego – surrendering to sound, rhythm, movement, being. By entering into a state of full presence, an effervescent energy flows out to the audience.

Take for example the Rolling Stones. Their film *Shine a Light* covers a live concert in the US, where Bill Clinton and his entire family – even his mother-in-law – are present in the audience. The Rolling Stones have not polished the music in any way. But, what is important here is not whether they play "correctly" or "incorrectly"; it is, that their energy flows unhindered. This is apparent regardless of whether you like their music or not. They are present and therefore exude energy. I'm speaking particularly about Mick Jagger, who runs un-choreographed around the stage and sings freely, while Keith Richard, his opposite, plays his guitar solos as slowly as it suits him, as his eyes glisten in a deep, meditative happiness.

To some people Sound Healing feels like coming home. They have a natural talent for it, and easily find the Note from Heaven.

If you feel uncertain, then proceed carefully. Seek and you shall find. The results will speak for themselves. In general, ask your client for feedback during the Sound Healing session.

Here are some of Dr. Karl's guidelines concerning words of advice on how to be the best possible instrument for the spirit world:

The need for control is probably what is most damaging for your ability to have contact with those like us.

The right way: You have nothing to prove – what you have is something to share.

Examine your inner motive carefully. If it is essentially to prove that you are right, or doing the right thing, all of your energy and the effect of your performance will be marred by the energy of your need to achieve, and the result will be that you will be working against the advancement of mankind.

The energy that manifests itself through you is given to you with the intention of providing assistance. In some cases, that energy will result in a swifter destruction of the human form.[104] The most effective would be if the healer could dissociate him/herself completely from the ego and put it in a bucket throughout the healing session. This would be a great advantage. Unfortunately, this is not humanly possible.

"What you need to be conscious of is whether you are activating your own thought process or you are following your intuition implicitly. In most cases it is a very fine line, and impossible to tell the difference. However, bearing this difficulty and limitation in mind (the fact that it is difficult to know the difference between intuition and ego), our instructions are as follows:

Follow your intuition, for if you do not, you will contribute injustice to the world. The chance of the impulse coming from your own mind, and therefore not being genuine, is so slim that it is worth taking the risk.[105] So, therefore: Follow your intuition, no matter how stupid it might seem. This is the point. It is with the fear of appearing stupid that the human brain has its biggest problem."

Graham B./Dr. Karl, recording February 2007.

A comment from the author: Common sense and keeping one's feet on the ground are conditions for the above being true. If one's Sound Healing doesn't seem to work, I would say that it is immaterial how intuitive a practitioner one claims to be.

In my experience, the ego is involved when:

Someone feels the need to make themselves appear noteworthy/to bolster their self-esteem by exaggerating when speaking about themselves and their achievements.
Someone judges another person in a treatment situation.
Feelings of insecurity occur.

Fear of intuition

Feel your own power. Don't be swayed by the judgment of the masses. Walk calmly forward.
Bertel Thorvaldsen to Hans Christian Andersen

The prerequisite for trust in one's intuition is grounding and faith. Grounding because you are the hands of the angels, and need to stand on the ground in order to serve on Earth. Faith because you need determination to purify yourself. The fear of not being good enough, not belonging, not being wanted and not wishing to be here are the basic feelings, that stand in your way of getting access to your intuition. The four basic feelings have many variations, and they are all excuses for your choice of being safely more or less jailed in your pain body. It needs faith to rise up from the mud by abandoning the role of the victim.

Through self-examination you can regain faith in yourself and start a purification process with unknown duration. The necessary faith for this process cannot be decided or wished for. It happens. One day you suddenly feel the urge for walking your path and release the burden of other people's demands. Your intuition is calling you to reunite with the one you truly are, but you do not know what that means.

The fear of following the intuition is a natural part of the healing process.

When the other side sends us inspiration, how can we be sure that these powers are good?

Our sensory system receives signals. These signals are usually interpreted by the reptilian brain through an unconscious, instinctive process, that activates the nervous and hormone system and thus creates certain reactions in the body. Throughout life we humans have, thanks to our consciousness, the possibility to gain knowledge by training our awareness of these sensory signals. Many people choose not to listen at all, with the result that they in the end can hardly feel themselves. When you exclude listening to your dreams, your feelings, emotional and physical sensations and thereby your intuition – you exclude the higher energies in yourself.

How come humanity in general mistreats animals, each other, the sea, the Earth, the sky, the air in the name of growth (gaining money) when we have the knowledge we have? Because the majority of human beings have disconnected themselves from listening to their intuition. The urge for growth and greed is an expression of an underlying fear animated by an instinctive feeling of being incomplete.

"Woman, your faith has healed you." The moment you start listening to yourself, day by day you learn how to recognize and have faith in the messages that are sent to you. As your faith grows your fear fades.

Intuitive listening reunites you with the frequency that resonates with the sound matrix which you are and always will be.

The moment you start to communicate with your Soul through the original sound matrix, you lift yourself above the emotional state and get in contact with your heavenly source. Gradually you reconnect to the spiritual Oneness level where truth is resonance in the right frequency at the right place at the right moment.

Through conscious and playful listening to the intuitive signals that you pick up with your senses, spirit can guide you to such an uplifted experience of truth. Humbleness and gratitude overwhelm you.

The Ego and the Soul in fruitful cooperation

The Complementarity Principle, formulated by the Danish quantum physicist Niels Bohr, is based on a concept of life as a *Oneness divided into two separate forms of awareness: Observing and being.* For example, an artist can be so caught up in his painting that occasionally he must take two steps back to observe his work. He then continues his work based on his observations and the understanding these give him. The ego is the observer and the Soul is "being".

To allow intuition to fully flourish, the ego and the Soul must cooperate. The Soul does its part in complete surrendering, but it can only do this when the ego releases all of its usual barricades. Back in its normal state the gates are again closed, so that the ego can examine, control, and evaluate the results – like a sentry, watching out to monitor how grounded we are. The question "Am I good enough?" has a nourishing, ethical meaning here: "How good have I been in letting the Soul work undisturbed? Is there something I can do better next time?"

It is a misunderstanding to try to fight the ego, because it is an integral part of us – our bodyguard.

A balanced ego is priceless.
An unbalanced ego is damaging.

The ego is the Soul's active organ on the Earthly plane.
Lars Muhl

The Nature of the Soul

It feels liberating to cast aside responsibility and "serve" a power that you perceive as higher than yourself. The moment the anchor is hauled in, it is the ego that lets go, because it feels secure in the situation. The Soul loves to be free because its nature is infinite.

Mum, when you are dead, you can fly to any planet you want to, just like a rocket.
Ghil Ben-David, four years old.

The Nature of the Ego

Introspection and evaluation. A wounded ego becomes tense and overcontrolling driven by fear. Fear blocks the energy flow, and the whole organism becomes fragile. The contact to intuition is restricted because of alertness. Surviving and protecting the instrument is number one. When the Soul is imprisoned by fear or anxiousness for a longer period, access to dreams often closes off.

To shut out possibilities is to be blind. To open yourself blindly is seduction.

The role of the ego is to cooperate with the Soul.

The art of life is to constantly maintain a balance between being and observing.

It is only at the point of balance between ego and Soul, grounding and spirituality that consciousness is lifted up by the fire of transformation. When this happens, a deep gratitude manifests in the heart.

When Dr. Karl, during our first meeting in 2001, calmly predicted that my son's kneecaps would be found, I wanted to believe him. However, it wasn't until the specialist found them – to everyone's surprise – that my logical reasoning began to trust. As already mentioned, it would take more evidence before my ego was ready to surrender.

Robert Johnson's seesaw

The American Robert A. Johnson wrote a gem of a book: *Owning Your Own Shadow*. The author studied with Jung and worked as a Jungian analyst his entire, long life.

Johnson describes the psyche as a seesaw. One side of us is in the light. That is the side that we like to show the world, and which is our positive and cultured perception of ourselves. The other side is the shadow, a prerequisite for the development of ethics, because the shadow's existence makes it possible to consciously differentiate between good and evil. Our subconscious lives in the shadow, and it contains all that is forbidden and everything we repress in ourselves.

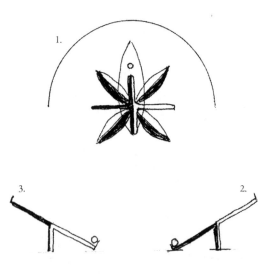

The seesaw in three positions. 1. Balance between dark and light produces a rainbow, a symbol of the higher state of consciousness. The Oneness level is made visible. 2. A weighed down shadow/low self esteem. 3. Delusions of grandeur.

Robert Johnson makes an important point: There is no trash can in our psyche. For example, it is impossible to discard your sexuality, sense of guilt, traumas, jealousy, hate and so on. Regardless of how much time you spend in a monastery, the repressed and unresolved feelings will live on in the shadow, if you do not deal with them. When too many emotions are repressed and the hard disk is full, the seesaw is weighed down, and the shadow swells like a boil. As a result of pain, the shadow grabs the ego's full attention. One's perception of reality becomes twisted. A classic example of this is when a person is convinced that everything is always someone else's fault. The shadow is so weighted down that there is no reach for any inner reflection.

Robert Johnson gives advice on how to avoid burdening the shadow: Give your shadow attention. Accept it like a small child. Listen when it calls. Sit down with it for five minutes: "Yes, yes, little shadow. The guests stayed for far too many days. I am irritated and angry that I haven't managed to get everything done." (An example given by Johnson.) Give your negative feelings full attention while embracing them with unconditional love. After one minute, pressure from the shadow is alleviated, and you avoid taking your pain out on your surroundings. In addition, I would, of course, sing myself free.106 It only takes a few minutes, and can be strongly recommended if you have the chance of going into a room by yourself, going for a drive, or simply finding a spot where you feel unrestricted and can freely let your voice out.

Vocal Prayer

When you sing the Note from Heaven, you raise your level of energy. This literally means that you connect yourself to the Oneness level which is a pure impersonal energy. The entrance for this energy can be found through a general cultivation of the senses. For example fasting will not only train you to control your sense of taste and desire for food. It purifies your sensitivity in general. The same thing is true for cultivating your listening ability. When you sing the Note from Heaven you reconnect to the Oneness level, in the moment your hearing sense is adjusted to sense a higher and finer vibration. When Sound Healing with the Note from Heaven, you pray for these high vibrations to resonate through you in order to heal and retune the receiver.

The Note from Heaven lifts you above the pain body. As the pain body's nature is a victimizing and complaining one, you need to remind yourself with all your power that it is your responsibility to pray. The pain body which is distorted will pity you and tell you that praying is in vain. Then remind yourself of the following words:

Any heartfelt prayer is heard. You are not your feelings. You are your thoughts. Take responsibility for yourself. Sing your prayer.

You will know that your prayer is heard, when the Note from Heaven appears. Soon you will feel relieved and your pain dissolved.

Inflation of the ego

Inflation of the ego is normal in all activities here on Earth, and is in my opinion one of the most difficult challenges mankind faces. We all have blind spots when looking at ourselves.

When a heavy shadow is released, it is followed by an inflation of feelings. This inflation process functions similarly to when a pendulum is released after being held at a sharp angle. The pendulum will begin by swinging powerfully to and fro, but the oscillations will gradually reduce in size.

We are talking about a law of nature. The pendulum can on one side swing from a lack of self-confidence and patterns of self-destruction, all the way over to arrogance and delusions of grandeur on the other side. The further out on the periphery you have been, the greater the possibility of a manic contrast. You can protect yourself from this phenomenon by being conscious of its existence. Therefore, as a Sound Healer, be aware that there is a chance you will become inflated, cocky, and yes, even get a superiority complex the first time a significant Sound Healing occurs. The ego will celebrate its bet with the Soul as if it had been the first horse over the line at the Grand National. During this celebrating, the connection to higher energies will be lost, because the power can only work through you when the seesaw is in balance. But enjoy the celebration, the enormous abundance of energy, and just carry on once you've recovered from your hangover and are sober again.

A person who has lived for a long time under the monstrous spiritual pressure of a concentration camp will, after being freed, and precisely because of being freed, be exposed to certain spiritual dangers. These dangers (in terms of mental hygiene) are nothing less than the psychological equivalent of decompression sickness. The diver's bodily health is threatened if he suddenly leaves the diving chamber (in which the air pressure is abnormally high), and, similarly, someone who is suddenly released from an extreme spiritual pressure can, under certain conditions, be damaged both spiritually and morally.
Viktor E. Frankl, Psychology and Existence

Viktor Frankl's example of decompression sickness applies to the development of both the therapist and the client. To be cured is a radical change that normally has to take place over a period of time, because of the client's usual need to gradually accustom him/herself to the idea of becoming well. In cases where a client is mentally prepared, however, healing can occur spontaneously like a miracle.

How to create a healthy relationship with the ego

Thomas: "Sir, could you please tell us how to get rid of the ego?"

Dr. Karl: "Let us say that this is the magic wish that many people would like to be given the solution to. Again, there is no single correct way. It is again unique. Though there are certain generalities that can assist one to move forward in the process. The first is very simple:

To be able to contain in your mind a combination of being proud of what you can do, but, at the same time, understanding that this does not make you any better than anyone else. That is the first state of mind to achieve.

This is a big problem in the human field. Priority, value, and importance seem to be placed on everyone and everything. What has to be realized is that *value and importance are absolutely transitory and are, therefore, of no value.*"

"Hmm. For instance, my dear, if you need a pair of shoes, what use is it to go to a fruit shop? Yet it could be said that fruit is important for your existence – much more important than shoes. Yet if you already had fruit and you had bare feet that were being hurt by the stones in the street, then the shoes would become important. And this can be said for all aspects of mankind. Not one thing of mankind can actually be said to be more important than the other. They are totally variable. Therefore, it is understandable that it is right and proper for a human being to be able to appreciate – you might say be proud of – that which they are able to achieve, and at the same time to realize, that that *only* makes them more satisfied inside, it does not make them a better or more important person."

(Graham Bishop, recording from the Sitting with Sound and Science, February 2007)

When the ego takes on the role of the Soul

There are charismatic people in the world who, according to their own statements, possess supernatural powers that enable them to work miracles. For example, they can according to what they say make objects materialize out of thin air, cure the sick, levitate, awaken the dead and so on. Their radiance can be likened to that of Jesus. I have sat in my chair, mouth open, and listened to such people and, at the same time, wondered what these fantastic people wanted from me, a very ordinary human being.

Following a session in which I had hardly begun to carry out Sound Healing, because the client's need was, first and foremost, to have an audience in order to boost his/her self-esteem, I felt completely worn out and unhappy. With hindsight I can see that this was largely due to the fact that I had disregarded my own responsibilities.

Lars Muhl has made it clear to me that the light such people radiate is a Luciferian light.[107] A human being can become addicted to the conviction that they are enlightened, and have been a master for so and so many incarnations. There is no back door in such a role, because how does one allow oneself to sink lower than the very top? A person that has adopted the role of being enlightened, radiates enlightenment, and can appear very charismatic. That person either becomes elevated to guru status, or the world cannot cope with them, and they feel excluded. The light they bear resembles that of the Soul, but it is the light of the Ego – a light which spellbinds the world, but which is built on unstable ground. It is a deception of the self, which in the end lets down the possessor of the light.

What if the point is that you should be nothing, in order

not to live in the shadow of everything? – That it makes no difference if you are enlightened or not, as long as you simply do your best?

Why proclaim yourself to be "enlightened" when the light is self-evident in the dark?

It is not the lamp, but the light of the lamp, that attracts the insects.

True healing is to give the individual that which they require – not that which they wish for.
Dr. Karl

The above sentence was emphasized time and again in the séance with Sound and Science.

Distinguishing between ego and intuition

When you listen to a person's voice, whether during singing or speech, it's possible to feel the energy level of that voice. The development of the hearing sense is closely linked to the development of intuition, which is latently connected to the inner ear and the development of the ability to listen consciously on all levels.

The conscious use of the ability to listen is my primary tool when I support people singing themselves free and surrendering themselves to the Note from Heaven. The body resonates to sound stimuli with physical signs, and the Listener can identify the right energy frequency for stimulating a certain part of the body by listening to the quality of the sound.

The form of energy concerned is not a physical excess or deficit in the normal sense; rather, it is an energy that touches the heart, mind and body. It's the same energy that touches you when another person has something genuine to say. When this energy is expressed, the mood in the room is raised to a freeing, vibrant level. It's hard to explain, but easy to demonstrate, because most people instinctively know when a person's voice is resonating freely. Some of the most common physical reactions to genuine expression are yawning, tears, lips quivering, a feeling of being deeply moved in your heart.

By refining your ability to hear the difference between ego and intuition, you can find a reference point, a physical navigation sign,[108] and thereby feel secure when you Sound Heal. You can train this ability by listening for hours on end to your own breathing via its vocal expression as you surrender to the Note from Heaven.

Don't be fooled by your own politeness. This is all about genuine energy, without the slightest hint of pretension. The Note from Heaven awakens devotion, tenderness, spontaneous joy, hairs standing up on the back of the neck, yawning, a physical opening of the heart, goosebumps and so on. The spontaneous reaction is laughter and/or tears at the same time. In the wake of the energy, deep gratitude, love, and happiness flow.

Signs that your intuition is working:
A pleasant tingling in the hands and scalp. It can feel as if you are wearing a hat, a ring around the crown of your head, the heart overflows with gratitude and the body is filled with well-being. What you do feels right, easy, light and playful. The wind is puffing you from behind and you are carried forward. A sense of compassion, deep calm and love arises naturally in connection with Sound Healing.

Signs that one's intuition is blocked:
Insecurity, nervousness, sweating palms, perspiration, heart palpitations, stomach pain, restricted breathing, stress, boasting, a lot of talk about yourself, self-reproach, a lack of grounding, general imbalance, etc.

Abstain from Sound Healing if these symptoms occur prior to

or in connection with a Sound Healing session. Check whether performing the opening ceremony can get you in touch with your higher state of consciousness. If you feel energy tingling in your hands, body or scalp, and your vocal light is working, then you can safely carry out Sound Healing, regardless of your private emotional state.

Pitfalls

Be aware of the difference between the physical sensations in your body when you Sound Heal another person, and when you are releasing your own emotions.

Take responsibility for listening attentively for this difference.

The pain body is always ready for action in various guises. It can initially seem liberating to blurt out the nastiest, devilish and violent sounds and who knows, perhaps it is easier to do this in someone else's name? Whether the release of one's own emotions can have a healing effect on another person, I leave it to the reader to judge.

In Sound Healing with the Note from Heaven, no chances are taken in this respect.

I am aware that some shamans/Sound Healers work with the dark forces, and that these are recognized as just as legitimate as all other forms of expression. My viewpoint is that it is fine to capture a heavy, dangerous fish from the darkest depths of the inner oceans, but the fish will break free sooner or later, only to disappear back into the darkness if you don't haul it up on land. Storming around in your own darkness provides no release on the spiritual level.

The shadow gets the attention it yearns for and this can give the body a swift kick of energy. However, if the weight of a heavy loaded shadow is not shifted to the light side of the seesaw, no problems will be solved in the long run. It can provide an immediate sense of self-confidence to have dared to overstep your own boundaries of propriety and be "nasty", just as it can feel liberating to allow your anger free rein.

But! The root of the anger must be exposed and rendered harmless in order for development to occur. Without a thorough search, the outburst of sound will remain at a pubescent level: A teenager, whose unconscious objective is to demonstrate that, "I do what I want to, because I dare to."

In reality, it is all about a person's failed attempts to resonate freely and authentically in the world. Fair enough. But this sort of expression doesn't belong in Sound Healing: *The manifestation of shadow energy has nothing to do with the Note from Heaven.*

By a conscious acknowledgement that the "ugly sounds" can, and must be taken up into the light, in order to "land a catch", a big step forward has already been taken. We may stand there with a fishing line and play at healing. However, when there is a tug on the line, we are fishing for real. The moment the fish is landed, the energy level in the expressed sound rises and the most glorious overtones and undertones occur; making the sound overwhelmingly strong, pure and beautiful. The fish is transformed when it sparkles brilliantly in the light.

Eliminating the influence of the ego in Sound Healing

1. Prioritize your shadow and pay attention to it as soon as it calls you.

Take it seriously. Just like a parent that takes care of their child's first complaint before bigger problems occur. Sit yourself down and care for your shadow, even if you don't understand what is wrong. If you notice an imbalance, take care of yourself. No one is perfect. Everyone swings on the seesaw.

It is the urge for perfection that makes a person shut their eyes to their own imbalances.

Accept your imbalance as something natural. We are all affected by the movements of the stars in the sky, and by hormones and chemicals in the inner organs, the glands and brain.

A stable path to balance is found in the loving acceptance of your own weakness. With repression, the shadow is forced to take control. It gains weight and sits so heavily on its side of the seesaw, that it obscures the powers of consciousness on the light side. You and your principles have become featherweights, worthless. The solar plexus closes and the subconscious can now rule without any restrictions, while the higher forms of consciousness are made powerless.

2. A dominating shadow sucks on the energy of the listener. No development occurs in a vocal expression that goes around in circles. If you are consumed by your own world, unable to listen to the Recipient's body, it is your shadow that is singing. *Tear yourself free from personal emotions by becoming aware of them and repeat the introductory ritual, in which you lift up your hands and ask for love and light to be sent through you.*[109] Regain your humility in being an instrument that is simply producing the sounds that the Recipient's body is calling for. Step aside and trust spirit to work through you in a present state of openness. When the seesaw is in perfect balance, the higher dimensions literally manifest as a rainbow of overtones. The gate to the higher spheres within you is opened, and the healing power of spirit will flow liberally through you.

Sound scanning is a steady listening intention, in which the empathic consciousness prevents the personality from interfering.

Spirit communicates through the overtone signals, which only can manifest when the ego withdraw.

Interference from the ego will immediately close down the communication. Therefore Sound Healing first and foremost is about training the ego to step aside during Sound Healing.

The results of your Sound Healing will gradually build a bridge of trust to the other side, and when the bridge is stable "I believe" is replaced with "I know". From then the contact with Spirit will be a part of your life. You will be at hand whenever spirit needs you. Spirit will be at your side whenever you need them – they will work on you through your dreams and help you in any way, whenever you ask for their help – even for getting a parking place in an impossibly crowded city.

Part 5:

Vocal Sound Healing

The signature sound of the voice

One should always keep in view that one must not sacrifice the natural quality of one's voice. For every person must know that there is no other voice like his; and if that peculiarity belonging to the voice of a soul is lost, then nothing is left to it.

The effect produced by singing depends upon the depth of feeling of the singer. However artificially cultivated a voice may be, it will never produce feeling, grace and beauty unless the heart be cultivated also.

Hazrat Inayat Khan, Sufi master, classical Indian musician

As earlier mentioned every person has his/her own specific inaudible sound matrix/frequency. People that resemble each other in terms of vibration are in *harmony* and get on well together.

With awareness of each person's individual frequency, you can begin intuitively to open yourself to your sound family.

It is possible that during the course of your life, you have tried to adjust your frequency in order to improve communication with your surroundings. The result can be fatigue and illness, because *it is taxing to be out of alignment with your fundamental frequency*. The transformation of negative primary emotions into positive ones supports the restoration of your original signature sound: "I am good enough, I belong, I want to be here, I am wanted and welcome." The energy body unfolds, and you get in touch with your healing abilities, because you stand more and more in your light. We train to find our way back to the true self, to resonate with the frequencies that flow freely through us. This is why regressive cell-singing is an integral part of becoming a Sound Healer. So many of us are held back by our pain body's perpetual statement: "You're not good enough," our frequency becomes contorted, and twisted like a crippled child, whose limbs have not been allowed to stretch out fully.

The vocal light

When you carry out Sound Healing with love and compassion, you unfold your energy field by surrendering to the Note from Heaven (the natural voice). Therefore, when Sound Healing, you will likely be able to produce sounds that would normally be beyond your range. The manifestation of these sounds occurs through, what I have chosen to call, "The Vocal Light".

By chance, when singing the Note from Heaven, I discovered that the vocal sound changes character and color, when it is aimed at and slides slowly across a client's body.

Again, this is a phenomenon that needs to be experienced in order to be fully understood.[110]

The following is an attempt at an explanation:

A sound flows from the mouth like a cone of light, whose form expands or contracts depending on which vowel the singer is forming with the lips. In most cases, it's easier to produce the sound if an "H" precedes the vowel. Just like when a ship with the wind blowing on its sails is pushed forward, the windy "H" increases the level of energy/light in the note. Follow the light to the area where it gains in strength and becomes more intense. The sound expands and becomes rich in overtones, when a resonant opening occurs in the energy field.

Before you begin, it is worthwhile to practice the vowel sounds in the next section.

"Vocal Light" is an expression for the sound that occurs in the resonance between Sound Healer and Recipient.

Vowels

Vowels reflect feminine consciousness – being present in the moment, a circle.

Consonants reflect masculine consciousness – a point of departure, direction, a dot.

Of the consonants, "H" provides the softest and most open point of departure, when setting a tone, like a tender wind that doesn't tug unnecessarily at the sails. "K" or "T", for example, take more energy at the point of departure, as they attack the note with a small explosion.

Vowels can behave differently, depending upon the person you are singing at and the consonant that is eventually linked to it. The following explanations should therefore be read as a general rule, as there will always be exceptions.

The Danish pronunciation of the vowels "E", "O", "Ø" (ö), "Y" (ü) and "Å", are not found in the English language, so please watch the demonstration and training video on https://www.youtube.com/watch?v=zYUa9Wz1SG0.

"Haar" (Father) is the most open vowel. It creates high overtones and covers large areas of the receiving body. The "Aaar" is the entrance and exit to life and is an expression of total surrender to the wonder of life. It can work remarkably over the stomach in Sound Healing, and is easiest to sing in the chest register.[111]

"Håår" (Call) is a closed version of "Haar". It is darker and creates a deeper overtone. People who restrain their light, unintentionally sing "Håår" when being asked to sing "Haar".

"Ho" (**(Hoe) Ho ho ho** – laughter of Santa Claus) can resemble the sound of a bell when sung in the middle register, and produces a deeper overtone than "Hår". "Hoe" is a narrow, ringing sound that can work in all places, and from my experience it is often effective around the throat area. The sound becomes centered when the "Oomm" form is used, as the "m" increases the singer's inner focus. The "m" collects the sound's resonance inside the singer's cranium and places a focus on inner peace and balance. By using a "Hoomm" sound with an open feeling inside the mouth (lifted palate), it is possible to produce a resonance that is heard from inside the head and vibrates in the entire cranium. In the beginning, you might hear the sound solely in one ear. It is a very pleasant experience.

Used with undertones, which is related to the reptilian brain and the autoimmune system, "Ho" or "Hu" happens, through my and many of my students' vocal expression, to change into a sound expression like a chord as a very deep and coarse vibrating sound whenever a trauma is detected by the vocal light. Using undertones I can thus scan a body and map the physical reaction related to trauma: illness, abuse, fractures, shocks in a body. I cannot express the trauma sound if you ask me to do it. The sound only appears as a resonance in the healing situation when there is a trauma which needs attention. This phenomenon is one of the most basic tools I use when Sound Healing with the Note from Heaven.

"Huu" (You) produces a narrow cone of light that can be focused, so that the light becomes directed, intense and strong. "Huu" has the second deepest overtones of the vowels. My expression of "U" is giving me good results. It is precise and useful for sound scanning with real tones, and it is my primary vowel.[112]

"Høø" (Hö fur is close to it) is pronounced with a pursed mouth. This vowel is leading to and supporting the overtones of "Yyy".

"Hyy" (Y – ou) – pronounced with a pursed mouth pointing slightly upwards (like a monkey trying to whistle); can sparkle in an overtone series from "Huu – øøø – yyy – iii", where the pursed lips are drawn back and down and out in a smile on "iii" (He).

"Hii" ("ee-sound" like in **He**) is physically the most horizontal and smiling vowel. The penetrating sound of this vowel, when used as a vocal light, can function like a sound surgeon's scalpel, whose cut is uncompromisingly sharp and accurate. Sometimes the receiver has felt the "Hee" sound like it's vibrating right through the spine. In many cases "Hii" has managed a high pitched tinnitus. Some people love it. Other people cannot stand that sound. Normally "Hii" belongs in the higher pitch of the vocal range and can be used to purify people's "antenna" – the silver thread in the top of the head.[113]

"Heei" (like in "**it**") purifies the other vowels. Experiment by thinking "Hee" (Heei) while you sing a high note using "Hii" (H**e**). The "Hii" sound will more than likely open up. "Heei" makes the other vowels sparkle when you think of it in the background. "Heei" is like the invisible salt of the tonal sea.

"Hææ" (p**e**n – **e** lefant) is a transitional vowel leading to "Haaar", one of the pearls on the string of overtones: "HIiEehÆææAaaar".

Exercise I: Vertical and Horizontal Movements with Vowels

Vertical, inward curved movement:

a) "Haa ææ ee ii ee ææ aaar." Close your eyes and feel the gentle movements inside the mouth, while you open and half close the mouth (like a dreaming crocodile).

Vertical, outwards curved movement:

b) "Haa åå oo uu oo åå aar." Close your eyes and feel the fine movements inside the mouth, while moving the mouth silently between the vowels (like a fish chewing water).

Horizontal volcano shaped movement:

c) "Hii-yy-øø-uu-oo-uu-øø-yy-ii", a line of vowels which, when sung with power from the diaphragm, can cut through bone and marrow with very high and stimulating overtones. "Hyy" works generally best together with "Huu" and "Hii".

Exercise II: The Gate of Life

This exercise can bring you back to an embryonic stage – the tadpole phase. The key is in the opening of the mouth, which is the entry and exit point of life and therefore also the gate to the "other side". Close your eyes and open your mouth in super slow motion on a silent "Aaar" – so slowly that you notice the lips part and the lower lip gradually slide down over the front teeth.

When you have opened your mouth as far as you can with the help of the weight from the lower jaw, slowly release the hinges of the jaw, which are located directly under the ears.

When the mouth is completely open, you will have opened your gate to the higher plane – the gate that you literally pass through when you pass in and out of life – the first scream, the last sigh.

To be completely relaxed, the lower jaw needs to slide back slightly again. Notice how the opening and the gradual closing affect your state of mind. Play with the movement and experience the feeling of being a tadpole that dwells in the embryonic fluid, and pick up its imperceptible movements in the consciousness of the lips.

When your mouth feels completely open and relaxed, you can mentally transfer this opening to other parts of your body. You can imagine the opening as the first circle in an eel net and collect the body's chakra wheels together, just as you would collect the rings of the net, so that they become one.

After some time, try to gradually close your mouth. The lower lip will have become so heavy that it will be difficult to close your mouth completely. And because the state that comes with an open mouth is so blissful, it can take some time to collect yourself and close your mouth again. I have tried to fall asleep in this position and woken up with a feeling of having grown from a tadpole into a codfish. My body was completely recharged.

Exercise III: The Great Breath

A full breath is called "The Great Breath" in Taoist philosophy. This exercise is fundamental when working with the Note from

Heaven, as it awakens the Hara/Sacral/Chi chakra which is located a hand's width under the navel and is the energy center. In Book I, The Note from Heaven, you will find several related exercises, expanded explanations, and illustrations.

Breathe in through the nose and focus on the movement of your stomach. Your exact posture is not so important, as long as your stomach expands outwards on the in breath and is lightly drawn inwards on the out breath.

Notice your stomach. Give it your full, loving attention. Gradually allow the inward movement during exhalation to be prolonged. Maintain a playful attitude and remember to thank your stomach for breathing; however big or tiny it might be, thank it for being there, through the thick and the thin. The more evenly it moves inwards during exhalation, the easier it will be to glide on the notes during Sound Healing. The wave movement of the stomach (diaphragm) when you softly press it inwards during exhalation and release it to expand outwards during inhalation, it's a caress – a total acceptance of the stomach and your gut feelings – a trampoline in slow motion. The stomach is worth its weight in gold, when it is allowed to move in and out in a relaxed and free motion. It sets your breath, and therefore you, free. Stomachs are beautiful when you accept them as they are.

Exercise IV: The Vowel Circle

a) Without using sound, practice gliding from vowel to vowel so slowly that you are aware of even the smallest movements in the cavity of the mouth. Move in this way gradually around in the vowel circle. Slow movements activate the muscle memory of the reptilian brain and cause deep relaxation.

b) Once you know the vowel circle by heart, close your eyes

and repeat the exercise, still without making a sound. The change in the vowels can sometimes be felt and/or seen in your mind's eye like a kaleidoscope, whose patterns remind one of crystals, that gradually change their shape.

c) Find a suitable note and let the voice go for a journey of discovery with the vowels and the transitions between them. Close your eyes and listen carefully while singing. Search for the places where the sound is especially rich in overtones. In these places, the sound will expand like an intensified light, and you will be able to experience a pleasant ringing in your ears, and possibly even hear several notes at a time (clusters).

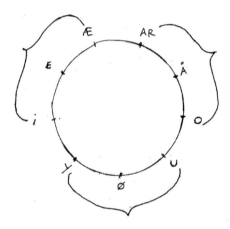

Exercise V: Sound Scanning

My dear, you cannot hear the resonance of the human structure. What you are hearing is our guidance. What happens is that those in our world who are working with you bring themselves down to a frequency level which is audible.

Dr. Karl

a) The Primary Vowel

Aim your face towards the stomach of the recumbent person (or animal) that you are practicing on. Sing *one* relatively low note and search around the vowel circle until you find a vowel that gives resonance. You will most likely experience that one of the vowels feels most natural for you to scan with. The vowel that feels best for you is called the primary vowel. Always use your primary vowel as your starting point when commencing sound scanning.

When you find a point of resonance with the primary vowel, then try the other vowels, and stick with the sound that stimulates the vocal light the most in that particular place of the stomach. The most commn primary vowels are "Aar", "Uu", and "Oo".

b) Scanning the Energy Body

In general, the more slowly you move your head during a treatment, the more precise your sound scanning will be. Fast movements in the energy field can make scanning difficult, and can be unpleasant for the Recipient. *Use only slow, gliding movements.*

Examine the layers of the aura field by singing a few centimeters away from the stomach and gradually move your head vertically through the body's energy fields. You will experience that the quality of the sound changes. What you should be listening for are luminous overtones that are more or less twinkling like stars. In the point or area of resonance, the sound will expand and radiate more than in other places on the body. This is where the strongest effect is, as the area is open to energy transfer. It feels as if the sound is almost pulled out of you.

Move yourself slowly out of the aura field and back in towards the stomach again, until you have mapped out the place that is the richest in overtones. Stay here until you feel that you should move on (do not sing the same note in the same place for longer than 2-3 minutes).

In the event of there being several vowels that enlighten a

certain place, the Recipient will in most cases be able to give you a direct response about which vowel works best. For example, a powerful "Hee" can create a completely different effect from a round sounding "Huu".

Before you speak to the Recipient, step consciously out of the contact to spirit, and when you continue, step consciously in again. It is as easy as opening and closing a door.

c) Scanning the Stomach

The primary aim of this exercise is to learn how to make *a slow gliding movement with your head*, horizontally in the air, from the pelvis and up to the stomach area with *one fixed scanning note* (a relatively low note in the stomach area). The vocal light is directed towards the Recipient's body. Feel free to come as close as a couple of centimeters, if it feels all right, and be prepared to change the distance in the direction the sound leads you.

When the sound finds a point of resonance, it intensifies and expands the sound of the vocal light. The Recipient's body can be seen as an invisible map that you are scanning. Move yourself in and out of the resonating point until you have no doubt where the resonating point is located. *Remember to maintain the shape of your mouth.*

It is possible for every hearing person to learn to find a point of resonance.

If you are unable to experience the point of resonance, do the following:

1. Try again.
2. Change vowel.
3. Move slowly further up or down the body.
4. Move slowly around the torso.
5. Move slowly to another deep note – follow your intuition.
6. Adjust the distance between you and the Recipient. Do not be afraid to go very close to the body in appropriate places

(let the Recipient be covered with a blanket). Be aware of keeping your spit in the mouth, and do not sing directly at the receiver's face, unless they wish you to do so.

7. Ask a helper to listen to you and let you know when you are approaching a breakthrough for resonance.

8. Notice if your stomach muscles are actively being drawn inwards when you carry out Sound Healing. If not, you should practice alone, and delve deeper into the exercises in Books I and II, and investigate if the breath is blocked due to traumatic experiences.

9. Stick with just one note when you are registering resonance, and don't rush.

10. Some people have difficulty hearing overtones in the sound. If the Recipient or others in the room hear the overtones in your sound and you don't, then keep in mind that through practice, you will begin to register them. First note the physical reaction in your body to the changes in sound. In some people, the upper lip begins to vibrate involuntarily, or maybe you will notice a feeling of warmth, an opening in your heart, a tingling in your fingertips, forehead, or crown, when you find the precise area where your vocal light resonates.

Which sound is the best sound? It is the sound that is correct in relation to a specific ailment.
Dr. Karl

If the Recipient Doesn't Feel Anything

If the Recipient doesn't feel any effects of the Sound Healing, there are two main explanations: One is that the Sound Healer is not in touch with the Note from Heaven. The other explanation is that the Recipient has raised a wall around their sensitivity. If they have experienced steady emotional stress in their early years, the body can have found it necessary to shut out emotions.

You will notice that approximately 15-20 percent of people cannot feel any sensation in the body during the first Sound Healing. These people often have a hard time feeling themselves in daily life. Do not panic if you belong to this group. Sound Healing awakens emotions softly, layer by layer, but it takes time. With patience and trust, you will sense the energy sooner or later. Listen to the body's signals after the Sound Healing. In some cases, they might first appear a couple of days after the treatment.

After a large course with 150 people, I received a comment from a participant that she thought it was boring to meditate on the breath and sing "Haar" for an hour nonstop. It had also felt boring and mechanical when she carried out Sound Healing. In addition, she had found it very unpleasant to be Sound Healed by the others, because they had transferred their bad energy to her.

An intellect or ego that stubbornly maintains control, without allowing higher consciousness to enter the mind, will become excruciatingly bored. It will sit and judge its surroundings and thereby separate itself from the Oneness level. If one is also paranoid about the "bad" energy of others, then one will actually end up manifesting one's own little version of hell. Like attracts like, and indulging in judgmental fears creates negativity and saturates the body with negative feelings. In this way, thought processes are self-fulfilling.

In the experience of "being present in the moment", knowledge is transformed into wisdom. A wisdom that we take with us when we die. We must find the courage to go on a journey of self-discovery. That is why we are here.

Exercise VI: Glissando Exercises

1. Practice a slow glissando[114] with your voice. Close your eyes. Imagine your spine. Glide from down and upwards while singing "Haar" and push the abdominal muscle slowly inwards

like an accelerator on each exhalation. Allow your hand to glide upwards together with the exhalation, with a graceful flex in the wrist. Let them fall each time you inhale. The slower the tonal glissando, the more details you will discover. Next step is, to try if you can glide between two fixed notes that are side by side on the piano (a second). When you slide very slowly between two notes that are close to each other, the microtones will be audible and expand your listening ability. At the same time, the very slow glissando will bring you into a light, meditative state, because you are listening inwardly to micro movements.

2. Slide downwards the small interval on "Haar" and note that the abdominal muscle (stomach) is still active, but that it works less when going downhill. Let your hand follow the movement.

3. a) Slide slowly now, in one exhalation in a semicircle from the top (the highest note for example Re) down to Sa on "Haar". The stomach moves inwards during the entire process. Draw the semicircle with your hand while singing. b) Then draw the other half of the semicircle from down (Sa) and upwards (to for example Re), while singing. c) Draw a full circle, while gliding on "Haaar" (Sa-Re-Sa) in one breath.

4. Imagine the sound as a light flowing out of your mouth. Glide as in Exercise I from a low note and slowly up to almost your highest note on "Haar" while you imagine that you are singing on a tree. In this exercise, as in exercises 5 and 6, a hand movement is unnecessary.

5. Slide slowly from a high note and down again, while you imagine that you are healing the tree with your sound.

6. Slide around in a circle while you imagine that you are painting a circle of light through which you heal the tree.

7. Make up some of your own gliding exercises if the inspiration strikes you. Dwell on those exercises that feel good. Where there are "holes" in the path (where the voice is weak), try to use soft and slow glissandi to fill them in.

Exercise VII: The foundation for Sound Healing with the Note from Heaven

Sound Scanning exercises 1-5

In these exercises, carried out with a Recipient present, both the tone and physical movement of the Sound Healer's head is variable. The goal is to find the frequency that resonates with a specific area in the Recipient's body. To carry out these exercises, you must know how to breathe correctly,[115] have practiced glissando and learned how to open yourself to the Note from Heaven.

1. Using your vocal light/your voice, slide over the Recipient's torso. Start at the pelvis with a sound in a relatively low register, and raise the pitch gradually as you move up the body. The feeling of where the low, middle, and high notes belong on the body is developed with practice. The first step is to learn to slide slowly up and down. The vowel that works the best at a certain location is individual – both for the Sound Healer and the Recipient. You have to feel your way. Start with the primary vowel.

2. Listen carefully to the sound. The place, where the vocal light expands/rings with overtones, is the place you should seek out and remain at. Points of resonance appear where a halo of ringing sound occurs around the core of the sound. Stick with the note that resonates and try different vowels, until you are in no doubt as to which ones give the most light.

Allow the vocal light to resound in the same area until the

sound fades in resonance, or until you feel that it's enough – maximum three minutes at the same place. The head is held still and the mouth and sound are directed towards the point of resonance. Place your hand lightly on the place at the same time. Slide a little up or down with the head, so that the vocal light slowly moves to the next resonance point and return back later, if the place you have found is insatiable. (In some cases the body can suck in the sound and attract you like a magnet.)

3. Glide slowly higher up with the vocal light so that both the sound and head move. Through a very slow glissando with the vocal light you are connecting the old point of resonance to a new point of resonance. When you have found the new point of resonance, remain there and load the place with sound/light. In this way, the whole body can be scanned with sound, from resonance point to resonance point. If there is a place that draws in sound for more than three minutes, go on small sound journeys nearby the area and then return to the place.

4. Tonal glide in an ascending direction: The vocal light/head is moved upwards over the body. Tonal glide in a descending direction: The vocal light/head is moved slowly downwards over the body. The starting note must be adapted to the starting point. If you start on your lowest note and then try to slide further down, it will be impossible, and you will then need to find a more suitable note.

5. Exercise in precision.

While gliding, if you hear a beautifully clear overtone, that only occurs as a sporadic, radiating glimpse of light, which swiftly disappears again during the glissando, do the following: Slide extra slowly over the area, while you sing the vowel in combination, with the note that resonated. Try different distances. When the overtone reappears in the vocal light, take a note of the area with a finger/hand. The location is sustained by imagining a beam of light from the Sound Healer's mouth to the point of resonance. The Sound Healer slowly moves the position of the vocal light without changing the shape of the mouth in any way. Note that the overtone will disappear and only recur in the position that you have marked with your finger.

Undertones

The lower and rougher the note, the further down the body it will usually resonate. One way to envision over- and undertones is to compare them with a solar system, where the base frequency is the sun. The over- and undertones that are closest to the sun are the easiest to hear. Further out, an infinite number of planets exist in the form of overtones and undertones that can be difficult, even impossible, to distinguish with the human ear. Regardless of whether the tones are audible or not, they affect our acoustic solar system, and it is their very existence, which makes live sound so much more effective than recorded sound.

The relationship between recorded sound and live sound is like tinned food in comparison to fresh food.

Regardless of how high or low your vocal register is, you will still be able to create a sound that affects the fundamental frequency of cells, because the different overtones/undertones affect each other just like planets do. However, the notes that are vibrating close to the fundamental sound will be the easiest to feel physically. Triads often resonate in the same place. For example, notes in a major chord correspond to overtones that are close to one another in the fractal structure of overtones.

Unfortunately, we didn't have time to ask Dr. Karl about undertones. According to Graham Bishop, Dr. Karl has emphasized the undertones' great importance in several other sessions. The undertones that Graham Bishop produces sound like a whirring tractor engine. The sound is created in the nose and throat, and corresponds to the more inward sounding undertones which are used in "Hung Song".[116] Undertones normally sound coarse and unruly until the pure signal appears as a deep note, much lower than the notes you normally will be able to sing. There are basically four kinds:

1) The outward sounding undertone can be expressed by a guttural creaking sound in different vowels, where "O" and "U" create the deepest undertones. Within the field of sound scanning with the Note from Heaven, undertones created by open, guttural, creaking vowels are normally used for sound scanning from the feet to the solar plexus and for identifying traumas. As the undertones have an autonomic nature, an experienced Sound Healer will surrender to the undertones and listen for the changing resonance in the sound, which in about 80 percent of the cases will communicate a message from the receiver's body.[117] When you are experienced, you recognize certain outstanding signals showing you the physical placement of a trauma and/or imbalance.

2) The inward sounding undertone is created by a closed nasal cavity on "Ng". Try to close your ears with your palms while expressing the sound: "Nggg". It should sound like a mixture of the singing of cicadas, a purring cat, a drill machine and the sound of a beehive. It is the purring or drilling part of this sound that you can hear loudly inside your head. A clear regular note sung in "Nggg" is not what we are looking for. It is the energy brought forth by the undertones that is in focus. The undertones support the autoimmune system, so you need to accept the animal sounds in you in order to get in contact with your inner purring cat.

For some people the "Nggg" sound can be expressed right away, for others it is harder to express than the outward sounding undertone. Tensions and good manners leave traces and have shaped our voice. If the "Nggg" sound is hard to express, then practicing the Note from Heaven surrendering to "Haar" will support your voice to return to its original matrix.[118]

This inward sounding nasal undertone is very useful for self-healing, especially when expressed as "Hunng, Honng, Hinng or Hanng" it can vibrate/energize any part of your body. Focus on the part you wish to vibrate and sing the undertone of for example "Hunnng".[119] I am especially using the "Hunng" sound to purify the pineal gland and the endocrine system. This method can balance the hormonal gland's secretion of endorphins and kick-start the body's natural detox system (melatonin and heparin sulphate). "Hung Song" (inward sounding undertones) is the central sound tool used to support the body in detoxing toxic metals. The method of "Hung Song" is described in detail in my two books Help and Heal the Pineal.[120]

During brain-scanning with undertones I mostly use inner sounding undertones from "Hunng, Honng, Hinng or Hanng", as they cover different areas of the brain. The open outward sounding undertones cover bigger areas and are of great use when healing the corpus. The inner undertones penetrate deeper than open undertones and are as precise as a dentist tool. From my experience the "Hung" undertones have a purifying effect, whereas "Hong" undertones heal and round off, "Hang" seems to influence the autoimmune nerve system as it stimulates the brain stem and cerebellum (reptile brain) through the back of the oral cavity. The undertones of "Hing" (heeng) seem to me to stimulate the lobes of the brain – and can also be used to consciously eliminate unwanted parasites, tumors… But this is all on its way. For the last years I have mainly concentrated on uncovering the healing properties of the inner undertones of "Hung" and "Hong".

3) Uninvited undertones can appear in the middle of the most beautiful sound when sound scanning with normal notes. Please receive the uninvited guests as visitors from above. Repeat

the vocal expression without adjustment, and if the uninvited undertones continue to appear, then invite the undertones in by letting them unfold their sound totally as it is. If the undertones appear during a Sound Healing of another person, then direct your vocal light[121] to the area of the body where the undertones first appeared. Examine if the receiver's body is truly resonating with and calling for this undertone. If it does, the undertone will reappear exactly where it is needed. *We are truly all devices who receive signals. The question is whether we are aware of listening, because the signals will only be consciously received if we hear them.* Remember we are made up of electromagnetic patterns and are therefore born with a potential to receive any signal. Awareness of who we are leads us to focused listening. You are light. **Turn on your inner radio and start tuning your self, so that you can serve a higher frequency and thus purpose.**

4) Trauma sound is an undertone signal appearing when your vocal light meets a trauma. A classical trauma sound is a jumping donkey sound, which cannot be expressed in any way unless it appears in resonance with a receiver's body.

Instructions for outward sounding undertones

The outward sounding undertones resemble a cracking sound, which is a basic exercise used in classical singing to relax the voice. The undertones manifest through the cracking in the remnant of an unclear radio signal. When you hit the right frequency, a deep note, much deeper than your voice normally is able to express, can appear.

Babies produce undertones while they are exercising the sphincter muscle[122] around the mouth, the muscles of their eyes, feet and hands: Open, close, open, close.

Therefore, this cracking sound, resembling a cat's purr, is retained in every human being's subconscious mind, regardless of nationality.

Pretend you are a baby and lie down with your tongue relaxed in the lower part of your mouth, while you growl, creaking like a door. Think of a scary movie and let the door open slowly. Or open your mouth completely and imagine being a crocodile. The demons come forward. Sounds like these stimulate the reptilian brain and therefore activate the autonomic nervous system. To feel embarrassed about sounding rather nasty and not nice is natural – persevere nonetheless. The sound is doing you good. Babies love it.

When my youngest son lay as a baby, outward sounding undertones were his favorite bedtime song. Each time I sang traditional lullabies to him, he responded with a reproving, growl, "Ahrrrrrh." It was only when I sang undertones that he smiled and peacefully fell asleep.[123]

When you sing undertones in general, it's important to relax your jaws. Let yourself feel lazy, with an open mouth, and the tip of your tongue resting behind or on top of the lower teeth. Open your mouth slowly and relaxed and find a dry sound which has no tonal ring. One or more undertones will gradually occur if you are relaxed enough, and yes, it is not at all about looking intelligent! Many singers can produce undertones immediately, while singers with tension in their neck and jaws will have difficulty. The reason is most often that the vagus nerve is out of balance. Practicing the Note from Heaven will gradually resolve the imbalance and this tension.

If the undertones are hard to express, try hanging your head, moving it slowly from side to side between your knees while you growl. Play lightly with the undertones, because if you put pressure on yourself, they will not occur. If the undertones don't come through, try visualizing a slightly higher position of the note inside the head.

Slowly shift between different vowels and you will find that some vowels are more suitable for creating undertones than others. Just as the colors of the rainbow have different frequencies, the same thing is true for vowels. *"Uuu" and "(H) Oe" are the vowels that create the lowest undertones. "Aaar" and "(H) Eh" tend to be the easiest vowels for a beginner to practice undertones with.*

If undertones still do not occur when moving through the vowels, try to gradually change the angle of your neck while purring. In the beginning, the sound is dry and crackling, like an unclear radio signal. Suddenly, a very low note can appear out of the signal. Remember, this is not singing, this is growling and purring!

On the CD *Rising*, I sing outward sounding undertones on the last track, *Roots*.[124] This is an example of how undertones sound, and it can be a good exercise to sing along to it. To distinguish your own sound, either when singing in a group or together with *Roots*, it's useful to make "elephant ears". This is done by placing your cupped hands behind your ears.

Sound scanning with outward sounding undertones

When you have played enough with the growling to be able to produce undertones, then try using them in sound scanning. If you are free of tension in the jaws, it will be much easier to sing them in a Sound Healing situation than if you sing for yourself. You may find that strange sounds, unknown to you, appear, just like if you caught a foreign radio signal.

Now and then, undertones can occur by themselves (uninvited undertones),[125] as a normal sound can begin to growl over an area that is calling for undertones. In this case, follow the growling of the sound and let the undertone unfold. During a course eight participants lay on the floor ready to experience the effect of undertones on their bodies. I sang at them one at a time. Fantastic undertones were produced with certain participants, while it was difficult to produce undertones with others. It was easier to sing undertones at the pelvis area on some participants, but certainly not at the feet, ankles and knees. The phenomenon repeated itself when I alternated between people: It was the same participants and physical locations where the undertones wouldn't appear, and the same where they did appear. I changed postures, but it made no difference.

The Recipient's body seems to draw sound that it resonates with out of the healer's vocal light. During sound scanning in general, it can feel as if the sound is being pulled out of you, and it can be difficult to stop singing, because the experience of the energy is a blessed feeling of uniting with the Oneness level.

Some people have a special flair for undertones, but not all are adept at creating them in the beginning. If outward sounding undertones do not occur, try to make them resonate in another place in the receiver's body, at the feet, the legs or the stomach. If you succeed here, then try again in the original place, which then might have softened up. If you cannot make the undertones at all, just accept it.

Outward sounding undertones, produced in the resonance of a Receiver's body, have an autonomic quality. You cannot control which notes are produced, just as it is impossible to sing resonating undertones with the slightest amount of performance tension.[126] Therefore, intuition plays a remarkably powerful role in the world of undertones. Be aware that the types of undertones we are singing are not the same as Tuvan throat singing.

True healing appears when you listen to another person and express what his or her organism is calling for.

I consciously avoid methods of training harmonics, because as already mentioned, the goal is to give space to the higher powers to communicate through the sound signals. *An artificially practiced over- or undertone is not produced on the basis of listening to another person's resonance/the higher powers assistance. It is based on the healer resonating with themselves* while performing harmonics, for example, when the tongue is pressed back and pharynx/the throat is closed. It is comparable to pressing a button which is set on a particular radio program. When you are in control you stop listening for other signals.

The approach in Sound Healing is to listen, and let the sound grow out of resonance with the Recipient. This makes a world of difference, even if both cases are about overtones and undertones. *The intention should never be to perform, because when it is, you inflict your ego's energy on the Recipient. You are the hands of the angels, and angels cannot work in an energy calling for applause.*

The outward sounding undertones belong in general to the toes, ankles, knees, thighs, pelvis and stomach. These limbs make up the root of the body.

Like the root of a carrot is under the ground, undertones are a tonal mirror of the subconscious part of the body. In order to express the lowest level of vibration and achieve the strongest effects with Sound Healing in general, the Sound Healer must work with undertones, because they represent the subconsciousness.

The first time I expressed outward sounding undertones, they occurred by themselves during a Sound Healing full of beautiful overtone-rich notes. Suddenly my voice began to sound scratchy, as if static came on the radio, and the low undertones flowed through. My first impulse was to feel embarrassed for the client, and I tried to keep the sound nice by entering performance mode. But I didn't succeed. The undertones' growling sounds kept on coming spontaneously. When the client told me that the deep tones felt genuinely good, I stopped trying to prevent the signal and allowed the ugly sounds to ring out. After using outward sounding undertones, the Sound Healing increased and became much more effective.

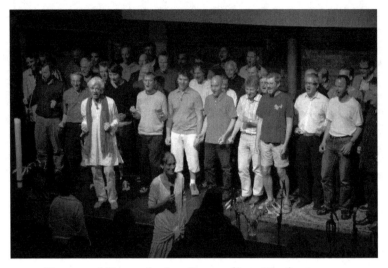

Personal Boundaries Regarding Undertones

The first time making guttural, growling outward sounding undertones in front of other people can feel embarrassing.

However, when ordinary people experience Sound Healing with undertones, they usually[127] get so absorbed by the pleasant, calming, softly swirling vibration in the body, that they do not bother to judge whether the sound is strange or not. Some clients have told me it's like the fizz in carbonated drinks moving up their legs, others say they get very warm from it, and many fall into a deep sleep. As a Sound Healer, stay mindful of the fact that even if you can't feel the effect of undertones yourself, they are nevertheless very effective indeed, more powerful than you might think. Undertones – Unconscious.

A professional female clairvoyant that received Sound Healing asked me to stop singing undertones, because she simply couldn't cope with them. This surprised me, because the tones burst clearly through, and that kind of resonance usually means that the client needs and/or is receptive to them. Afterwards, she explained that the energy from the notes had accumulated in her genital area, which had embarrassed her, as she and her husband had not been sexually active for ten years.

If the client doesn't feel anything, and that makes you feel uneasy or ridiculous for having sung undertones, then listen to the client's stomach:

If and when the Recipient's stomach begins to gurgle or rumble, it's because the autonomous and sympathetic nervous systems are getting rebalanced.
Jonna (student in Sound Healing)

Sound Healing exercise with outward sounding undertones

The Recipient sits on a chair, lies on a couch or on the floor. If the Recipient lies on the floor, you can improve your working posture by sitting on a chair with the Recipient's bent legs resting on your thighs.

1. Ask for love and light, and reach out your arms with palms turned upwards. Lower the arms and turn the energy collected in your palms towards the Recipient. Place the second and third fingers (the healing fingers) softly on the Recipient's big toes.[128]

An alternative is to hold very lightly with your hands. The touch must be light enough that the energy can jump between the healer's hands and the receiver, as if they were two poles. If you hold too tight, the energy cannot be felt.

Then, sing undertones and find the correct distance and the right place by moving the Vocal Light over the toes; closer up and further away, while trying out the undertones with the different vowels. Stay with the vowel that gives the clearest outward sounding undertones. In some cases you have to get very close to the toes. I sometimes sing with my mouth directly on the back of my own hand, so that the undertones are transferred directly through my knuckles to the Recipient's feet. From the big toes (represents the head) the energy flows through the meridians, the electrical lines of the human organism, all the way up to the brain. If you know the reflexology points, it is possible to stimulate them with sound too. For example the ear area is under the fourth and fifth toe, the eyes under the third and second toe.

2. The Sound Healer gently touches the Recipient's ankles with their hands and scans as described above. Alternatively, you can hold the right hand between the ankles, if you need to collect energy down through the left hand.[129]

3. The knees. The same procedure as above.

4. The hips. Gently hold the sides of the hip joint and don't go too close to the genitals, unless you know the client well. In one case, when a cancer stricken woman with an egg-sized lymphoma in the groin came to me for Sound Healing, I asked if it would be okay for her if I could sing directly on the tumor. In general, it's a good practice to ask the client before the treatment starts, if they are comfortable with you touching them.

5. The stomach. It can feel good for the receiver, when the Sound Healer lays the whole hand cautiously on the stomach. Let it float so lightly that the breath is supported by the hand following the movement of the stomach. Move the hand slowly around as if on a thin pillow of air, following the vocal light and marking where the biggest access to the sound is. From here, isolate the point of resonance with the vocal light, as previously mentioned, by testing whether it is more difficult to sing undertones at other places nearby the point of resonance. In some cases, undertones can cover large areas, in other cases a very specific area only. Undertones are also effective without the use of physical touch. When a place is saturated with outward sounding undertones the sound will be less energetic and the eventual trauma sound vanishes. Before going on, I suggest to

scan with inner undertones (I use mostly "Hung" or "Hong"), to see if there is further imbalance deeper inside the body. If there is, test if it is "Hung, Hong, Hing or Hang" that is needed, and apply the sound until the area is saturated with energy.

6. Undertones can be useful to loosen up tense, tight areas, like for example a stressed solar plexus. If the Recipient has specific parts of the body that are tense, it is worthwhile to apply undertones. *As a general rule, I advise to be careful using outward sounding undertones in the head area.* If you have trained inward sounding undertones and can express them, you can apply for example "Hung Song" to specific areas of the brain. Otherwise use the real notes and overtones at the head area. Nonetheless, there are some people who like to receive outward sounding undertones around their head and for example a humming tinnitus or a tumor will from my experience often benefit from inner and outward sounding undertones.

Undertones and tumors

I have experienced brain tumors being diminished by undertones from my own130 and from my students' experience. Interference between two voices singing almost the same note on purpose will create deep undertones, that also might be helpful in diminishing tumors. However, this hypothesis needs to be tested scientifically. I have experienced swollen lymph nodes diminish in a few minutes by applying undertones.[131]

Undertones and tinnitus

Tinnitus with low notes can be diminished by undertones sung over the ears where the hearing center is placed, in about 70 percent of the cases. The students and my experience show that the vagus nerve in many cases is involved in tinnitus. Undertones can loosen up the vagus nerve if it is tense. For example, a student recently found that when she sang undertones on a man's jaw his tinnitus disappeared.

I myself have worked on hundreds of tinnitus clients and experienced that the undertones help against a deep whistling in the ears. The high notes are eliminated by finding the exact frequency with the overtones of high Huu or Hee notes, but the background noise of general whistling is almost always eliminated by undertones. This is especially true if the tinnitus is caused by sound. Here we have the highest healing rate (70 percent over 1-12 treatments).

It is a great feeling to be able to help people suffering from tinnitus, but there is a minus: People come to be fixed, and this attitude can close down the higher energies' work. Therefore it is beneficial always to start by teaching the client the Note from Heaven, so that their cells open up, and they hopefully can learn how to sing down their own tinnitus.

Often the healing manifests easier when a client is taken by surprise. For example I was shopping and the shopkeeper was complaining about her tinnitus to a customer. I interfered and asked if I should fix it.

Before Sound Healing a tinnitus I always ask if it is a high or a low note and about which ear is the worst. In this case it was a deep whistling in both ears. When sound scanning the shopkeeper with undertones, at the hearing center placed over the ear, a clear trauma sound appeared. I stayed with the trauma sound until it disappeared after about one minute's singing.

"Is the tinnitus gone?"

"Yes, it is completely quiet inside my head now!" The shopkeeper and the customer stood with their mouths open and I left with a light feeling of getting help from angels.

In general it is important to teach the recipients how to sing their own tinnitus away. Some are too shy to try it at first but they are surprised when they succeed. Instead of being on the edge of suicide (some people are on antidepressant medicine because of tinnitus), the client's situation is now changed. The feeling of powerlessness is taken over by self-responsibility. I have seen many of these kind of cases. As a Sound Healer you must know that they can do it in order to persuade them into Sound Healing themselves. If the cause of tinnitus is radiation or some other form of stress, tinnitus will return as long as the root cause of the tinnitus is not removed. Therefore, you should if possible teach the client how to sing down tinnitus themselves – or train a relative to release their tinnitus with sound.132

Undertones and broken bones

An American study showed that daily Sound Healing with a cat's purr heals broken bones approximately three times faster than normal.

Because human undertones are similar to a cat's purr, and also vibrate through the skeleton, I am convinced that undertones can stimulate the healing of broken bones. A client told me about a child who had asked her parents to sing for her broken leg morning and night. They sang dutifully, thinking it was all very sweet and innocent until the doctor, just 14 days after the cast had been put on, proclaimed that it must have been a misdiagnosis, because there was no sign of a fracture! However, the old X-ray showed otherwise.

Something similar happened when I sang on a woman who had been diagnosed with a concussion and a broken arm a few hours before I came to sound scan her. The concussion vanished after two days. At the two weeks checkup the doctor surprisingly found that the fracture was healed. So my theory is, that the more fresh an illness, a trauma or a fracture is, the stronger and faster effect the Sound Healing will have.

Sound Healing recreates order in the body and thereby supports the immune system.

Undertones and trauma sound

When I was filmed for a program about healers in Aalborg University Hospital, the scientists tested a person who sang herself free. In this test they saw that the vagus nerve reacted positively. After the test, the producer Lasse Spang Olsen wished to try a short sound scanning. I started up with undertones and got the sound I usually get, when there is a trauma of abuse or shock. This sound has a giant vibrato, which I can only express if it appears as a signal. It seems to vibrate between a very low and a high note. I have the idea that the trauma sound which moves between undertones and overtones tries to bridge energies between the subconscious and the consciousness level in order to repair imbalances in the organism.

This sound usually would appear only in a certain area, but in this case it appeared on the right foot, then in the left ankle, then one of the knees and so on. There was no end of trauma sounds. Lasse asked me to point out all the places I could find, and then in the end he reminded me, that he had been a stuntman for years. All the places the trauma sound had appeared there had been fractures of the bone. He asked me about other areas, and I was baffled to experience how precise the scanning with the trauma sound was.

Undertones and colic

A young couple with a baby suffering from colic were present at a Christmas lunch. I was discretely asked if Sound Healing could possibly offer some relief. In a location away from the group, I began to feel the baby girl. It's important that the child cooperates and that a positive feeling is generated between you and the baby, before you start. Listen to the child and mimic their sounds. If the child fiercely resists, then you should hold back. However, I have never experienced a child resisting, as it feels pleasant to have undertones sung on the stomach.

After approximately 20 seconds, the girl relaxed and became

calm. The parents called the next day and told me that the consistency and color of her stools had changed, and her colic seemed to have disappeared.

After this case, I healed several other babies with colic. I met the majority of babies with colic out in public places, where the parents sat in misery with dark shadows under their eyes. Be aware that it can feel like an encroachment for some mothers, that someone else can "comfort" their child, where they cannot. The mother is often weighed down and tormented by her powerlessness. Therefore, it's important to point out that what you are offering is the possibility of removing the child's stomach pains.

I have often felt awkward offering to sing on a stranger's child; but in a train carriage, on a beach or similar such places, where everyone suffers from the baby's wailing, I can overcome my awkwardness. I normally mention my experience with colic, and say that if the parents would like my help, they are welcome to let me know. The colic has disappeared when I have sung on babies with this affliction. So do give it a try yourself. Remember to be completely calm, and if possible, hold the baby close to you, find a deep sense of stillness and love while you hum, support the neck with one hand and lay the other on the child's lower back/over the stomach. You can also lightly lay your hand on the baby's stomach, while it is lying in a pram [carriage]. By the way, men's low voices, with their wonderfully vibrating sound, are irresistible to all stomachs.

Undertones and hernias

My eldest son suffered a hernia when he was eight years old. We were encouraged to have him operated on, but I was afraid of a general anesthetic, because as an infant he had been close to dying in a hospital environment. As the hernia in his pubic area came and went, we dared to decline the operation. One day the hernia wouldn't go back in. While my husband rang the hospital, I sang undertones directly on the hernia, in a desperate effort to ease our little boy's pain. After 30 seconds, the hernia had vanished.

For a couple of years, we managed like this, singing undertones to the hernia. Please note that I do not wish to prevent anyone from having surgery for a hernia. I only wish to inform the reader that it is possible to affect an acute hernia with undertones.

It later turned out that my son's hernia was caused by one of his testicles. It had been floating around in the groin and hadn't found its way down into the scrotum. My son was operated on and everything went well.

Undertones and leukemia

In the treatment of leukemia there is a paradox because the immune system attacks its own white blood cells. A woman named Bente, who received the hardest possible chemo treatment, according to the hospital's test still had cancer cells in the body and was given up. Her husband asked me if Sound Healing could be helpful.

I have always hesitated to treat leukemia cases, because it is an illness caused by an autoimmune reaction linked directly to the white blood cells. Sound Healing strengthens the immune system in general, so I was doubting whether to just trust the Note from Heaven as usual. When meeting the couple I understood that they believe in Jesus. Therefore I asked Jesus for healing, love and light for the woman while surrendering to the Note from Heaven. Since the new white blood cells (T-cells) are primarily matured in the bone marrow and the thymus gland, I sound scanned Bente's skeleton with undertones because undertones vibrate especially strong in bone. Trauma sound appeared all up along the spine and in the thymus. The energy was very strong and water streamed out of my eyes. We both felt the presence of Jesus and were overwhelmed by unconditional love and gratitude. After a few minutes the trauma sound disappeared and the resonance sounded normal. I then sang real tones and scanned with overtones in order to add new fresh energy to support Bente's body.

The day after the treatment Bente had blood tests taken at the doctor's. Her blood tests were surprisingly great. The part of the immune system that should be kept down in order that she could heal was kept in place, but the other part of it was working perfectly. Her blood percentage was normal and even though it was wintertime Bente did not catch any cold or flu. After the fourth treatment Bente's hair started to grow and her blood tests were still great. No more trauma sound was present. Every day Bente sang the Note from Heaven and "Hung Song" for one hour. She said that she felt it filled her with a genuine life force. Bente is today cured of her leukemia.

The Feeling of Sound Healing

It is a precondition for becoming a Sound Healer to exchange Sound Healing sessions with a practice partner, so that you can feel the effects on your own body. The Sound Healer cannot feel what happens physically inside the Recipient, when their complete attention is focused on listening to the resonance in the sound. While laying hands on the Recipient during healing without singing, most healers can sense a fine energy vibrating in their fingers. For about 80 percent of Recipients, Sound Healing feels like a pleasant bubbling, slightly tingling sensation, but the Sound Healer can normally only notice the resonance. When you close your eyes, your other senses become more acute, due to the reduction of sensory input to the brain. In general, closed eyes improve the Sound Healer's ability to concentrate.

An inexplicable phenomenon

Sometimes during Sound Healing with the Note from Heaven, the sound will only ring in one ear. It feels like the auditory canal is being massaged on the inside, it becomes warm and starts to tickle.

Other sounds ring in both ears. The times when I have heard the sound, for example, in the right ear, the Recipient has usually also heard the sound in their right ear.

I use this phenomenon when Sound Healing people with hearing loss, because I assume that the sound affects the ear that resonates. Note that the source of the sound that is heard in one side only can be sung even from quite a distance away from the ear – for example the feet, stomach or pelvis.

When you Sound Heal at the brain be aware that if a trauma has its roots in the reptilian brain (cerebellum), then the treatment must happen in the same side as the trauma is located. This means that a neck pain in the right side will be related to the right side of the brain. If a trauma has its root in the big brain (cerebrum), then it works the other way around and a pain in the left arm will be related to the right hemisphere. When we work with undertones we work primarily with the reptilian brain (cerebellum) and therefore a right side problem will be located in the right side of the brain.

Physical reactions of clients during Sound Healing

During Sound Healing, some people see colors[133] and in some cases also images in their mind's eye. It is natural that sudden twitches can occur in the body. In more rare cases, the body will begin to twist in spasmodic movements. This is due to a reaction in the autonomous nervous system. Ask if everything is okay if the Recipient looks uncomfortable. As a general rule, though, the client is completely caught up in the movements, and needs first and foremost support through that process. The Sound Healer can later explain that the sphincter muscles in the body are working together, and that the reaction is a natural part of the healing process that is taking place.[134]

It is a common phenomenon that the Recipient experiences the Sound Healer's touch in several places at once: "I thought you were down at my feet, but you were up at my head." The explanation of this phenomenon could be that the sound from the Sound Healer starts an energy process that is similar to lighting a fire. You light the fire, and then it continues to burn by itself.

Another possible explanation is that spiritual energies are present during the Sound Healing session. Sometimes the Recipient notices several hands on them, even though only the therapist's hands are present. The author, singer and healer Lars Muhl and I once carried out Sound Healing together on a large group of people. During the session, a woman felt that she was being massaged over her entire body, from her feet upwards. I had only touched her lightly for a few seconds on the head and stomach with the tips of my fingers.

When the big toes are Sound Healed, the energy can easily work in a different part of the body and have an effect there. For example, some clients notice energy affecting the forehead while having their toes Sound Healed. It's also possible that the Recipient notices certain points in their body being activated, and they can then even describe a meridian pathway, without any prior knowledge of such things.

It is a natural and normal reaction to fall into a deep sleep during Sound Healing. Some Recipients sleep very heavily and considerable effort must be used to awaken them after a treatment. Others drift to and fro between states of consciousness and perhaps cannot remember that they have been "out of it" even if the Sound healer has heard them snore. And then, there are also those that are awake during the entire process.

Three Personal Experiences as a Recipient of Healing/Sound Healing

A) I experienced healing for the first time during my four-year stay in Israel. After a student, Daniella Segal, opened her voice for the Note from Heaven, she proclaimed that she could clearly feel that the voice work had set energy in motion in her body.

Daniella explained that she was a professional healer, and since she offered to give me a healing, I thought it would be interesting to try and laid down on the floor. During the healing session, I was surprised to feel the movement of her hands on my body without her actually touching me. Waves of energy put me into a completely new state of consciousness, and to my surprise, I noticed my body levitate a couple of centimeters off the floor. It lay there and pulsated pleasantly. When she put her hand on my stomach, I wished that it would go on forever.

B) That experience of healing[135] led to my ex-husband and I educating ourselves as healers in Mystical Therapy – a method founded and developed by Master José from Spain. People there were generally dressed in white, and it was quite a formal atmosphere. Alejandro was our teacher. The energies spoke for themselves. Several of the 50 participants had intense reactions with tears and spasms. Despite very little experience with meditation, we experienced an internal feeling of twirling in the air during the meditation. After several meditation courses and a compulsory three-week detoxification program, we were ready to take the healing course. During this course, we learned a healing technique – the form of which will be covered in the following section as an example of how to do a Sound Healing session.

When my husband stood for the first time and carried out the newly learned movements above me, it was just too comical. I quickly forgot about suppressing my laughter though, because contrary to everything we had learned, he roughly grabbed my big toe. It hurt. We Recipients had been told to shut our eyes. I suddenly felt my body float high up in the air. During the whole time I felt a firm grip on my left big toe. It continued like that.

Alejandro rang the bell. We were meant to gather and talk about how it had gone. But my husband was still holding onto my toe, and I didn't dare to open my eyes in case I fell down. It was so embarrassing that we just kept on like that.

The others carried on with the lesson. Finally, I opened my eyes in order to say that now it was enough. And there I lay, completely alone on the mattress.

My husband was sitting together with the others in front of the teacher. He had not once touched my left big toe!

C) Many years later, at the conclusion of a course with the Note from Heaven, it was my birthday and I was surprised by the entire group of 30 participants who wished to give me Sound Healing. I don't normally get Sound Healing from the group at my courses, but because it was a birthday present, I agreed. Two helpful and caring women flanked me and each took one of my hands in theirs. A third lightly touched my feet. The two women on either side were so eager to give, that they took my energy. I felt their desire to be "good enough", and, just as Dr. Karl had said, it is the energy carried by the sound that either gives or takes. The overly good attitude drew energy from my hands. From the woman by my feet, who was discreetly giving, the energy was streaming beautifully in. It was difficult to be aware of the rest of the group, because the two "over motherly" women suffocated the energy with their good intentions. However, it was an excellent birthday present, because we are many overly motherly types that walk this Earth – and in this way, I was made aware of that fact.

Sensitivity to sound

When a client is oversensitive to sound, the Sound Healer will need to be particularly empathic or possibly even heal without sound in the first session. Another possibility is for the client to sing with you as you Sound Heal. In this way, it may be possible for you to get close enough to the client to be able to sound scan in the normal way.

A client with Ménière's disease – an inner ear disorder which gives symptoms of constant dizziness – was so scared of getting worse that she became stiff whenever I started to sing. But when she tried singing at the same time, it was as if a curtain had been drawn back and the dizziness disappeared at once. In cases like this, I constantly keep an eye on the client's breathing and sing only when they sing. The length of the séance in this case is decided by the client, who has an express need to control the session.

Sensitive people have quite a hard time in today's society, and first and foremost, they need to be treated with care and consideration.

On one occasion, I guided a sound-sensitive woman to open herself vocally to the Note from Heaven, in order to experiment with the level of Sound Healing she would be able to cope with while singing herself at the same time. It was a fantastic session. The woman and I found a resonance that was difficult to shake ourselves loose from. Completely new sounds were created through the interference[136] which occurred during the Sound Healing with the woman lying and singing spontaneously together with me. The energy was extraordinarily high.

Men who are sensitive to sound

For some rare Recipients, Sound Healing can seem overwhelming. If a Recipient is used to holding their emotions back, it can seem like a type of indecent exposure when the sound awakens these emotions and brings them forward into the light.

A young man who studied in the university came for a session and claimed that he had no problems but just wanted to try Sound Healing. Everything went fine until three weeks after the session, when he called and accused me of having abused him with my song on his solar plexus. Following the treatment he had a hard time sleeping at night due to fear. He also accused me of having sung high notes over his head against his will. Yes, he had even received mild tinnitus because of it.

Before and during the Sound Healing session I had, as I usually do, asked the man to let me know how things were going. At the time he said that he enjoyed it. During the phone conversation with the man, I offered him a balancing treatment free of charge, possibly only laying hands on him without sound, but he declined. My clear feeling was that the man, in general, had psychological problems.

As a Sound Healer, it is easy to lose faith in doing Sound Healing when you get such a response. The accusation of having harmed another human being easily activates a sense of guilt. The investigative part of the ego needs to analyze and evaluate the situation for a couple of days, before it is able to let it go again. If you've done your best with compassion and love, then you do not need to blame yourself. Thank God for having a good lesson.

You need to be careful when carrying out Sound Healing on a person who has "no" problems. Never give a treatment to a person who just wishes to try the effect of Sound Healing.

Frank Lorentzen,[137] the model for several of the pictures in this book, received Sound Healing during the photo session. Here he saw energies being present in the room, and noticed a clear physical contact with these even before the Sound Healing session began. Regarding the young man's problem with fear, Frank thought that the student might have had an experience similar to that of Frank's and that may have frightened him.

Duration of Sound Healing

The duration of a Sound Healing session varies because there are many factors in play. When I have sensed the presence of a strong entity, and the Receiver has had enough faith, then people have been cured for serious illnesses in a few minutes. I know a Sound Healer in Norway who is overweight. She can only manage to do Sound Healing for ten minutes at a time. Despite this, she has had an effect on and cured several cases of tinnitus. When Dr. Karl and The White Brotherhood carried out Sound Healing on my son through Graham, it lasted a full hour. Sometimes I've also taken that long when giving Sound Healing. Nowadays, however, I restrain myself, because the effect of Sound Healing seems to be just as good after both short and long sessions. A complete Sound Healing session takes between ten to 30 minutes. Afterwards, half an hour is set aside for the client to rest, so that the energy can work in the body. For some very sensitive clients, a rather short session is all that is needed.

As previously mentioned, it can take up to six treatments before a result is observed. If no results have been felt after the sixth treatment, the treatment is not working and should be stopped. In acute situations, Sound Healing can be given several times a day in serious cases, but generally it is recommended to have *four to ten days between treatments*, so that the healing process can be integrated and continuous.

Preparations for Sound Healing

Avoid eating half an hour before the session, milk products create mucus. Clean your teeth with dental floss or toothpicks (bad breath comes from between the teeth, unless of course you have an infection in the adenoids/throat). Brush your teeth. Wash your hands, and maybe use a light fragrance from pure ecological oils on your wrists such as rose, lavender or orange flower oil.[138] Strong odors can have an unpleasant effect on sensitive types. Make sure there is a duvet or blanket, extra cushions, and preferably a knee roll or large pillow to place under the Recipient's knees, if they are lying on their back. In my experience, the sound works through anything, even duvets. The most important is that the Recipient feels secure and comfortable, so that they can open themselves devotedly to the situation.

Prepare chairs at both ends and at the sides of the treatment table for the Sound Healer to sit on. If the healing is taking place on the floor, make sure that there is a soft surface to crawl around on, or use knee protection, so that the mucous membranes of the knees are protected.

Drink a glass of water with the Recipient upon their arrival. Water increases the healing process, and when adding lemon juice, the water structure is optimized and balanced.

Have a short conversation about their expectations and explain what will happen. Tell the Recipient to say if they feel anything unpleasant, or if something feels particularly good during the Sound Healing session. This is especially important for tinnitus, where the Recipient can clearly notice when a specific note makes the tinnitus disappear. If you make a combined treatment including instructing the Recipient in breathing methods, the Note from Heaven and/or regressive cell-singing, then you always start by doing an Interview: Primary feeling, Wish, Code words and Tension. See page 174.

Protection
When you surrender to the consciousness of love and light, you will draw love and light towards you. If you are afraid of negative energies, you will attract negative energies.

If you want to protect yourself from temporarily taking on possible ailments from which the Recipient suffers, it is first and foremost a matter of eliminating any tendency to pity them.

Pity carries negatively charged energy with it because you separate yourself from the client by judging them as being in a bad position. Dr. Karl explained that at our first meeting: "Pity" – or in other words to feel sorry for someone – creates an opening in the energy field to take on the Recipient's ailments *temporarily*. It will last one-two days.

As mentioned, this feeling can be eliminated simply by being aware of it. Push it to one side and replace it with compassion.

If you manage to unlearn feeling sorry for someone

and replace it with compassion, you do yourself and your surroundings a big favor.

When a person is bound to his pain body, he gets nourishment from pitying those around him or by lapping up the catastrophes of the world and sharing them. Such thoughts create a vicious circle that ends up negatively affecting the person having those thoughts. Therefore, eliminate pitying yourself and others!

In my experience, if a Sound Healing session is interrupted by conversation – whether it be with the Recipient or another person in the room – it can create a similar opening in the energy field, just like "feeling pity" does. One example of this was a man suffering from cancer, who had a sizable tumor in his large intestine. Together with his wife, he travelled 350 kilometers for an acute Sound Healing treatment. Because the wife had a good voice, I gave her a crash course in Sound Healing, so that she could continue the treatment on her husband at home, in case the effect of Sound Healing on him was positive. While healing her husband I therefore eagerly explained the Sound Healing process, while trying to maintain my focus on the man's energy field with my sound.

When I came home I went to bed, doubled over with violent pains in my large intestine. It was not until several hours later when my husband wanted to drive me to the hospital, that I realized which disease I had just been confronted with.

If I feel weak or tired before leading Sound Healing courses, I sometimes sing a short self-composed song that protects me from being drained of energy. I encourage you to compose your own song or verse if possible, because the considerations you make when doing so will be beneficial. I have not protected myself for many years, and I don't normally do so now either, because I trust spirit full heartedly.

But if I feel in need to strengthen myself in a challenging situation I sing the following words eventually while walking, dancing, sungazing (barefoot for grounding):

I am surrounded by angels and protected by
The Note from Heaven
Unconditional love, unconditional love…
That's what I give, that's what I get
That's what I radiate, that's what I spread

Let my heart be filled with your light
Let my soul shine freely and bright

The Structure of a Sound Healing Session

When you carry out Sound Healing, working within a set framework or structure can give you and thereby the Receiver a sense of security. The structure is not the main issue. What is important is that you, the Sound Healer, feel completely secure, so that you are able to surrender to the Note from Heaven without having to think too much. There are important details regarding Sound Healing in this chapter, so do not skip over them, even if you already know which structure you work with. The following structure is inspired by the Spanish Master José's system, Mystical Therapy. It can be used with or without sound. The participants in my Sound Healing courses also learn to heal without sound. Silence is a part of the sound picture.

Opening Ritual

Introduction

You give the client your hand and welcome him/her by saying their name. Candles are lit. Water is poured.139 You and the client define a clear wish for the session. If it is their first session, explain what is going to happen, and tell the client that it is their responsibility to interfere if he/she feels anything is not comfortable. In a combined treatment the Recipient will be instructed in breathing with the stomach and how to sing the Note from Heaven. Depending on the problem it is an option that the Recipient can sing themselves free. After this it is time for Sound Healing.140 Ask for permission to touch him/her lightly and to hold him/her under the neck and close the ears with the roots of your thumbs, when you Sound Heal around the head. The Sound Healing takes place with the Recipient lying on a couch or on a mattress on the floor. Make sure the Recipient is lying comfortably. Briefly, see if the Recipient needs an extra pillow under their head, a cushion under their knees, maybe an extra duvet and that their feet are tucked in.

Practical Information

If the client has a hearing aid or glasses, ask them to remove them and put them in a safe place. Let the Recipient know that they can say anything to you at any time, if they feel like it. They are welcome to go to the bathroom during the course of the session, as Sound Healing can increase pressure on the bladder in some cases.

Opening Ceremony

Tilt your neck slightly back and widen your arms out to the sides with hands open, palms facing upwards. Ask to receive love and light down to the Recipient. The Recipient's name is mentioned and the specific wishes that the Recipient has asked for are spoken out loud, for example: *"I ask for love and light for Peter who wishes to dissolve the root cause of his cancer."* Or: *"Jesus, we call upon you to heal Bente's leukemia so that she can be totally cured."*

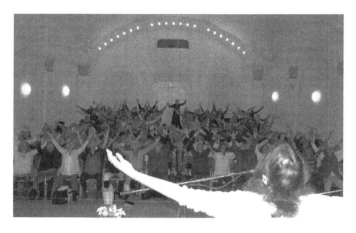

Lower your arms slowly, still with open hands, palms facing upwards. On the way down, you will feel light pricks of energy in your hands. The main opening for the transfer of energy from the universe is in the hands and the head.

Sound Healing the Energy Field

Hum softly while improvising a lullaby with gliding notes while the Recipient's energy field is stroked with soft, slow movements that resemble caresses in the air.

Kinesiologists have noted that it is best to stroke in an upwards motion over the body, when you are working in the aura's layers. For me, either way feels good. During the stroking, you can move from 80 cm down to 2 cm away from the body, in the various layers of the aura. In the same way, the hands can outline the aura's oval shape around the body, as it is stroked and rounded. The same procedure can be done at the halo around the head, marking it with soft, shaping strokes. For some, the humming can be the most pleasant of all. There is something extraordinarily balancing, subtle and invigorating about being hum-healed.

Sound Scanning the Energy Field

Open the Antenna/Silver thread

As some people get a headache when the energy in the body rises during the session, I usually start a Sound Healing by opening the energy field in the top of the head, so that the pressure of energy can be released, when it is rising to the head.

Position yourself behind the client's head and sing approximately 60-80 centimeters away from the crown of the head and find a high note that resonates here. The vocal light should be directed towards the middle of the crown. After having sung out in the edges of the aura, the top of the crown is touched lightly with the second and/or third finger of the right hand. The right hand is the masculine and giving hand. The left represents the feminine side and primarily receives energy, but it can also be used during Sound Healing. I then scan the crown and find a high sound that resonates here. If you are weak in the high register, find a register suitable for you. Use of the correct support will strengthen the development of high notes in your voice over time.

Slide now with the vocal light over the body in a soft, descending improvisation, finishing in low notes at the feet.

Sound Scanning the Body

When you are sound scanning the vibration can be passed from your body by a gentle touch. The lighter the touch the stronger the energy will pass from you to the client. Imagine that the electric receivers of the system are very sensitive and are lying just under the skin. If you press them the slightest, they close, but if you connect with a gentle touch as a butterfly wing, then the energy flows.

1. Sing undertones/low notes 60-80 centimeters away from the feet. "Huu" and "Hoo" will create the deepest undertones.

2. Sing directly on the toes. Gently hold the big toes with the healing fingers (index and middle finger). If the undertones resonate well in the big toes, then stay there for a while. As a general rule, if the notes are difficult to produce in a certain area, go on to the next point. The area may open itself during the Sound Healing of other parts of the body.

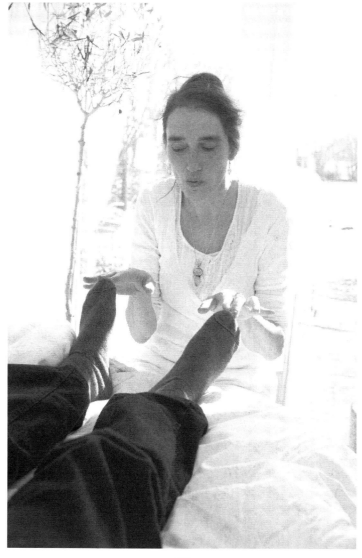

3. Undertones are sung on the ankles.

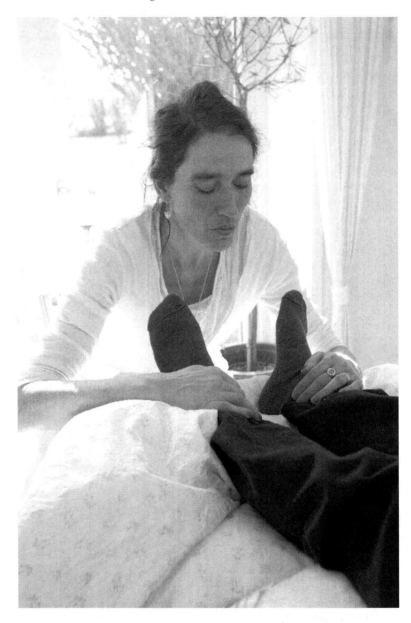

4. Undertones are sung on the knees.

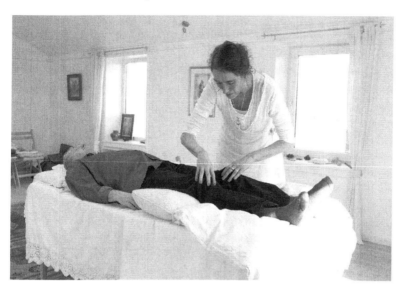

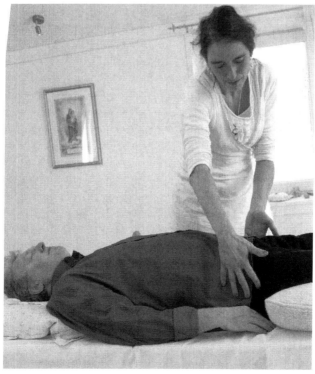

5. Undertones are sung on the hips, where both hands are laid lightly on either side of the pelvis. You can also abstain from using your hands. The vocal light can be directed at the genitals with discretion/at an appropriate distance. If a point of resonance can be opened in this area, then there is a possibility for tonal ascension through the spine from the base of the torso. (We are not talking about a kundalini release, but a flow of energy.)

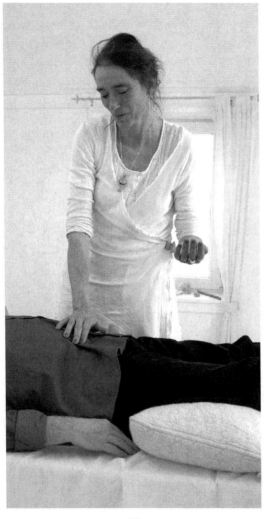

6. There may be a need for undertones or low notes at the stomach area. Judge this for yourself, based on which note resonates the best with your vocal light. The vowel "Aaar" is broad and can work well at the stomach, because there is a large area with fluid here. Experiment with the different vowels and use the one that resonates the best.

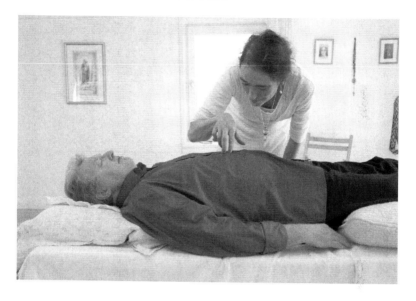

7. Solar Plexus. Sound Healing using "Huu" tends to resonate very precisely here. Be also aware of the stomach, kidneys, adrenal glands and the pancreas placed in – or close to – this area. Experiment with vowels and distance as previously described.

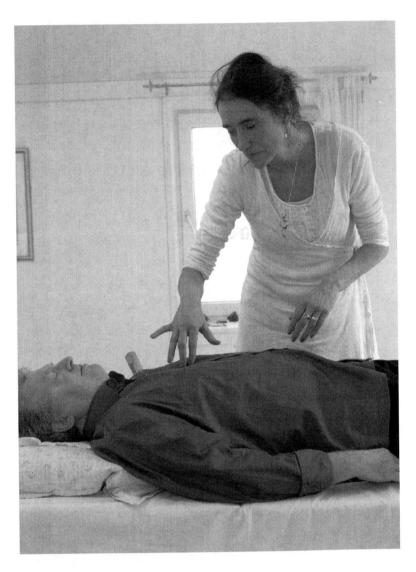

8. The Heart Chakra. You can lay your hands on the middle of the breastbone or also touch the breastbone lightly with the fingertips. Follow the sound of the vocal light in an examination of the chest area. If the Recipient becomes moved, ask them to let go and sing on the cry notes if he/she is tensing/holding back the tears. A light hand on the forehead and/or a clear and comforting

"Huuu" sound on the third eye (middle of the forehead) will calm the client as the higher consciousness is animated, and feelings are balanced. If there are strong emotions, the Recipient can sing them out supported by the Sound Healer. Some clients enjoy singing together with the healer during a Sound Healing treatment. This is fine, unless it makes a precise sound scanning impossible, in which case I ask the client to refrain. I then let them know when they may sing again.

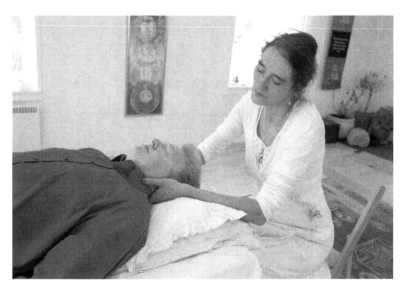

9. The Throat Chakra. The transition from the chest voice to the head voice. Never put your hands directly on the Recipient's throat. The healing fingers/fingertips are laid discretely in the middle of the collarbone. Alternatively, position yourself behind the head and from here lightly place a hand on either side of the throat. It's difficult to get close with the vocal light in this position, as you then breathe directly in the face of the client. If it is necessary to get close, hold your hand over one ear and sing from that side. Then change sides. Another alternative is to shield with the left hand so that your breath doesn't blow directly onto the client's face. It is pleasant for the Recipient,

when you lay a hand on each shoulder, as it lifts the burden of emotional stress away.

Yet another method is to place your hands carefully under the neck and hold them in a bowl-shape with your two index fingers in the two recesses found under the edge of the cranium, on either side of the middle. In this position, you can close the Recipient's ears with the root of your thumbs, when needed. I do this for the sake of safety, in case the sound is very powerful and penetrating. The "Iii" sound has especially strong and cutting overtones. Some clients sleep obliviously during the Sound Healing.

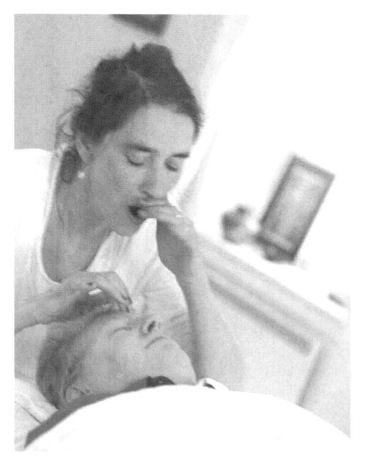

10. The Third Eye. A relatively high note. A discreet third finger or index finger is held lightly on the center. Another possibility is to lightly hold your right hand over the forehead. Follow your intuition. Contact with the energy field in the forehead gives peace and clarity and can advantageously be combined with the other chakras, for example by holding the left hand lightly at the solar plexus while holding the right hand on the forehead. In this way overwhelming feelings can be calmed.

There can be a lot of energy in the third eye, and sometimes your fingers or hand can lightly quiver with energy.

If you do not experience energy in your hand, raise the left hand up in the air, while you Heal with the right hand. You will collect extra energy like this. A part of Indian ayurvedic therapy is to pour warm peanut oil in a thin, constant stream onto the third eye. It has a very gentle, deep, and relaxing effect. You can do something similar by blowing warm air onto the third eye. You will need to go very close, though, so that the air doesn't cool down. Try doing it in the palm of your hand.

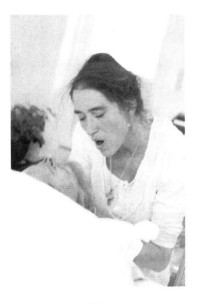

11. The Crown Chakra symbolizes the "spiritual hole" through which communication with intuition takes place. It is here that you, in the introduction to the Sound Healing, found a point of resonance with a high note. Now the cycle is closed. If the Recipient has been able to open up in the root chakra, the crown chakra will most likely also be able to open. If there is still plenty of heavy baggage hidden in the shadow, the organism may be vulnerable to the strong light from the crown chakra. In that case it can be difficult for the Sound Healer to find resonance in the high register. The organism must be able to bear the weight of its baggage in a cleansing process.

The organism is so wisely designed that it always protects itself. A gradual cleansing is preferred in order to avoid strong side effects. Each of us have our own limitations, which are expressed through individual physical reactions. In this way, the Sound Healer's voice will not be able to reach further than the Recipient's body allows, as the voice will simply shut down. However, this will not occur if the Sound Healer transfers his or her own feelings to the Recipient. This is why it is so important to Sound Heal with scanning and listen as much as possible to the Recipient's signals.

12. Now you are free to Sound Heal as you see fit. A possibility is to glide slowly along the main row of chakras to create flow along the spine. Or there may be particular places that require extra attention. If in the beginning there was poor resonance at the feet or in another place, go back and try to see if the situation has changed. It does usually change when the whole body has been scanned, because the energy from an open area finds its way to the closed areas and has been affecting them.

13. One possibility that can be applied to the entire session is to start an energy flow between two points of resonance. This can be done by holding the fingertips with the palms of the hands

facing one another on their own points on the body. With one hand here and one there, glide between the two points. (See the image below.)

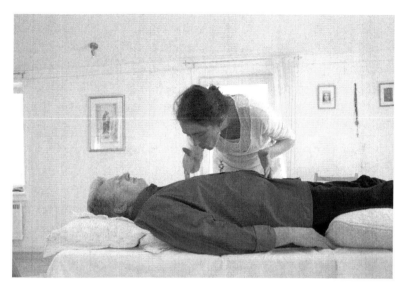

The hands work like plus/minus in a magnetic field and the voice supports the current, as it glides from one resonance point to the other. Gliding between resonance points demands that you are an experienced sound scanner, because you will need to remember the tonal interval between the two points. It is an advantage to practice ear training/note names order[141] to be quick to hear where the resonance points are as you pass them. A sensitive Recipient will clearly be able to physically feel a slow gliding note between two resonance points.

14. If you have read my books Heal the Pineal and or Help, you will know how to scan the endocrine system by focusing the inner undertones of "Hung Song" on the Pineal gland, hypothalamus, pituitary gland, thyroid gland, thymus, adrenal glands and the ovaries/prostate. Any anatomical knowledge is great to have because you can be exact and pin pointed. For

example, in cases of stress and shock-related trauma, I would stimulate the amygdala and hippocampus in the brain because the amygdala is our body's traffic light. The light may flash red even though the danger passed a long time ago. The hippocampus then processes the alarm signals from the amygdala as if there is still a danger situation. The signals from the amygdala and hippocampus are directly related to the adrenal glands. In case of stress, it is therefore beneficial to stimulate an energy flow between the amygdala and the adrenal glands using the method described in point 13. If undertones appear, use internal undertones in "hang, hong or hung" depending on the resonance of your vocal light.

Another important piece of information is that if someone is seriously ill, it is crucial to sound scan the liver because it is the largest detox organ in the body. In case of trauma sound around the liver, saturate it with undertones. As described in my book Help, sound healing of the liver can be supported by a wrap of warm castor oil at night, as castor oil (Ricinus oil/Christo's oil/ American oil) supports the release of the toxins that the sound healing may have loosened. The more anatomy you know, the more accurate the spirit can be in the communication through you.

Rounding off and concluding a Sound Healing Session

While humming, stroke slowly with flat hands in a line approximately 20 centimeters above the body up over the row of chakras, which are thereby closed down to their normal level. If the chakras remain wide open, the client can be hypersensitive to the impressions around them. The energy centers are closed down by consciously thinking: "Now I am closing the energy system back to normal condition."

Then, as in the intro, the entire energy field is stroked with soft humming.

Finally, a couple of spirals are traced with the fingertips, from the forehead and upwards in the air over the third eye. This ritual is done to bring the Recipient's consciousness back to reality (some are far gone/sleeping deeply). Most often, the Recipient is lying and cuddled by/lingering in the pleasant, soft energies after the Sound Healing.

After the agreed relaxation time, the Sound Healer rings a bell. Strike the bell carefully three times and let each note ring out before the next strike. I have experienced that a pure bell sound has made my entire energy system pulsate with the bell's frequency after having received healing. It is a very pleasant sensation.

Gratitude Ritual

As the final closure to the Sound Healing session, I lay both of my hands on my heart chakra and give thanks for the love, energy, light and healing that we have received. This ritual should not be confused with a forced feeling of piety. What is essential is that the ritual awakens a feeling of deep affection and gratitude in the heart for the healing that has just been taking place. The veil leading to the Oneness level is closed.

If the Recipient is moved by this gesture, the ritual will be twice as powerful, because a genuine feeling of gratitude manifests itself by the organism acknowledging that a healing has occurred.

I find this part of the healing process to be among the most important. Sound Healing is an exquisite gift, as both the Healer and the Recipient receive the healing energy. If the feeling of gratitude feels unnatural, you can practice it, simply by placing your hands over your heart. The energy that occurs in this gesture can be surprisingly moving, and awaken a natural gratitude in you.

Deep down in every person there is a longing – a longing for higher dimensions – the miracle in ourselves. A miracle can only manifest if the Recipient accommodates it with gratitude.

After Sound Healing the Recipient is usually thirsty and needs a glass of water. You should drink too.

Water strengthens the effect of healing.

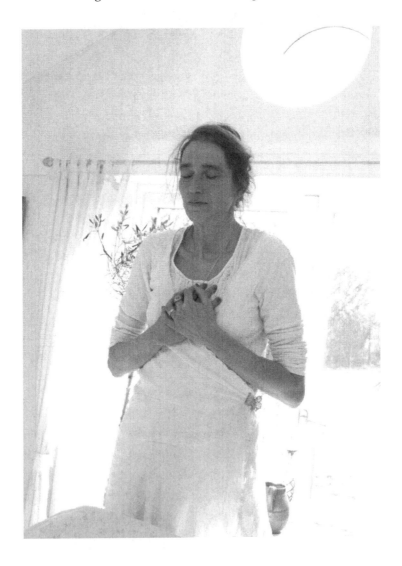

The Structure of a Sound Healing

I. Opening ritual presenting the wish

II. Stroking the aura while humming

III. Opening at the head and feet

IV. Sing up through the body on the seven chakras along the spine

V. Sing on areas that need special attention

VI. Stroking the aura while humming, as the chakras are closed down again

VII. Gratitude ritual

Examples of Special Sound Healing Sounds

Dolphin sounds

From the Recipient's cheekbones and upwards, dolphin sounds can occur. These are sung at the top of the short register, using "nngg-iih" sounds. Maintain your focus on a bright "ee" sound. These short, high, ng-nasal sounds can have a strong releasing effect and help people into a state of consciousness, that they would otherwise not have access to. In addition, a search around the short register can lead to a discovery of a super high note. The "nngg" sound opens the vault of the nasal cavity, and the "ee" on top takes the sound to new heights. Try also to supplement it with a cleansing "he" (i-nteresting). The dolphin sound can release the area around the third eye by means of a playfully light sensation. As a Sound Healer, if you have a hard time reaching the higher octaves, do not try to force the notes out. Contact with the higher notes will occur naturally during sound scanning when the voice is ready.

Singing low notes relaxes the vocal cords and therefore makes them more flexible when they are stretched in the high register. A good way to practice high notes is to play with your laugh up on a high nasal "nghi, nghi, nghi" sound. If it is easier to laugh "har, har, har", you can reach the top of your vocal register by letting the laugh increase in tempo and become a hysterical vibrato which goes over in furious, cutting Mongolian song (this is primarily for women's voices). There must be complete support from the diaphragm, so that the voice is able to resonate freely in the high register without becoming tense and pained. After having sung high notes for a reasonable amount of time, it is a good idea to limber up afterwards with undertones.

Silver thread notes

An imaginary silver thread is drawn from the crown of the head and outwards like an antenna which is being unfolded. This thread symbolizes the connection to cosmic consciousness.[142] The drawing of the silver thread happens at the same time as the voice produces an upward glissando in the short register, preferably with dolphin sounds, if they occur way up at the extreme edge of the voice's abilities. It's a kind of game mixed together with Sound Healing. The audience tends to smile when I pull the silver thread during Sound Healing demonstrations. Is this for real or a joke? The healing occurs in the meeting between humor and seriousness, where the energy has optimal terms to work freely. As a rule, the Recipient notices more effect than the audience realizes, so the Recipient often doesn't laugh. It can feel like a liberating cleansing of the mind when your antenna is extended. It is through the crown chakra, that our individual frequency resonates and communicates with the outside world/the universe.

Asinine sounds/Trauma sound

The closest I can get to describing this sound, which is a far cry from that which we in our culture perceive as aesthetically pleasing, is the donkey sound "Hee haaw". This sound is impossible to express consciously by the Sound Healer. It appears as a rather scary sound, which shifts between two or more notes in a vocal transition: A fast repetition of hiccups between the falsetto and chest registers. In my general experience, this sound occurs when the Recipient is carrying a trauma, which the body yearns to be released from. So you can say that this rough, pulsating sound is the body's cry for help. One Recipient once told me that this asinine sound seemed to express all the fear that she was not able to express herself. The sound transformed her. She felt like God knew her from within and had expressed her deepest feelings.

As a Sound Healer, I blindly trust that the sound is doing the job that needs to be done. If the client seems open to dialogue, I ask about the trauma connected to the sound. You need to be careful here, because some people's pain body will get nourishment from the suspicion that they possibly have been a victim of violent, psychological or sexual abuse in this or previous lives, without them having known about it beforehand. Don't give any fuel to the slightest sign of a glowing ember here. It is blocked energy that is calling to be resolved. We can never know the exact truth about what is the cause of a trauma, but we can sing forth a symbolic story and change it.[143] The donkey sound has a loosening up effect, that any other sounds or words cannot compete with, so receive it as a gift, if it occurs. Let the sound continue until the Recipient's body is saturated and the trauma redeemed. The Trauma sound will then disappear and a steady note replaces it.

Vibrato sounds

Wild vibrato sounds that swing rather evenly up and down can occur. These are sounds I would not be able to produce under any circumstances, even if someone asked me to. The art is to trust that the voice knows better than you do. Accept it and let the voice vibrate freely in any fashion it may choose. When an obviously completely foreign sound flows through you, it is normally followed by a high release of energy.

Your own sounds

Be aware that you may receive your own individual messages or signs connected to particular vocal expressions. If you are open and allow the voice to lead you, it will come naturally, when you are ready for it. When you gain experience and know how your voice normally sounds, it can come as a surprise that your voice begins tugging at the reins. So listen to your voice with an open attitude, and allow it to move freely while you follow along, astonished. Where are we going now?

The Use of Organ During Sound Healing

Inspired by the above and by Dr. Karl,[144] I have experimented with using organ sounds with individual Sound Healing. On an electric piano I choose an organ sound that goes well with my voice.

The organ sound has an embracing effect with its powerful vibration. During sound scanning I choose – if my intuition demands it – to amplify the vocal light with the organ. I then double my voice with fundamental notes and fifths on the organ, which are kept going with the pedal. The volume is kept loud in order that the Recipient can feel it in the body, but it should also be adjusted in relation to the power of the voice. An amazing overtone alchemy occurs when the sound of the voice melts together with the fifths in the organ. If you press the wrong keys, the pedal should be lifted, and you begin anew. The expression begins to resemble music, and most clients feel uplifted with the combination. During "organ" sound scanning, the organ sequences appear as small, refreshing breaths of fresh air. In this way, the Sound Healer moves from a pure vocal sound to organ/vocal and back again to the Recipient to sound scan them several times, if necessary. When the organ sound is stopped, it is faded slowly out with the volume knob.

It is my experience that around the heart area the F or F# often appears. Here the organ should only be played on the F/F#

without adding a fifth to it, because then it is easier to make interference notes with the voice sliding up as close as possible – just under or just over the F or F#. The fifth of the organ is a well-tempered fifth, and that already makes it work slightly against the Fibonacci sequency which is building on the Music of the Spheres – Natural Overtones.

Alternative Sound Healing Positions

In case of deep traumas from early childhood, it can be effective if the Sound Healer takes on the role of a mother/father:

If the Sound Healer and the Recipient have built up a close relationship, the Sound Healer can sit down on the floor and embrace the Recipient from the back, while singing and possibly gently rocking them. This can work well with children, animals, and also adults that have a need for love and contact. The Recipient sits on the floor with their back towards the Healer's stomach so that the Healer's voice will resonate from his/her torso into the Recipient's back. I will normally only do this with someone I am sure won't be offended, and when I know that it will not awaken any sexual undertones.

There are certain ailments in neck and back where it's an advantage for the client to be sitting on a chair. But in a sitting position, the Recipient will lose the feeling of deep relaxation they would otherwise gain by lying down. So there are both pluses and minuses by using the sitting position. In a quick, acute healing, it's alright if the Recipient is sitting. In lectures or workshops where I demonstrate Sound Healing it is normally done on a chair.

If you have a grand piano, you can experiment with having the (not too heavy) Recipient lying down (carefully) on the sound box covering the strings, which then will resonate into the body of the Recipient during Vocal Sound healing, maybe also combined with playing the piano.

If a Recipient has breathing problems due to acute stress,

they could begin the session by lying in the fetal position during Sound Healing. Here the Sound Healer gently can hold on to the sides of the lower part of the Recipient's back and support their breathing by drawing the hands outwards when the Recipient is breathing in.

About Offering Sound Healing

Jesus said:
Ye are the light of the world and that light should be seen, just as a town that is built on a hill can be seen from afar. A candle is not lighted to be hidden under a bushel. Nay, it must stand high and free so it gives light to all. In the same way, let the light ye have been given shine before people, so they may be inspired by it and glorify The Heavenly Source.
Matthew 5:14-16

Be honest and make visible who you are, and what you can offer.

The effect of Sound Healing speaks for itself. By all means, wear the cures/improvements you affect in people via Sound Healing as feathers in your cap. They will strengthen your authority and willingness to trust in the powers that work through you. If the Recipient is willing to write down the effects, give a review of the results or even give an interview to a camera. Your authority as a Sound Healer will be strengthened as long as you keep humble. Cures are easily forgotten with time. When a cure occurs, the Recipient is given a new zest for life and only wishes to move forward. As a Sound Healer you think that you can remember all of the details, but in reality you can't. So do write down any results and details.

The first time you experience the healing power of sound flowing through you, you can be overwhelmed with a desire to save the world. This is natural. However, in your enthusiasm, try to avoid convincing or forcing people to receive Sound Healing.

I have stepped over the line a couple of times and experienced that being eager gives no positive results, as it awakens the Recipient's defense mechanism, which then shuts the body off from receiving energy. The result is that you end up wasting your own energy, the energy of the Recipient, and the energy of the higher consciousness.

It's a matter of sharing sound with the Recipient, rather than convincing them of the effects of sound. Be careful with your family. It is the biggest challenge to withdraw from helping dear family members from serious illnesses, when they refuse to receive treatment from you. It is a natural reaction. Often family cannot see you as a healer, because they know you personally.

Let people contact you, maybe in the beginning from a poster where you offer free Sound Healing, and make it clear that you need guinea pigs and are offering Sound Healing.

But of course, in critical situations you should not hide and wait for people to ask for a Sound Healing, when they do not even know your abilities. You must help out in whatever way you can – always with respect for the Recipient – if the Recipient requires assistance, and if it feels right to do so. For example, in an emergency, like when a woman slipped down and wiggled on her ankle right in front of me, I sat down and put my hands on her ankle first in silence, and after asking her permission, I added undertones. The woman contacted me later and said that her ankle had healed and that the fracture had disappeared within two weeks.

But in general the Recipient needs to make contact him/ herself in order to be as open as possible. The same applies to well-meaning relatives that make contact on behalf of a sick person. Ask the sick person to make contact themselves, if they possibly can.

Sometimes, a long journey can work miracles. The fact that

a client has invested time and money in coming for a treatment is a testament to their belief and willpower, which creates an opening in their energy field, making them receptive to Sound Healing. The question of whether the healing should cost money or not is a classical issue. In some cases, the treatment will lose its healing effect if it is free, because money is about value. In other cases, if you surprise the Recipient by rejecting money, it can awaken a deep gratitude within the Recipient which can strengthen the healing. At the same time, there is an energetic balance sheet to be taken into account, as the Sound Healer's time and energy must be offset. Everything is a question of balance.

Too few clients

If it is hard for you to attract clients it may be due to a deep rooted fear, an inner fight with your ego: "Am I good enough?" If you take on the role of Sound Healer instead of being one, the power of the sound is impaired, because it is the ego that takes on the role.

It is impossible to get around this. And if you have read my story, you know a little about the process. It is about opening the voice, open, open, and leaning back into your innocence. – About being able to be a blank piece of paper, whenever it is needed. The desire to do Vocal Sound Healing feels like a burning urge to serve in this field.

I have trained Sound Healers that, despite good results, still don't believe that they are good enough. The ego will not allow them to take on the role of Sound Healer. The fear of being made an outcast in the local, tribal-minded society is very powerful. A great number of healers have been burned as witches throughout the history of mankind.

We all have our own path in life, and it is therefore of great importance to develop the talents we have been given. If you repress yourself, the repressed powers will make themselves known sooner or later, often in an uncontrollable and or twisted form.

One stands strongest by being oneself. If you feel the sound calling you and if it feels right and natural for you, then go for it. It is an art to be a Sound Healer, and like any other art, some people are more skilled than others. You know that you are a Sound Healer the day you get a healing result and at the same time know that it was not you that did the job. You might have sound scanned hundreds of times without big results, and then all of a sudden Spirit starts to work through you and you stand baffled with the knowledge that for sure this was not you doing this. This is the paradox: Sound Healing works when you have gained enough humbleness in knowing that you have passed the test of being worth to be nothing.

The moment you get convincing results, the rumor will spread. And if you ignite your light and let it shine from the rooftop, so everyone can see you, then people will surely find you.

Too many clients

As a practicing Sound Therapist, you must listen carefully to yourself; because if you don't, sooner or later your body will force you to. Following an appearance on a popular TV show, I was called by hundreds of viewers in need of Sound Healing. My diary was soon booked several months in advance by people from near and afar.

The thought of the many treatments to come made me feel nauseous and my enthusiasm sank dramatically: How could I follow up on each client should they need several treatments? And I knew from experience that they would, if I was to treat them properly. It was a full house. Success, or the opposite? My voice gave me the answer: It disappeared. It was not until I cancelled everything that my voice returned.

I write this book in the hope that perhaps you as a potential

Sound Healer can help me to Sound Heal the many people who are interested, and who will sign up once the amazing healing potential of sound becomes known to the man on the street.

There are some therapists who, without warning, suddenly can't cope dealing with people's problems anymore. To avoid this happening to you, listen to your body. It should remain a pleasure to Sound Heal and never become an exhausting duty. Take care of your time. Some people like to get personal attention. It is not your job to give attention – it is your job to let Spirit heal people through you, and that happens normally within five to ten minutes, when you are a well-trained instrument.

Sound Healing Combinations

Sound Healing Two Recipients

If possible, the Recipients are positioned with their heads in the same direction, because the energies at the head and feet usually have different frequencies. If the Sound Healer is working with touch in combination with sound scanning, the Recipients will need to lie with enough space between them, so that the Sound Healer can easily reach the seven primary chakras on both of them at the same time.

The big toes can be touched lightly with one hand between each of the Recipients' feet. A hand is placed between the ankles of each Recipient. With outstretched fingers, a touch of the ankles is implied, depending on how widely the Recipients' legs are spread. Sometimes you can almost feel the sparks jump from the little finger and thumb when touch is only implied.

The same applies at the knees. At the hips, one Recipient at a time is touched, or both at once in the air over the root chakra. On the hara, solar plexus, heart, throat, the third eye and crown chakra, one hand is used on each Recipient. Here there is no differentiation between right hand and left hand energy.

As far as the sound is concerned, your focus alternates from one to the other. It is optimal if you can get the same sound to resonate with both clients at the same time. The position of the hands will need to be adjusted, so that they mark the resonance points that have been found. After a general going through the seven chakras, each client is given Sound Healing on specific areas.

All of this is just a guide. Follow your intuition first and foremost. Sometimes the sound that you thought had healed one of the clients will have healed the other. The body absorbs the sound that it requires.

Sound Healing of Groups

When you Sound Heal bigger groups of people you need a strong faith in Spirit.

At the beginning of a Sound Healing session I always ask to receive love and light for the Recipients. After that I open my voice up to the Note from Heaven. This can happen unaccompanied or with a tanpura, Tibetan bells, bowls, guitar or piano/organ accompaniment.

The prerequisite for a successful Sound Healing of a group is that the Sound Healer is open and unprejudiced, as this gives Spirit/the higher powers the greatest possible latitude. When the higher powers connect with the Sound Healer, he or she glides into a state of being that radiates a natural authority.

The preparation for Sound Healing a group is based on the inestimably important work with the Note from Heaven that you do on your own, and in the practice of sound scanning in one-on-one situations.

When you express a true openness, you resonate with devotion and pass this on to the Recipients. The role of the Sound Healer is to call on the higher healing powers and support the participants in opening themselves up to these. Your merging with the divine will inspire the participants to a similar merging.

If fear-of-failure takes over, the divine power will be cut off and you will stand there like a fairy without power in your magic wand. The participants are dependent on your ability to channel devotion and affection – to surrender yourself to the higher powers. You are their channel – the one that builds the bridge between the worlds. You will only feel an urge to heal groups, when you are ready to bear this responsibility.

In my International Education of The Note from Heaven, the students are learning an alternative to free Sound Healing: "Song for deep relaxation and healing" which can be used safely for healing of groups. In this song each part of the body is dedicated a verse – for example: "Your feet are merging into an infinite darkness, sinking deep down, leaving all tension behind. Your feet's light body is lifted high up above blessed by heavenly light – blessed by heavenly light."

The Sound Healer sings themselves through the body while sending healing to the body part described in the specific verse. The recipients are lying down and relaxing for 15-20 minutes while the Sound Healer walks around among them and sings for them. People love it because it reminds them of a lullaby. I myself am very fond of listening to the recording of this song,[145] as I get the energy of about 2-3 hours' sleep in 20 minutes.

Sound Healers on the Same Wavelength

When two people sing together in harmony, a third, elevated energy is born.

As Dr. Karl expresses on page 347, it is only advantageous to carry out Sound Healing with another if there is harmony between you. This harmony cannot be desired or learned. It occurs when two or more people are on the same wavelength.

We are each born with our own fundamental frequency. It doesn't pay to try to change your fundamental frequency in order to adapt to your surroundings. Your fundamental frequency is you. If you run away from it, you lose yourself. The prerequisite for meeting true resonance in another person is that you completely uphold your own sound. If your fundamental frequency is wrapped up in dissonant diverted notes that have occurred in an attempt to adapt to your surroundings, you resonate with people that have corresponding dissonances.

When you become aware of the dissonances, your resonance will gradually change, and new frequency structures will occur in your social relationships. Despite the unpleasantness of change, you will give everyone a gift by seizing your own clearly ringing bell and tolling it out over the continents. Like the Pied Piper, you will attract kindred spirits, and the resonance that your innermost longings call for will occur.

Resonance awakens unconditional love.

A person who has the full courage of his/her convictions will shine like a sun and inspire everyone, regardless of resonance level. Everyone will be able to hear or notice the quality of the bell's sound, as it will nourish and inspire its surroundings. If two such clear bells ring together in resonance, a miracle is born. The gate to the heavens opens, and the Holy Spirit descends as a third configuration.

Sound Healing as a Duo

Both Lars Muhl, my eldest son and I have worked together on Sound Healing a client. The advantage of being two Sound Healers is that interference tones occur when you sing similar notes, but not at exactly the same frequency. If you have an ear for these interference notes, which are very low and can feel like a vibrating insect or a dry rustling sound in the ear, you can produce them together. We are talking about much lower notes than the human voice normally can produce.

I don't know much about the effects of these notes, but it feels good inside the ear, and Recipients give positive feedback. The founder of BioAcoustics, Sharry Edwards, used specific interference tones on her son's smashed knee and it resulted in the growth of a whole new kneecap.[146]

So these support tones seem to be able to build up new cells.

Experiencing resonance with a Sound Healing partner, you feel connected on all levels. You feel free and whole and breathe a sigh of relief. There occurs a natural listening, a state of being within the mutual improvisatory Sound Healing expression. Harmony, happiness. You open your mouth, and the overtones flow out like a bubbling brook without you knowing where they come from.

The acoustics in a room are also important. When Lars and I have Sound Healed groups together, there have occasionally been situations where we were not able to hear each other properly. The psyche reacted immediately with sadness when the upper, lightly hovering communication lost its glow and fell to the ground.

The chemistry between two people is fine-tuned through sound work. The harmony is as fragile as the finest, thinnest porcelain. You cannot be too careful with how you treat resonance. The smallest amount of dirt on the "sound" surface creates discord and therefore sharpens the practitioner's attention in the name of Sound Healing.

The Fifth

When singing more people together you can work with the harmony of the fifth. The fifth is the fifth tone from the ground note of the major scale. The distance between the first two notes in *Can't Help Falling in Love "Wise men say..."* and *My Favorite Things* is a fifth. The reason why this tonal interval is creating harmony is that the fifth is the first clear overtone to appear after the octave in the fractal structure of overtones. So by singing the fifth, a Fibonacci spiral can occur and rebuild cells that are out of balance, by reminding them the natural sound shape they originate from.

Choral Sound Scanning

It is possible to carry out Choral Sound Scanning with a group of four or more people. In some cases, this form of Sound Healing has a strong effect. When I had weekly Sound Healing courses in Copenhagen, we experimented by asking the Recipient about the difference in sensation with being sound scanned by me and receiving Choral Sound Scanning by the whole group.

The feedback was the same with respect to the sensation: When I Sound Scanned by myself, it had an isolating and precise effect. When the group sang, the effect was a broad spectrum, and the Recipient felt as if they were being illuminated from several sides on the area in question.

As far as the effects were concerned, there was mixed feedback: Some were attracted by the precise effect, others by the broad spectrum effect.

Choral Sound Scanning is a nice way to sing together, which develops the participant's listening abilities. At the same time it is a moving gesture, because one person gets the full attention of the group.

The Recipient lies in the middle and is evenly surrounded by the rest of the group. One or two participants stand at the feet and sing undertones. One or two participants, who are good at high notes, stand at the head. The rest of the group stands at the sides. The conductor of Choral Sound Scanning stands inside the circle near the Recipient and conducts with standard hand gestures: The conductor can cut off, wave the sound on, show weaker or stronger dynamics, close parts of the group off and bring forward, for example, the basses (undertone singing).

Procedure for Choral Sound Healing:

1. As in a normal Sound Healing, the arms are raised up with open hands facing upwards, while the participants surrender to becoming channels for love and light.

2. The group softly stroke the Recipient's aura on all layers while humming.

3. Choral Sound Scanning typically starts with the undertone singers at the feet. It is important that they sing undertones and not real tones, as these can inhibit the scanning.

4. The conductor gradually scans the Recipient from the feet and upwards over the body. When a point of resonance is found on the Recipient, the conductor keeps the vocal light here and gives a sign to the rest of the group to sing along. If the sound is very low or high, the conductor can choose to sing a triad, so that the participants are able to choose the sound that best suits their voice.

5. When the group has a good grip on the sound, the conductor can choose to signal the choir to continue, while she improvises further up on the Recipient's body and finds a new point of resonance, which resonates with the sung harmony. If there are experienced Sound Healers in the group, others from the group can begin to sing melodic phrases, and a beautiful choral work unfolds its wings. It is the conductor's responsibility to stop the group song when a new note is to be scanned, or if chaos occurs in the choir's expression.

6. When the Choral Sound Scanning is over, the aura is carefully stroked/the energy field is closed during soft humming with calm movements.

7. Gratitude Ritual: Hands on the heart.

Sound Healing based on the Sound of the Heart

During Lars Muhl's and my cooperation in Sound Healing individuals, a method arose which is based on the sound that resonates with the Recipient's heart.

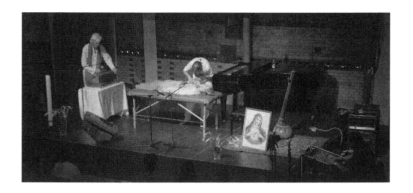

Lars is sitting by the harmonium, while I sound scan the Recipient over the heart area. When the resonance of the heart is found, Lars amplifies the sound with his Indian organ (if the sound resonates with microtones which are not found on the organ, I try to find one which does).

The music that follows is improvised, and we work with the Recipient's heart sound as a fundamental note. Lars improvises with his voice and harmonium, while I sing on the Recipient and find sounds and expressions here. Sometimes Lars stops using the harmonium and sound scans together with me. The process happens in the now, which we must submit to in consummate listening. During these Sound Healing sessions that we have done in front of an audience of up to 450 people, the entire audience is affected by the treatment. The musical key can change during the process if certain points of resonance show themselves on other parts of the body.

Communal Sound Healing

In Communal Sound Healing, the participants are divided up according to time, space, and number of mattresses. Let us say that there are 30 participants and that there is space for ten to lie in parallel in a long row. The ten lying down are positioned so that their heads are facing the same direction. The other 20 carry out the Sound Healing.

If you have 30 minutes for the session, there will be three rounds of healing at approximately six minutes each, with four minutes set aside for awakening/alternating. The Sound Healers stand together in front of the Recipients like a choir.

Guidelines for instruction:

1) The Sound Healers comfort the Receivers. If anybody looks like they need a blanket or a pillow, they do their best to support them.

2) "Sound Healers, lift your arms, tilt your head back slightly, ask to receive love and light for the Recipients, lower your arms slowly and now give the energy you have collected in the palms of your hands to the Recipients."

3) "Recipients, ask that the Sound Healing be sent to where it is most needed in you."

4) The choir now intuitively find one common note in the group and listen into the sound.

5) When the group feel safe and the Note from Heaven has manifested, the fifth (Pa) can be added. Then the third (Gha).

6) When the harmony is incorporated in the Note from Heaven, it is time for one by one to throw a flower of sound into the sound-sea. The group will adjust to the new impulses and will gradually start to modulate in harmonies (some groups learn to add a small seventh (Ni komal), which invites to change chord – or a fourth (Ma) to create tension).

7) When the group feels safe by throwing flowers of sound impulses one by one, they move, still singing, out in the room and encircle the Recipients lying on the floor.

8) All Recipients get attention. Some of the Sound Healers will sound scan and throw their notes as flowers into the sound of the choir. Others will adjust to the choir's sound and find the resonance in the Recipients' bodies. Another possibility is to touch the Recipients lightly on the feet (if

they have agreed about it beforehand) while surrendering to the intuitive Sound Healing.

9) The degree of healing is equivalent to the degree of listening. In Communal Sound Healing the single voice only has a meaning in the context of the group, because it is the listening harmony in the group that heals. You should only throw a flower, if you feel it is pulled out of you and will add to the beauty of the Sound Healing.

10) When the healing is over often the group spontaneously stop. Other times the leader gives a sign to Humm and close down the healing by stroking the energy fields of the Recipients.

11) The leader instructs everybody to put their hands at their hearts and thank for the healing we have received.

During a Communal Sound Healing, the Recipient's body absorbs only the sounds that it needs. It is not uncommon that people fall into a deep state of relaxation, some even sleeping heavily, when a healing session of 10-15 minutes is over. Therefore I strike a temple bell, and we swap. In some cases people need to lie down for several rounds, in other cases there are Sound Healers that prefer to heal for the entire session. It tends to go up in a higher unity with the numbers. Each group healing takes between ten and fifteen minutes, because people need to take their time afterwards. The course leader controls the clock, and is active as a Sound Healer in each round.

There only needs to be one person present that doesn't listen to the others and acts as a soloist for breaking the magic of a Sound Healing. This is the same as a single link breaking in a chain. The whole chain loses its strength and meaning, and the links fly everywhere. People who think they are good singers and wish to show this to everybody; or their opposites, tone-deaf people that are afraid of making mistakes can create panic reactions which will make them switch off and forget to listen. When this happens I stop the group and ask the soloist to remember to pull back and give space for everybody. Tone-deaf people can very well be aware of listening to the group and noticing the moods of the group expression. It is the fear that creates havoc. The most important thing is to LISTEN and react to the sound impulses. There is no "good" or "bad" singer. Sound Healing is all about being present through attentive listening.

A soloist that is consumed by their own performance doesn't listen.

The energy level falls to its lowest level as soon as an ego appears on the arena.

The Recipients feel it instantly when it happens. Let your voice out, but do it within the boundaries of the group. It is pleasant to let it out with a long note. You feel carried by the other voices, like a small twig which is carried by a strong wave – a wave that can also arise when one person dares to throw themselves out in full surrendering and is followed by the rest of the group.

Another possibility is that the entire group join each other in a Communal Sound Healing and heal each other while doing it.

Remote Sound Healing

During the COVID-19 pandemic, I have used Remote Sound Healing for treatments with excellent results. During around 30 webinars, I have used Remote Healing and scanning with undertones and even my international training of the Note from Heaven has been done online. So in this way, the pandemic has been a great gift to expand the field of Remote Healing and thus our consciousness: Energy follows intention. We know it when we experience it.

For example, a woman, 48 years old, mother of two, with terminal cancer (twice admitted to hospice) called me. She had cancer in the bones, breast, intestines, liver, and could only take nourishment intravenously. When I felt her faith in the Note from Heaven, I made an instant Remote Sound Healing on her using mostly inner undertones with "Hong, Hang and Hung" song. I imagined her body and sound scanned her: The kidneys were in a rather good condition, the liver was, according to the trauma sound scan, only attacked on the right side and quite superficial. This gave hope, because then her body would be able to cope with a detox of cytokines from stomach and bones. During the scan of the woman's small intestine, it turned out that it was the entrance from the stomach to the small intestine (duodenum) and the exit of the small intestine to the large intestine (ileum cecum junction) that appeared to be blocked by infection/cancerous tissue. I also scanned the brain to find shadows of the root cause of the cancer. It turned out to be located on the right side of the frontal lobe.

The woman relaxed after the remote treatment and slept with a packet of castor oil on the liver the first night, the next nights also on the small intestine.

Three days later she called me and said she had had the best weekend in years. No pain, more strength.

I gave her another Remote Sound Healing and eventually she gently tried to fill her lungs completely. She could breathe fully without pain. When I asked her to sing the Note from Heaven, it manifested itself overwhelmingly strong, so strong was the expression that all the signal disappeared from my phone (a good sign). We were both overwhelmed by surprise and happiness. Now the woman sings daily as much as she feels good about, and in my experience, the Note from Heaven will help her as she is open to energy work.

My experience with remote healing is that it works in the same way as when you heal a person present. Your faith and the recipient's faith are what matters. If it's hard for you to imagine the person, you can use a doll or a folded blanket.

Both the recipient and the giver must usually both be aware

that the healing is happening as it is sent between a "sender" and a "receiver". You can heal through the phone, but you can also do it without the phone. The energy will pass if there is faith at both ends of the electrical communication. Distance has nothing to say. Just as you can call anyone in the world, you can heal anyone in the world. But you usually need to have a conscious connection. In case of unconscious people or people you cannot reach, you can heal them with distant healing through the Grail Meditation.

Grail Meditation

This meditation is very deep and can have a profound impact on people. The Note from Heaven is a bridge to "the other side/Heaven". In this meditation we literally move our souls up into the front yard of Heaven where unconditional love and profound wisdom are present.

The group first connect to the Note from Heaven and sing until a higher energy level has manifested in the room. One way to feel it is that the temperature rises remarkably and you feel lighter in your forehead.

The grail is shaped with a round foot, symbolizing duality (in the radius of the circle) and Oneness in the center of the circle. We now enter the center and glide up through the stem of the Grail, and travel through a tunnel of light while meditating in silence. If you feel you cannot get up, make yourself small as a tadpole.

There are five rounds:

1) You will enter the front yard of Heaven with any request you may have. Often people meet beloved ones, and sometimes participants are surprised to meet a person that they have disliked, embracing them with unconditional love, as if all of what has happened between them was just part of an act. Forgiveness takes place. Questions are answered.

Everything is possible. All living beings have their complete matrix in the heavenly level. This means that you can meet the sacred forms of both living and dead people.

2) You descend to support one or more relatives to enter the front yard of Heaven. Help them to travel through the stem of the grail. You are not allowed to wish anything for anybody else, but the blessing of unconditional love, everybody longs for, so it is allowed to bring that up. It might surprise you to see your relatives' reactions. If they cannot get up, please make them tiny as tadpoles.

3) You descend to support one or more important public persons/politicians/speakers to enter the front yard of Heaven. Help them to travel through the stem of the grail. You can ask for a blessing of unconditional love for everybody.

4) You descend to support a group of people, it can be a group of scientists you wish to have inspiration from or a larger group, for example I wished to bring Muslim women, but they sent their men up instead. If you have such a huge group, you need to make them really tiny, in order that everybody can join you to enter the front yard of Heaven. Help them to travel through the stem of the grail. You are still only allowed to wish them a blessing of unconditional love in the front yard of Heaven.

5) You descend to support a part of nature to enter the front yard of Heaven. For example all the pigs from the industrial farming, or chickens. Some participants have blessed the sea, the Earth and so on. Send them up to receive unconditional love.

In the end you help everybody to descend and return back to the Earthly realm. Make sure to make them all their natural size, when they are safely back.

We thank for the beautiful journey and the unconditional love we all have received.

It is very unlikely to happen, but if anybody has a hard time being grounded, when they return to Earth, let them walk barefoot outside and/or find a tree or a root of a tree, and let them touch this with their feet and hands. Finally a cold shower can be helpful.

Sound Healing as a Profession

Sound Healer is not something you call yourself – it is something you are.

You can practice Sound Healing and call yourself a Sound Healer. But you only become a true Sound Healer on the day that the other side manifests a miracle through you, without you having done anything special. Then you stand agape with your dismantled ego in your arms: "I had nothing to do with that."

Being a Sound Healer consists in trusting the benefits of being nothing. You only have to listen for the right program just like tuning an old radio. When you find the right program, and you experience that the higher powers are ready to work through you, then respectfully submit yourself one hundred percent to their service.

Through courses and education you can gain tools, feedback and help to improve your skills. But the real education occurs when the barrier to the other side is removed.

I can therefore not teach you to become a Sound Healer, but only share my experience, ethical guidelines and inspiration. Some course participants need to go through a longer process of transformation while others will have immediate breakthroughs. The common thing that I have experienced from pupils that are getting good results is that their nature is humble, grounded, straight and honest.

Practice is necessary to gain experience, yes. But just as no teacher of meditation can guarantee Nirvana for their students, no one can pave the way for you to your higher consciousness. That path is yours and yours alone.

Part 6:

Selected Case Stories

Written Feedback from Recipients

Edema on the retina – Jan-Helge Larsen, Practicing Doctor[147]
"While we sang for the full hour, I directed the energy I received up to the area of my right eye where I suffer from an edema on the retina. I experienced the entire area growing at the same time as it became more and more hollow. After a while some clicking sounds started inside my cranium, and it felt as if the entire area opened up, and the edema disappeared. When I came home I tested my sight, and my image formation had become normal, which is a sign that the edema was gone – and it still is today thirteen years later." (2021)

Asthma – Inger Gustafsson, Nurse
"I have had asthma since I was a child and have always had problems with my breathing.

Several years ago I learned how to breathe with the stomach muscles. It was difficult and I only succeeded when my attention was fully focused on it while lying down. The diaphragm and stomach musculature shakily expanded in an unsynchronized way or pulled together again. It felt like being constricted around the middle.

On Tuesday evening (after the course with Githa) I discovered that my stomach was breathing for me. Calm and secure as if it had never done anything else, both when I was standing (which had been worse) and sat down. My lungs waited, as if they had never been used for anything else except for delivering air in time. Today is Thursday, and it is still like this!! The fear, which until now has had its unconquerable kingdom in my stomach, must have been sucked out in the powerful air stream, together with the rage and sorrow in the voice. For the first time my entire body has had a collective drive – one voice – one cry. Feelings have found their place in the body again. They are being heard and seen in full view and with a new identity. Hidden resources. I cry a lot and cry now, without my dinosaur skin. But everything is so good, and I am enjoying my newborn breath, and the tears are a long awaited rain falling in a dry place."

Whiplash, Back pain (compressed discs), neck, tail bone, fatigue – Lene Finn Lauritzen, Teacher and Singer

Feedback following participation of a Sound Healing seminar in January 2011 (115 participants):

"My back pain that I had had for 18 months due to a fall with compressed discs as a result is GONE. The blockage of my tail bone is GONE. My neck pains after having not been able to function for three months because of fatigued suprarenal glands is GONE. The rest of my body feels as if it has been run over by a steamroller, and therefore I lay completely still on my bed today. My head is somewhat thrown about. I sang all afternoon yesterday – everything I love to sing – notes that have been lying dormant for years! I am very emotional today. During the morning I have had some powerful, releasing sobs from a level I cannot identify. They came all the way in from the depths of me, and were followed by a feeling of happiness/ deep laughter."

Cancer in the right breast, right lung, bones and spine – Birte Madsen Trolle, Dentist

"In the Summers of 2001 and 2004 I had an operation for cancer in my right breast. Both times I opted for no follow-up treatment because I was newly married and wanted to be able to become pregnant. In early 2008 I was told that the cancer had spread to my right lung and basically all of my bones, especially my vertebrae.

All that the doctors could offer me was life-prolonging chemotherapy every third week. It would give me up to six more months to live.

My philosophy was that I would survive by strengthening my immune system as much as possible, at the same time as I would need a form of treatment – especially for the cancer in my right lung – but it would have to be as gentle as possible for the body.

I read about Githa Ben-David in a magazine and contacted her. Githa taught me 'to sing'. I howled for my life twice a day for half an hour at a time in the car on my way to and from work. I also received Sound Healing from Githa once a week. The sound scanning caused violent pains caused by my right lung expanding, at the same time as the last of the fluid in the lung disappeared. Before I started treatment with Githa on the 19th of November 2008, my PSI number was 900. When my PSI was measured again on the 15th of December, it had fallen to 151.

I could have walked on water.

It is now 2012. I still have not received any systemic chemotherapy. My life has never been better."

Chronic pain in the left shoulder, knuckle on the left foot – Dorthe Lynderup, conflict mediator in the Danish police (excerpt from film interview)[1]

"I broke my shoulder when I was thirteen years old and it has given me a lot of problems. The last half year I have not been able to lift it. I sang myself free in regressive cell singing and got sound healing. Now I can move my arm freely, it sounds crazy, but it is a fact. I can move it even to my back now. I have had problems sleeping at night because of the pain.

Beside this I have had a knuckle on my left foot. I would not believe this, but it is a fact, that I have been looking at this painful knuckle for two years, and now it has disappeared after a sound healing with deep undertones.

If you believe in miracles, then this is a miracle, because the knuckle is gone. It disappeared within 24 hours after the Sound Healing."

Examples of Sound Healing of people with hearing loss/deafness

Otosclerosis – Sofie Vejby Lindquist, Falster

Sofie's mother contacted me because Sofie had been using hearing aids on both ears since she was five years old. As an eleven-year-old, Sofie had serious difficulties keeping up in school because of her poor hearing. I remember that Sofie lay down on a mattress in front of the lit fireplace in the living room, and that I gave her Sound Healing for approximately 20 minutes while her mother watched.

After just a few minutes, Sofie fell asleep even though I was singing strong overtones quite close to her ears. I always ask people to take off their hearing aids before a Sound Healing, because they can give disturbing feedback, especially if you cover them with your hands. When I sing closely to a client's head, I hold my hands gently over the Recipient's ears and never sing directly into them.

After the first treatment, Sofia stopped using the hearing aids in order to train her hearing, which seemed to have improved. But it was not until the second treatment that her hearing seemed to be normal.

Six months later Sofie's mother called and asked for a third Sound Healing just to be on the safe side right before Sofie had her yearly ear test by an audiologist. After the Sound Healing, the hearing test showed that Sofie's hearing had become normal. The doctors concluded that it must have been a misdiagnosis. (At the hearing test the year before, the doctors had given up any idea of operating on her.) Today in 2021, Sofie is 28 years old, has graduated as a midwife and her hearing is still normal years on.

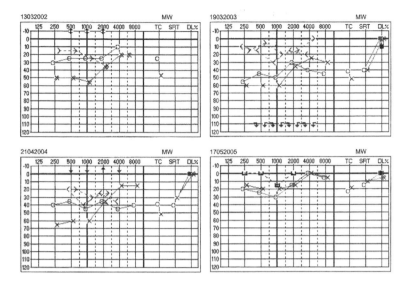

Complete hearing loss – Paul Simon, Lyngby

I received several neatly handwritten letters written in ink on thick, yellowed paper from Paul Simon – an 89-year-old man who had lost his hearing completely as a 75-year-old. Since then he had lived in a retirement home and communicated with written notes.

Paul Simon had a strong belief in the metaphysical, and had seven marriages behind him. We ended up meeting in Copenhagen three times after my weekly courses, where I gave him Sound Healing. Paul Simon always lay with open eyes when I Sound Healed him. The healing worked well, despite the fact that he didn't submit himself to it or fell asleep. After the third Sound Healing session, which was taken as a Choral Sound Healing and also filmed,[148] Paul Simon was able to communicate when you spoke to him with raised voice.

We celebrated at a restaurant afterwards. Paul Simon did not receive further treatment, but I met him some years later at a holistic event where he said that he moved out of the retirement home immediately after his partial hearing had returned. The audiologist had told him that he would have to live the rest of his life stone-deaf. But Paul Simon said, with his hoarse, compassionate voice, "They don't know any better..."

Infection in the skull – Helle Galsgård, Århus

Helle had suffered hearing loss because of an infection in the skull, that was caused by an ingrown flap of skin. She had once had an operation for this phenomenon. Now the flap of skin had grown again and the situation had worsened. A difficult divorce had increased the infection that seemed to be connected with psychological stress.

At our first meeting when Helle began to sing herself free, the infection started running out of her left ear. This had never happened to her before. She kept singing with a napkin on her ear. Afterwards she received Sound Healing. We agreed that she would sing daily.

The result of the first Sound Healing and her own follow-up singing was that two days later she got a high fever and panicked, because the hospital suggested an immediate operation which could very well damage her hearing as well as part of her brain. Luckily, she believed so much in Sound Healing, that she came to me to get acute treatment when she was on the verge of collapse. I am convinced that the fever was due to the cleansing process, that the Sound Healing/her own singing had started. As mentioned, it is normally the second day after a treatment that the effects of a healing are peaking.

After the second Sound Healing session the fever subsided, her hearing improved, and Helle felt compelled to sing low notes. After the third treatment (ten days later) her voice had opened completely in the low register. I noticed her whole stomach vibrate when she sang. Her sound moved my heart. When a physical reaction such as this occurs, I know that the Note from Heaven has broken through and gives all the help that is needed. Helle couldn't stop singing. "The sound does wonders for me. I can hear just fine now, have more energy, and

I am convinced that my infection has gone."

When she was scanned at the hospital, it turned out that the infection was gone, and that there was no longer any need to operate.

Examples of pain relief

Giving Birth

My youngest son began life with a singing birth that lasted one hour and fifteen minutes. The pain disappeared while singing the Note from Heaven (a powerful note on "Haaa"), but returned with shocking force the moment I stopped singing, which happened when the midwife needed to see how far we had come. Surprised, she said that the head was on its way out.[149] Some of my students have specialized in this field and help pregnant women to prepare for a singing birth.

Phantom Pains

When I carried out Sound Healing on two drug addicts with strong phantom pains, I played the CD *Sound of Light*. I had to be contented with humming to show consideration to the tourists at the hotel, where we were on holiday. After Sound Healing, the phantom pains disappeared in the male addict's amputated leg. He then went to the disco, where he danced with a prosthetic limb and drank all night long. The man's daily methadone consumption was six milliliters.

His female partner, also a drug addict, had an amputated arm. She told me before the healing that she was the person in Denmark who took the highest amount of methadone with a daily intake of 54 milliliters. After the Sound Treatment she reacted as if she had received an overdose of methadone.[150] She lay in her bed all day long with the curtains closed and felt awful. In the evening she returned to normal. The phantom pains slowly returned in both addicts after seven to ten days.

Examples of Sound Healing on cancer

Example 1.

Chili was in her forties and had been diagnosed with a melanoma that had spread to the lymph system. Since her family is predisposed to cancer and since Chili was the mother of three small children, she naturally felt powerless in this situation. However, she had composed herself and taken one step at a time on purpose. A lymph node on her inner thigh at the groin was the size of an egg.

During Sound Healing with undertones, the lymph node on her inner thigh faded rapidly after a few minutes, and became less than half the original size. We both rejoiced, but became also a little frightened at the thought that the cancer might have spread to the rest of the lymphatic system. Upon asking Dr. Audun Myskja from Norway, we were told that the lymph node had been drained, and that this was a good sign.

Sound Healing stimulates the body's lymph system. This does not lead to the spread of cancer. The cancer had weakened the lymphatic system – the sound had strengthened it.

As the lymphatic system is the primary organ of the immune system, the undertones had apparently stimulated the immune system.

Chili found her path to a cure through a combination of Sound Healing and healing forms supported by Health Creation – a combination of treatments that she is a mentor for in Denmark today.

Example 2.

A Young Man had a melanoma that had spread to the liver. He was close to dying after a heavy chemotherapy (IL2 cytotoxic therapy) at Odense University Hospital. After the treatment, the cancer had spread to his brain with several tumors there as well as tumors in the right side of his ribcage and lungs. He was given only a few months to live and couldn't drive because of dizziness. Every day he slept for several hours. The young man tried as much as he could to be a father for his small children, but was exhausted and frightened.

By contacting me he provoked his religious wife. He sang himself free and regained his normal breathing ability. Afterwards he received Sound Healing, to which he responded positively.

The young man sang daily in the days that followed, and told me that he made it through the day without needing to sleep. He had enough energy to create his own Facebook account so that friends and family could follow his sickness there instead of wearing him out with phone calls. The next time he came for a treatment he was happy and full of energy. He had auditioned for a serious chamber choir and had been accepted. In addition, he also had enough energy to be a father to his children.

Unfortunately, his family and he ate unhealthy food and the young man was crazy about sugar, which cancer cells live from (according to nutritionists and doctors open to Holistic views). The wife did not seem to be interested in changing their diet. There were religious arguments and divided opinions in the young family[151] about how cancer sufferers should approach their treatment process. The last I heard was that his family had persuaded him to be treated with chemotherapy at a private clinic, Humlegården, and that he could not sing there. While writing this book I tried to contact him but unfortunately found that his beautiful voice is no longer among us.

Example 3.

Annie was in her early seventies. She had pleural cancer and following a surgical removal of a cancerous growth in her diaphragm could not lie down any more. The doctors had only given her a few months to live, when she contacted me and explained that with her own life on the line, she wanted to be a sound pioneer because she was convinced that song can cure cancer. Annie's dedication inspired me to record the CD *Rising*[152] and to build it upon the relatively little scientific information that exists about the effects of sound on cancer cells.

Annie sang along with *Rising* twice a day despite having fluid in her lungs. Besides this she took two daily sound baths – in other words, sat listening to *Rising*.

To amplify the effects, she had positioned large speakers in front and behind her chair. During the entire process she measured her progress with an exercise bike. In one month Annie went from cycling 250 meters to five kilometers daily. After two years of tenacious work with *Rising*, Annie's diaphragm had improved so much that she was able to lie down in the scanner at the hospital. The scan showed that the cancer had reduced significantly in the right pleura – the side that she had felt vibrations in during the Sound Bathing. The left side on the other hand was slightly worse. We concluded that if you cannot feel vibration in a sick area of the body, it is useful to lead the energy there with your consciousness.

Annie did this now, and noticed that life also started coming into the left side. Annie's breathing was strongly inhibited because a lump in her solar plexus was removed and parts of her diaphragm were damaged during the operation.

Walking was also impaired, and the chemotherapy had destroyed the stomach's chemistry/created allergies to a wide variety of foods. Therefore, Annie through the entire process was very thin and weakened. Because the geographic distance between us was large, she only came to Sound Healing when she felt strong enough to drive – approximately once every six months.

We experimented by making recordings of my sound scanning of her for research purposes. She started taking Sound Baths in these daily. We concluded that the effects of live sound were the strongest, but she also got benefit from the Sound

Baths, she said. As Annie so courageously had tested the power of sound in such a determined and disciplined way, we had never spoken of the reason behind her illness. She had been the boss in our experiments, and I had listened to her and given her what she had asked for.

The last time we met for Sound Healing I asked her if she knew about the reason for the cancer. Almost three years had passed, and she had shown that she could survive through dedicated daily singing. Deep down she knew exactly what the problem was, but she concluded that she had no wish to change it. After this realization Annie tried another kind of healing for some time. Two months later Annie died from an additional blood disease.

Example 4.

Stine took part in a week-long course in song and Sound Healing in the South of France. She had cancerous growths in her brain, lungs, bones and liver and was weakened from a long chemotherapy treatment process, recent divorce, and the message that the hospital had no more treatment to offer her. Stine whispered because one of her vocal cords was paralyzed after the chemotherapy. We decided in advance that she wouldn't need to sing, and that I and the others singers would Sound Heal her daily throughout the course.

During the first morning song she was lying in the middle of the room being Sound Healed. I noticed a spark of life, tears in her eyes and red cheeks when she got up. On the second day, her paralyzed vocal cord started to vibrate. People could gradually begin to hear what Stine was saying. She took part in the song and experienced a full breath that activated the vocal cord which the medical doctors had declared paralyzed. On the third day her condition suddenly got worse. I led the group in giving her Choral Sound Scanning.[153]

Afterwards she felt much better. Stine was dripping with

sweat and the mattress was soaked. The smile returned to her face and her energy level rose. She walked eight kilometers in hilly terrain and climbed a steep hill. The tumor in her brain was measured shortly before she took the course in France. Four weeks after the singing course the tumor was measured at the hospital and found to be half the size.

Example 5.

Karen was in the middle of her 50s with a cancerous growth the size of a marble 1.5 cm across in her left breast. She refused all treatment at the hospital because she would rather die of cancer than go through chemotherapy, operations and radiation.

Karen took part in a week-long course with song and Sound Healing with me in the South of France. Two months before she had changed her diet radically to raw food (eating only fresh vegetables). Karen had a hard time relating to the emotions connected to the cancer. Only when she received Sound Healing from a male participant (a doctor), she got into contact with the source of the cancer. The whole night following, Karen struggled with an all-consuming fear.

At the end of the week, the cancerous lump was hard to find. It had diminished in size to that of a small pea. Her friend continued Sound Healing her breast after returning to Denmark.

Sound Healing of stress

At another week-long course in the south of France one of the participants was Anna. She is a female Steiner pedagogue [teacher] and was able to come due to a last minute cancellation. She had broken down a few days prior to the course due to stress. Anna had dark shadows under her eyes, dull hair, loose skin, and was worryingly grey in the face.

In the first lesson Anna began singing herself free at the same time as I loosened up her solar plexus – Sound Healing it with undertones. There are many possible combinations in

Sound Healing. Here, it was necessary to resolve the knot in her stomach caused by the stress. When the solar plexus began to resonate the knot loosened up. The woman gasped and her breathing suddenly opened up fully, which her powerful cry song clearly demonstrated.

The Note from Heaven stood like a column in the room. Every person present could feel its unmistakable power and we all became overwhelmed by gratitude.

After a couple of minutes in surrendering to the Note from Heaven, Anna's tears changed to echoing laughter which rang round the room, expressing her energy in staccato bursts of joy. The other course participants were jubilant too. Her release of energy blessed all of us.

Anna had found herself again, and her mood changed as if someone had waved a magic wand. It is normal that people become very beautiful when they have sung themselves free. The reason can be that they come into contact with something very fundamental within themselves and/or that endorphins are released. Anna's free singing was followed up by Sound Healing as well as daily surrendering to the Note from Heaven. She beamed like a ray of sunshine after two days. After returning home she changed her work and has not been stressed since.

Sound Healing for lack of sex drive
Anna Monter and a number of anonymous women

When I was reaching the final phases of writing of this book, I contacted Anna Monter asking permission to mention her "stress case". She reminded me then that she had also regained her sex drive, and that her family life had changed completely. Another woman sent me a text message following a week course, where she delicately wrote that she had had an amazing experience, and that the area below her waist had been brought to life.

Sound Healing ADHD

Johan Emil, 8 years old

In the local school there is a "C" class. This is where the restless ADHD boys are placed. Most of them are medicated with Ritalin (speed). Johan Emil became depressed and lost weight. In order for him to have a chance of gaining weight, he was temporarily taken off Ritalin. In that period, his mother gave me permission to Sound Heal him as an experiment. For over a month I gave the boy Sound Healing for five to ten minutes at a time, twice a week in a private room at the school. Johan Emil sang at the first meeting as well. His tongue always moved into the right side of his mouth. He had a speech impediment and spoke very fast. After the first two treatments, his pronunciation became clearer, he spoke more slowly, and I noticed that his tongue rested in the middle of his mouth. The feedback from his mother and support family is that Johan Emil had clearly become calmer after the Sound Healing. The mother noticed that it was easier to bring Johan Emil to public events compared to the past, where he used to be bouncing off the walls. One year after, Johan Emil was still in the ADHD class, but he had now permanently stopped taking medicine.

A Princess with ADHD

Jytte Johansen who is a pedagogue specialized in ADHD and Autism, asked me to do an experiment with her. We treated a 15-year-old girl with a serious diagnosis of ADHD who had beaten up teachers and repeatedly had cut her own wrists. She had been in psychiatric treatment and had been moved away from her family, but could not function in any school or anywhere else. This girl looked like a princess and also dressed in a quite sexy way. She was a wild one, drinking and sleeping with boys that were much older than her. Her father brought her to us against her will. She refused to sing, so I gave her a

Sound Healing where she wished to lie with a scarf draped on her head.

At the second meeting the princess fell asleep while getting sound healing. She slept deeply, as if she finally let her defences fall. ADHD children can fall in a deep sleep when receiving Sound Healing, which I as well as my students have experienced. The princess has a lot of energy and is a very sharp and intelligent girl. After one month she started cutting down on her medicine (not our idea), she stopped eating cakes and felt hungry for healthy food. At a lesson she wrote a song for her mother and we made a reunion meeting. Slowly, slowly she could sleep at night, and in the end of the two months, she went to an interview at a local school. She flipped her finger at the headmaster. We discussed with her how to handle it better next time. She succeeded to get into a youth school and stayed there for half a year. Today she is studying in High School.

Sound Healing struma/goiter (enlarged thyroid gland)

In several cases I have seen a goiter affected by song/Sound Healing. It is also common for people with bulbous eyes to have their eyes move back into place after sung with the Note from Heaven/Sound Healing. The condition slowly returns, but the eyes can be sung back in place again. The same applies to goiters. My hypothesis is that sound affects the hormone balance.[154]

Sound Healing a limb/leg

After a lecture, I, for a short time, sound scanned a woman who had lived with a severe tinnitus for 19 years. The tinnitus disappeared and everybody including me was happy. One week later the tinnitus had returned, so the woman drove a long distance to reach me so that I once again could Sound Heal her tinnitus.

The woman had agreed to be filmed during the session, as we at that time then were making the film: *The Note from*

Heaven. The cameraman was not very discreet and the woman got nervous, I could feel it. During the Sound Healing the most beautiful overtones appeared – but – her tinnitus did not move at all.

I was angry with myself, because the filming of our session obviously had weakened the healing process. Also the woman was disappointed. How come it worked so well, and then not at all?

After a few hours, when the woman had reached home she called me all excited.

"My foot has regained life! I can walk normally!" I had noticed that she pulled one leg after her, but we had been so fixated on the tinnitus, that we never got around to talking about it. The woman had lost her feeling in the foot after a mistake during an operation five years ago. Up to today her foot has functioned normally.

Other Sound Healers' cases

In Sound Healing groups around Denmark, participants have had a positive effect on/cured chronic pain, tinnitus, depression, cancer, stress and more.

Shortly before an operation, a course participant, Rose Lübich, affected a tumor on a teenager so much with Sound Healing, that it diminished in size from a tennis ball to a pea. The doctors decided that an operation was no longer necessary.

The Sound Healer Helle Westergaard has concentrated specifically on aphasia cases. The effects of Sound Healing here improve the aphasia sufferer's abilities to communicate considerably. The progress occurs gradually over a longer period of treatment.

Flemming Blicher, an engineer who participated in a weekend course, slept overnight in his mother's flat. He had not been able to speak normally with her for nine years after she had a stroke (a blood clot in her brain). Besides not being able to speak properly, her entire right side had been paralyzed. Flemming wished to show her, just for fun, the undertones he had learned in my course, and sang on her right hand. After the short Sound Healing, his mother could move her fingers on her right hand. Next morning Flemming decided to try to sound scan her head with undertones too. Then the mother started to speak, and Flemming send a text overflowing with joy, hearts and stars to me.

Jytte Johansen, who is educated by me, is known for being able to sing down tinnitus just as also Pia Fredløv a fellow student is. Both of the women are educated as pedagogues too. Jytte specializes in ADHD and the Autism spectrum. After the third treatment of a three-year-old autistic boy with no language at all, his mother rang her up and told her that he had said five words.

Another student of mine, Anne-Marie Gundestrup, is the owner of a private home for autists. She has been cooperating with Jytte, and is now able to do a wonderful Sound Healing too. Her/their results are so promising, that she is writing a book about Sound Healing autistic children (2020). One of the tools Jytte and Anne-Marie use is to Sound Heal the kids with a plastic sound pipe (you turn it around in the air and a sound is manifested). The kids hold one side of the pipe to their body while the Sound Healer sings in the other end. In this way the autistic children do not feel intimidated, they have fun and can move the pipe wherever they want to.

Martin Delfs, another former student of mine, yoga teacher and a professional within sports massage, is using Vocal Sound Healing while doing yoga. It is beneficial because the long exhalation soothes the pain from stretches and helps people to get deeper into the positions. The same thing is true for massage. Martin has obtained a lot of good results by Sound Healing joints, for example hips and knees while massaging.

There are so many results that I cannot mention all of

them here. The influence of Sound Healing on people with psychological issues, depression, stress and/or low self-esteem is hard to prove. But I can tell you, that a lot of students have had good results in this area.

Part 7

Research In Sound

Chromatic Toning of Cancer Cells

The following chapter is inspired from "Musical Medicine" by the Norwegian researcher and doctor Audun Myskja and by Fabien Maman's book: *The Role of Music in the Twenty-First Century* where you can see photos from the following experiment.

For more than six months during 1981, Fabien Maman, the French musician, acupuncturist and sound researcher, carried out nightly experiments together with the biologist Helene Grimal – a nun and researcher at the National Research Center in Paris. For approximately half a year, they worked together in the laboratories at the University de Jussieu in Paris – from midnight to five o'clock in the morning. At that time of the day, there was no noise from the metro or skeptical colleagues which could affect the results.

They exposed cultivated womb cancer cells (Hella cells in petri dishes) to sound from a wide variety of musical instruments. Singular notes were played chromatically ascending at a distance of 30 centimeters for approximately 30 seconds per note. A wide variety of instruments were used: Gong, xylophone, guitar, flute, bass, drums and more were experimented with. Afterwards when Maman sang up through the scale, the cell cores and cytoplasmic membranes began to disintegrate, after which the cancer cells exploded! See photo page 334.

The experiment made it clear that cancer cells were not able to tolerate a progressive accumulation of vocal sound frequencies. Destabilization became apparent after just three note impulses. When the sequence continued, the cancer cells exploded after a period of between nine to 14 minutes.

In an attempt to explain the phenomenon, Maman and Grimal came upon an observation that many physicists have made independently of each other: Elementary particles behave and work together like the notes of a chromatic scale. From this perspective, the explosion can be explained as due to an increased dissonance. The sound accumulates in the cells, but the cancer particles of the cells cannot contain the frequencies/ resonances. Therefore, they explode.

Cells from healthy tissue, however, survived the sound impulses, and easily received more scales without any sign of damage or disintegration. There turned out to be such a dramatic and constant difference between cells from healthy tissue and cancer cells, that the researchers concluded that healthy cells allow sound to pass through them and, in a manner of speaking, give this sound back to their surroundings.

Cancer cells on the other hand can neither integrate the sound nor get rid of it. When the frequency of especially vocal sound impulses was increased on the healthy cells, there were observed signs of a loss of the normal structures between the cellular elements – both in clumps of cells and inside individual cells.

However, this breakdown did not lead to an explosion when notes were played up through the scale, as it did in cancer cells. Instead, the cells responded by reorganizing their structures. They appeared to be stimulated or regenerated after having been exposed to sound impulses. This fits beautifully with Gerald Pollack's theory about structured water (see page 503).

The experiments also suggested the great significance of overtones for the health of cells. Overtones from acoustic instruments appeared to nourish the cells directly in a completely different way to synthetic notes, where over 50 percent of the natural overtones can be filtered out.

Maman and Grimal tried out their method on two volunteer breast cancer patients, who were taught to sing up and down the scale in 20 minute periods. In one of the patients, the growth disappeared completely (shown in a mammogram). The other patient had already been scheduled for surgery. During the operation, however, the surgeons found that the lump had withered up. The patient was followed up, and she has not had any relapse.

The Importance of the Vagus Nerve

The vagus nerve connects the brain with the inner organs and connects feelings and physical reactions. A new discovery is that the vagus nerve is responsible for registering the effects of hormones in the brain. In this way, the state of the vagus nerve affects the body's hormone balance and is crucial for controlling the level of oxytocins – the body's "happy hormones".

Excerpt from Sofie Langkilde's bachelor thesis about the vagus nerve

The following is an excerpt from an interview with the American professor and researcher in neurobiology, Stephen W. Porges, undertaken by Maria Lund Jensen, *Politiken*, 2007:

"Stephen W. Porges, the American professor and neurobiologist, has achieved good results using sound to affect stress, depression, ADHD and autism. Porges is a researcher with more than 200 scientific articles behind him and heads The Brain-Body Institute at the University of Illinois in Chicago. Since the beginning of the 1990's, he has worked with his theory, 'The Polyvagal Theory', which claims that our nervous system is dependent upon smiling, conversation, affection, friendships and love in order to function normally. We are mammals and have an inherent need to belong to communities where we feel loved and secure. The core of the theory is neuroception, which covers the autonomous nervous system's ability to decode our surroundings and the people we meet, and decide if they are safe or dangerous. Problems with this ability can lead to psychological suffering such as depression, ADHD and autism. 'Poly' means many, while 'vagal' refers to the vagus nerve.

Stephen Porges describes the autonomous nervous system like a traffic light with three main states – red, amber and green. An activation of the oldest and most primitive state (red) results in the body and consciousness being immobilized. We react with a slower pulse rate, slower breathing, and have a higher pain threshold. The body goes into shock or 'freezes' in dangerous situations, like a mouse that instinctively plays dead to divert the cat's attention. In state number two (amber), the nervous system prepares us for a 'fight-or-flight' reaction.

This should be understood literally, as a fleeing/fighting situation with an enemy, but also as a defense against sickness and trauma. In this state, our hearing of low and high frequency sounds is improved, while the downside is that we find it more difficult to concentrate and cannot receive or understand normal conversation. The third and most advanced state (green light) is only found among mammals. It is especially well developed in apes and humans, and makes it possible for us to communicate with advanced facial movements and language. It is therefore known as the communicative state.

According to Porges, our nervous system's ability to switch between these three states helping us to adapt to our surroundings is central in our mental and physical health. In the short term, the eldest two defense mechanisms are there to increase our chances of survival in dangerous situations. However, if we remain in these states for too long, sickness will occur.

The reason that neuroleptic problems occur is, according to Porges, because we are always surrounded by background noise, that stresses our autonomous nervous system, rather than giving us a feeling of security. In addition, the technological development of mobile phones, iPads, computers, chat rooms, and so on means that we have less face-to-face contact with other people and therefore lack well-rounded communication.

'Quite simply, we have a harder and harder time believing

that our surroundings are safe. The consequences are sleeping problems, learning difficulties, nervousness, fear, eating disorders and other psychological problems, all of which are connected to the autonomous nervous system,' explains Stephen W. Porges.

The good news is that the American has developed a sound treatment therapy that can help the nervous system to rebalance.

The thought behind the therapy form is The Polyvagal Theory, where neuroception is not functioning optimally, but where the actual nerve pathways are assumed to be intact. In other words, it is not the 'hardware' (the nerves and brain) that is defective, but the 'software' (the ability to carry out neuroception).

Stephen Porges does not have an explanation for exactly why the software is broken in some people, but he believes he has succeeded in reestablishing its functioning in his experiments.

'We have carried out experiments on 150 autistic people, divided into a test group and two control groups that only hear regular music. The people in the test groups that are very sensitive to sound – which approximately 60 percent of all autistic people are – experience the best benefits of the treatment. The control group showed no sign of improvement,' explains Stephen W. Porges. The treatment had a significant positive effect on almost half of the test subjects. Porges does not like to use the word 'cure', but in reply to the question, as to whether he has cured some of his test subjects with autism, his reply is 'yes', because their autistic behavior – characterized by a lack of eye contact, introverted conduct, concentration problems and monotone speech – gradually disappeared during the treatment.

Their physical state, according to Stephen W. Porges' theory, has been moved from fight-or-flight to the communicative state. In the scientific experiments with sound therapy carried out at the University of Chicago, test subjects listen to music with headphones for 45 minutes, once a week for six weeks.

The music is manipulated by the computer so that the

strength of the sound and stresses of the notes are constantly varied within the frequencies of human speech. The reason that sound therapy can affect a patient's psychological state lies partially in the function of the vagus nerve, which Porges' theory is named after. The vagus nerve is the biggest nerve center in humans, which, as mentioned, branches out from the brain to the small muscles in the face, the ears, and out in the body to the vital organs, among those heart and lungs. The nerve bundle has a large influence on the regulation of our hearing, speech and facial expression, which is necessary for social conduct. It also has a large impact on our heart rate and breathing, which changes when we are afraid.

The vagus nerve is the connection between the old defense mechanism and the communicative circuit. Therefore, by stimulating the vagus nerve with sound therapy, it is possible to activate the small muscles in the ears, and kick-start the other muscles in the face that regulate our facial expressions. Every person that has symptoms of defective neuroception – from people with depression to children with ADHD, soldiers and refugees with post-traumatic stress and chronically stressed people – will potentially benefit from the treatment."

Nerve Impulses are Sound Waves

The Danish research team "Heimburg-Jackson" at the Niels Bohr Institute has found a new explanation about the function of the nervous system: Nerve signals are not electrical impulses, as previously assumed. Nerve signals are a particular type of sound waves, called solitons. Normal sound waves expand in all directions and become gradually weaker, but solitons distinguish themselves by moving in one direction only, and maintain their strength until they suddenly die out. Sound almost always expands as normal waves, but if these pass through matter with particular properties, they are changed to solitons. When nerves are in transition between their fixed and fluid forms their cell membranes possess the exact properties of changing sound to solitons.

It has previously been impossible to explain why anesthetic works poorly on alcoholics and patients with infections. The sound wave model explains why.

Thomas Heimburg, PhD and Andrew Jackson believe that the electrical signal is a by-product of the actual signal, which is a sound wave. When a nerve sends a signal, it emits heat, but sucks the heat back into itself afterwards, which should not happen in an electrical impulse. It breaks the laws of thermodynamics, which state that electrical energy cannot cause temperature to fall when resistance occurs. It would be the same as a light bulb drawing all of the heat that it had emitted back to it when it is turned off.

Researchers have previously observed that nerves actually change their thickness, when sound impulses flow through them. It is similar to when a snake eats a mouse that can be seen bulging out of the snake's body, as it slides further and further down the gullet. It has not been possible to explain this physical change based on the classical Nobel Prize-winning Hodgkin-Huxley model. The conclusion here is that nerve signals function like electronic charges. It is, however, a completely logical consequence of Heimburg/Jackson's new sound wave model.

This new theory is built on the fact that our nerve membranes consist partially of solid fat and liquid fat which can be compared to olive oil that has been stored in the refrigerator.[155] If you add anesthetic to the fat membranes of the nerves, the melting point is lowered which leads to an impedance in the signal. As infection and alcohol raise the melting point of fat, the anesthetic's lowering of the temperature is hindered, which makes it more difficult to impede the sound signal, and therefore the anesthetic has less effect.

A comment from the author: It would be exciting to examine if specific low frequencies impede or slow down soliton signals.

If exactly the same frequency is produced in two loudspeakers that are facing each other, all sound will disappear. So it should be possible to make soliton anti-noise and use this as an anesthetic. I am convinced of this after having seen many clients fall asleep during Sound Healing.[156]

Research on the Cat's Purr

Excerpts from an article by Elizabeth von Muggenthaler[157] and Bill Wright.

"In America, there have been extensive studies done on the cat's purr. Sayings such as: 'A cat has nine lives' and 'If you put a cat and a sack of broken bones in the same room, the bones will heal' (the latter probably coming from the US), seem to have some truth in them. The reason is the cat's purr.

The cat doesn't only purr out of satisfaction, but also when it is seriously wounded, eats, is frightened, etc. A wounded animal, in full possession of its instincts, will normally avoid wasting precious energy on making a useless sound in a pressured and maybe life-threatening situation. As the cat's purr has survived the passage of hundreds of generations of cats, there must be a survival mechanism behind the sound.

The cat's purr has been shown to relieve human suffering both acute and chronic in 82% of cases. There is much to suggest that the sound is also able to generate the growth of new tissue (25 Hz), heal wounds, improve blood circulation and oxygenation, reduce swelling and/or prevent bacteria formation.

Orthopedic veterinary surgeons have observed how relatively easy it is for a cat to heal after breaking bones as opposed to, for example a dog. In one research project 132 cases of cats that had fallen from high buildings, with an average height of 5.5 floors up, were recorded. The record height was 45 floors. 90% of the 132 cats survived, even though many were supposedly lethally wounded.

Cats don't suffer nearly as much as dogs from ligament

and muscle damage, and a cat's broken bones grow together surprisingly easily and quickly. Researchers, therefore, believe that self-healing is the survival mechanism which lies behind a cat's purr. There is extensive documentation to show that low frequencies, at low intensity, work therapeutically. Low frequencies can strengthen the bone growth, heal breaks, relieve pain, promote muscle growth, strengthen joint mobility, reduce swelling and ease breathing difficulties.

In one trial the world's lightest accelerometer, weighing 0.14g, Endevco model 22, was used to measure the purr frequencies of different races of cats. The cats were lying on blankets and were regularly stroked so that they purred. The result showed that the purring frequencies were between 20 and 200Hz. The frequencies particularly settled on 25Hz, 50Hz, 100Hz, 125Hz and 150Hz, which correspond precisely to frequencies with healing properties established in the most recent research. All the cats had frequencies plus or minus 4Hz from these frequencies, which are scientifically measured to have a healing effect on bone growth, healing of broken legs, pain relief, easing of breathing difficulties and inflammation.

Research has shown that if bones are exposed to the sound frequencies 25 and 50Hz, they will be strengthened 30% faster than normal. The same is true for the time it takes for a broken bone to heal."

Bioacoustics[158]

Sharry Edwards, USA, is the founder of BioAcoustics. Her interest in sound started in 1975, when she went to a hearing clinic to be tested for tinnitus, because she had heard very high-pitched sounds her entire life. When the test leader came into the soundproof room and asked what Sharry could hear, Sharry imitated the sound (a so-called pure tone, or sinus wave). But the human voice shouldn't be able to produce such a sound! And Sharry certainly shouldn't have been able to hear anything, because the sounds that were being played in the room were outside the range of normal human hearing. The test leader felt his blood pressure drop dramatically and was forced to drop to his knees. He later told Sharry that he had studied martial arts, and that he knew this sound was used by the samurai as an offensive weapon to lower an opponent's blood pressure. During a research project, it became apparent that Sharry could change a person's blood pressure just by using her voice.

In another experiment, Sharry found out that everyone emits a nonverbal sound that she gave the name signature sound, because it is as individual as a person's fingerprint or signature. The signature sound is connected to a person's psychological and physiological status so much, that imbalances change the sound.

In 1982, Sharry discovered, during further research, that the signature sound she could hear and produce has a connection with the "stressed" sounds in people's voices – stressed in the sense of breaking, doubled, disharmonious, or totally lacking frequencies. She did not have much knowledge about music and didn't know the names of the notes, but, when she reproduced the stressed tones in their pure form with her voice, the body physically took the notes in again. In this way, the body reestablished the original signature sound, and the person felt better.

When Sharry's 20-year-old son had his left kneecap crushed into 35 pieces, Sharry sat with him at the hospital and played his signature sound for him. At the same time she studied the periodic table of the elements. She discovered that the number of vibrations in her son's signature sound was almost the same as the difference between the atomic weight of calcium and magnesium. She knew that a note could be given indirectly with the help of brain-wave frequencies. If a note of 10 Hz is to be used, you can play 30 Hz in the left ear and 40 Hz in the right ear, and the difference between the two notes will manifest as a third note. So the brain forms a 10 Hz sound by itself. Sharry Edward's son received the sound frequencies that corresponded to the atomic weight of calcium and magnesium in his ears, and his whole body began to shake. Because it felt good, the sound treatment continued on a regular basis and after two months he was able to walk again. In the space of nine months a new kneecap had grown to normal size. This had never previously happened in an adult.

Another amazing result with bioacoustics: A woman had fainted and was brought to the hospital. She lay in a coma for three weeks and was kept alive by artificial means. The doctors declared her brain-dead and asked her husband's permission to use her organs for transplantation. Her husband had previously received bioacoustic therapy and turned again to Sharry Edwards. The correct frequencies were found and played for the unconscious woman. After three hours of treatment she regained consciousness and opened her eyes. Three weeks later she was discharged from the hospital.

In a YouTube film from 2019159 Sharry Edwards mentions a new organ found in 2018 called the interstitium, a network of fluid-filled spaces in tissue that hadn't been seen before. These fluid-filled spaces were discovered in connective tissues all over the body, including below the skin's surface; lining the digestive tract, lungs and urinary systems; and surrounding muscles, according to a new study detailing the findings.[160]

The interstitium flows like an "open, fluid-filled highway", because it contains interconnected, fluid-filled spaces that are supported by a lattice of thick collagen "bundles". This phenomenon can explain why Sound Healing can travel anywhere in the body, and therefore cannot always be felt in the particular place where you sing. The sound simply travels through the fluid-filled highways under the skin carrying energetic loads into the body. Who knows, maybe the sounds are transformed to solitons when resonating in the interstitium, and by this way stimulate our nervous system.

Research into the Relationship between the Immune System and Cancer Cells

Professor Mads Hald Andersen is employed at the Center for Cancer Immune Therapy (CCIT) at Herlev Hospital in Denmark, where he works with vaccines for cancer. Some years back he had an experience: "I had isolated a mysterious cell from the blood of a cancer patient. It did not behave like other cells of the immune system. It was very difficult to get it to divide in the laboratory, and this made it difficult to categorize. Therefore I concentrated on other tasks, but the mysterious cell has always haunted me in the back of my mind, and has appeared in my thoughts during long showers and during holidays."

Researchers have now revealed that the mysterious cell is a so-called regulatory T-cell. Its role is to shut down an attack from the immune system. Shutting down an attack is just as important as starting one, as otherwise the body can be drained of energy. So the regulatory T-cell is vital. However, it plays an unfortunate part in cancer.

Mads Hald Andersen and a group of scientists are the first in the world to discover that the regulatory T-cell has a specialized job when it comes to cancer cells. It can recognize a stress signal on the surfaces of cancer cells and go in to play the role of bodyguard for these cells. "This can be one of the reasons why a cancer cell escapes the immune system and survives," says Mads H. Andersen.

The laboratory tests have given clear indications: If the scientists mixed cancer cells with killer cells from the immune system in a Petri dish, all of the cancer cells were destroyed. If they added the regulatory T-cells to the mix, the killing of the cancer cells was impeded.

"The cells we have found are extremely powerful. They are one hundred times more powerful than other regulatory T-cells, and only 500 are required to fend off an attack from 50,000 killer cells."

Senior MD Henrik Schmidt from Aarhus University Hospital, a specialist in cancer and the immune system, agrees with this interpretation and is impressed by the results of the research group: "The trick in the future will be to encourage the heroes of the immune system and do away with its villains." Lasse Foghsgaard, *Politiken*, July 2009.

If a particular frequency can eliminate or change the stress signal that attracts the regulatory T-cells to protect the cancer cells, then there will be no more cancer. I have no doubt that the exact frequency will be able to heal cancer whether it be made mechanically, electronically[161] or vocally.

Structured Water

Dr. Gerald Pollack162 is an American scientist who has written: The Fourth Phase of Water. As the title indicates water exists not only as vapor, liquid and solid: It has a fourth phase (or face) which G. Pollack and other scientists call structured water. Our cells are formed by structured water with a jelly structure, and if we include this as water we are made of 99 percent water.

Dr. Gerald Pollack and his students have made a remarkable scientific study of water which shows that water has an exclusion zone, which appears when it meets a water-loving substance like for example air or gel. In the experiment Dr. Pollack adds particles to bulk water and shows how these particles are excluded from the zone close to the surface. The water in the exclusion zone he calls EZ water. This water shows up to be a jelly substance that gives the water a resistant power, which enables a small coin to float in a glass of water. The fact that water has this ability shows us that water by nature expels dirt and keeps a space for pure structured water, which is built up in hexagons reminiscent of a beehive structure.

The Fourth Face of Water is negatively loaded, whereas the

expelled water is positively loaded. In this way EZ water is H_3O_2 and not H_2O. When you apply light to water the exclusion zone will expand. So water is carrying and can restore electricity.

As sound carries electricity, sound must have an influence in the EZ-zone of our cells. I believe the Note from Heaven is strengthening the immune system by providing an energy, which is absorbed by the EZ-zone.

Imagine that the EZ-zone grows and the electrical level of the body rises. That fits with our temperature going up, when singing the Note from Heaven and with the fact that the interstitium could likely be in charge of distributing the vocal over- and undertones as solitons with the purpose of energizing the cells.

Postscript

In the beginning of 2017 I discovered that Vocal Sound Scanning can heal people through Skype, mobile phone or meditation, and during COVID-19 in 2020 that you can heal people from all over the world in online webinars. This is a huge discovery, which solves limits set by travelling, and can help the Note from Heaven (including self-healing with Hung Song) in reaching anyone who resonates with it. I myself concentrate on passing the knowledge of the Note from Heaven to as many people as possible. Therefore my students take clients, while I am writing books and educating Vocal Sound Therapists in the contents of this book: The Ultimate Book on Vocal Sound Healing.

In 2018 I discovered "Hung Song" as it healed my menopause symptoms including allergy to gluten from one day to the next. Hung Song is a self-healing method that I have described in two separate books: *Help* and *Heal the Pineal*. You can heal your pineal gland, kick-start a natural detox-process and rebalance your endocrine system with the help of Hung Song. This is very helpful in a world where we are surrounded by pesticides, vaccines, heavy metals, parasites and radiation.

My advice to you is that you keep your organism strong and healthy by singing the Note from Heaven, balance your endocrine system with Hung Song, walk barefoot in grass/ground, detox by daily fasting until 11am, eat and buy only organic food, drink purified energetic water and do sungazing.

Lars Muhl has created a film *The Note from Heaven* about my life and work.

This film and other films mentioned via links in this book can be found on my homepage: www.thenotefromheaven.com or can be seen at www.cosmoporta.com.

The challenges of life can be seen as the shadow of a wave of energy, which can drown you or lift you even higher up to embrace the light. It is all a matter of your choice. The Note from Heaven is a vertical power, that can lift you through the emotional clouds to see the light. It is a conversation with Spirit and this contact can give you and me just as much as we are capable to open up for. Open – open – open. That is what my Indian song teacher Mangala Tiwari said again and again:

"Open even more than you think you can. Open your voice to God, only then you will be God gifted."

Githa Ben-David, Højby, Denmark 2.02.2020

Endnotes

1. The fundamental note that a scale is based on and named after, such as C in C major. Each person has his or her own fundamental note. See page 454.
2. A sound-scanning method using the Note from Heaven is described in *The Note from Heaven* Book III, *Sound Healing*.
3. See page 34 concerning the Moon breath (Ida) and Sun breath (Pingala).
4. See Physical Exercises 12-15 (pages 103-105).
5. See Book II.
6. Regressive cell-singing is a therapeutic method I have developed and which I describe in Book II. Traumas dissipate when a person is in the state of Oneness induced by the Note from Heaven. My clients can actually sing themselves free of tensions within their cells while totally retaining their integrity.
7. This phenomenon is elaborated on pages 22-24.
8. In his 1997 book *Waking the Tiger*, trauma therapist Peter Levine describes this phenomenon as "the mouse playing dead to the cat". See Book II, page 140.
9. The soul's entrance is energetically the pineal gland. This subject is described more specifically in *Heal the Pineal – Detox with Hung Song*.
10. See page 45.
11. See page 15.
12. See page 149, Regressive Cell-Singing.
13. If you are suffering from a serious chronic illness you are recommended to read my books: Help and/or Heal the Pineal.
14. Download the practice CD free of charge: https://en.gilalai.com/the-note-from-heaven/
15. See page 39 regarding the root note.

16. See the illustration on page 118.
17. The vocal cords of a man are longer than women's cords and differ in length.
18. A shruti box is an electrical instrument that plays a drone similar to a tanpura sound in the key of your choice.
19. JAS, London.
20. See the drawing and explanation on page 118.
21. See pages 103-105, exercises 12-15, and/or the chapter on Breathing on page 32.
22. See page 262.
23. This subject is deepened in *Heal the Pineal – Detox with Hung Song*.
24. See my books *Help or Heal the Pineal – Detox with Hung Song*.
25. www.thenotefromheaven; http://githabendavid.dk/eng/pages/vocal-sound-therapists.php
26. Link to practice CD: www.gilalai.com.
27. See Book III.
28. See page 484 of Book III, *Sound Healing*.
29. The ego functions as a policeman. Anxiety activates it. However, when it is under control, the ego supports the self and is happy to do so.
30. The practice CD can be downloaded for free on the English page on www.gilalai.com.
31. On my CD *Sound in Silence* there is a sound meditation on colors, chakras and note names. *Sound in Silence* English and Danish version can be purchased at www.gilalai.com; https://en.gilalai.com/the-note-from-heaven/
32. See page 51.
33. A concept formulated by Eckhart Tolle in his book *A New Earth*.
34. A muscular reaction occurs in the heart area followed by yawning sensations.
35. See page 390, Book III.

36. See page 390.
37. See page 98 [Appendix] of *The Note from Heaven* Book I.
38. See page 90.
39. See demonstration page 33.
40. One of the participants that I stayed in touch with experienced a gradual opening up to being able to sing. She easily slipped back into the role of being tone-deaf, but she had become conscious of the illusionary character of her trauma.
41. The listener is bound by professional codes of confidentiality.
42. See page 277, Resonance with Domino Effect.
43. In the Oneness level you can activate photonic energy, which is a potential energy source flowing through the whole universe.
44. The therapist may shed tears in connection with the heart opening/yawning. This is not conventional weeping, but is a navigation sign indicating that the client is experiencing a release. See Navigation signs (page 177).
45. See Regression (page 244).
46. See page 153.
47. See *The Note from Heaven* Book III, *Sound Healing* (page 271).
48. See Navigation signs (page 177).
49. See page 171 for detailed guidance on formulating wishes.
50. See page 220.
51. A German title for a doctor trained in holistic medicine.
52. See ignoring (page 223).
53. See regression (page 244).
54. See example on page xx.
55. See shadow-singing (page 368).
56. See also *The Note from Heaven* Book I, page 87 [Part 3 under Children, Adults and Voices].
57. See page 195.
58. See changing the story (page 231).

59. See the singer's personal tool (page 239).
60. See page 231.
61. See Vocal Sound Healing in *The Note from Heaven* Book III.
62. See also page 306.
63. See Book II, Part 1, page 143.
64. A symbolic plane which provides a connection between the physical and spiritual worlds.
65. See page 132, Plus power.
66. See Emoto's film *What the Bleep Do We Know!?* and his books, such as *Messages from Water (Volumes I and II)*. Masaru Emoto died in 2014.
67. See Release of Guilt (page 255).
68. Red symbolizes a nuance in the realm of feelings. For example, it could be the ability to trust another person.
69. See *The Note from Heaven* Book III, *Sound Healing*.
70. In some cases, the singer acts as if in a trance and answers with nods and grunts. Here the listener needs to be particularly empathetic, because a deep transformation can occur. The singer's brain waves are fluctuating between beta, alpha, theta and delta frequencies, which is when the subconscious mind becomes receptive.
71. See Book III, Robert Johnson's seesaw (page 368).
72. Sound scanning is described in Book III.
73. In the Grail Meditation this kind of healing can appear. See page 464.
74. A howdah is a carriage placed atop an elephant or camel, etc.
75. A round dot (usually red) that can be painted or glued on as a blessing. It symbolizes the third eye and stands for beauty.
76. Compare to the ignored rice (page 225).
77. See page 213 for the manifestation of the energy of Jesus; also, Grail Meditation page 464, Book III.
78. This corresponds to the *ida* and *pingala* energy channels

described in *The Note from Heaven* Book I (page 14).

79. See my book *Help*.
80. The vagus nerve is activated by yawning. This nerve is playing a big role in the healing process caused by sound, see page 493, *Sound Healing* Book III.
81. Can be purchased/downloaded at www.gilalai.com.
82. This relates to my theories on the oral cavity described on page 264 (The gateway between Oneness and duality), as well as Paula Garbourg's theory on the mutual relationship of sphincter muscles (see page 229).
83. Dr. Karl learned English especially so that he could work through Graham without putting unnecessary stress on his system.
84. They call themselves The White Brotherhood – a name Graham Bishop begrudgingly divulged.
85. Further information in Book II, page 121.
86. Also mentioned in Book II page 244.
87. *Den Musiske Medisin* is not yet translated to English. It has been published in Norwegian and Danish.
88. Erik Hoffman, author of: *New Brain, New World* (Hay House).
89. See page 129.
90. See Book II page 121.
91. See Sharry Edwards page 499.
92. http://www.royal-rife-machine.com/
93. See case story, page 482.
94. See example, page 477.
95. Traditional Haka dance and singing in Australian Rugby.
96. See case story Bente (healed from terminal leukemia), page 414.
97. http://psrcentre.org/images/extraimages/41.%201211916.pdf
98. See page 491.
99. Dr. Karl is speaking on behalf of The White Brotherhood

(700 spirits) according to Graham Bishop.

100. See Hazrat Inayat Khan, page 77.

101. The direct experience of communication with the other side is creating a transformation beyond words.

102. The consequence of this must be that the magnetic field influences our general psychological and psychic condition.

103. I only listened to it three years later.

104. In case of supporting death help.

105. Later Dr. Karl mentions that if you are in doubt, the chance that it is your intuition speaking to you is about 80 percent.

106. See Book II, page 121.

107. Rudolf Steiner theory.

108. See Book II, page 177.

109. See page 425.

110. See YouTube Demonstration of Sound Scanning...

111. The chest register is the basic deeper voice which resonates primarily in the torso. The chest register gives way to the head register, where the voice by making a long slide upwards becomes thin/brittle or shifts gear.

112. See page 390.

113. Connect our soul with inspiration from above.

114. Glissando is a slide up or down the notes of a scale.

115. See page 388, Exercise III, The Great Breath.

116. See link to film Hung Song https://www.youtube.com/watch?v=O3R7w95oxqQ

117. See page 333, Book III, Part 3, Sound and Science.

118. Mentioned in page 385.

119. See link to film *Hung Song* https://www.youtube.com/watch?v=O3R7w95oxqQ

120. www.gilalai.com

121. A vocal light is the column of sound that is expressed through the healer's mouth. This imaginary column is directed to the place in the body where the healing is applied.

122. See page 229: Paula Technique, in Book II.

123. Undertones affect colic, see page 412.

124. Download is available on www.gilalai.com. Address in this link.

125. See page 400.

126. When using techniques to express undertones, you are not listening to the receiver, your intention is to perform.

127. About 80 percent of human beings can feel the undertones.

128. According to reflexology the big toes are related to the head.

129. Healing method where the left hand is raised to collect energy. See page 437.

130. See page 476, Helle Galsgård – case story.

131. See page 478 (swollen lymph node in the groin – cancer).

132. See link to film – the wife heals the pig farmer who has tinnitus (he is suicidal).

133. Sound in relation to colors will be treated in my next book.

134. See page 229, Book II.

135. The healer's name is Daniella Segal. She lives and works as a healer in Kfar Sava, Israel.

136. Interference: (wave propagation) the superposition of two or more waves resulting in a new wave pattern.

137. Frank Lorentzen is a composer, healer and works with crystal bowls.

138. I use DoTERRA oils, which are some of the purest on the market.

139. Water stimulates the process of sound healing. You can bring an organic lemon. Lemon restructures the water.

140. Some Sound Therapists and some clients prefer only to do Sound Healing.

141. See Book I, page 65: Sa Re Gha...

142. Further information can be found about this subject in my book *Heal the Pineal*.

143. See page 125, Book II.

144. See page 292.

145. www.gilalai.com link to Deep relaxation and healing song.

146. See page 499, Bioacoustics.
147. Medical Dr. J.H. Larsen is interviewed by Lars Muhl in the film, *The Note from Heaven*. Link below.
148. See the film at www.cosmoporta.com.
149. See page 263.
150. See page 477.
151. See page 325, the importance of the family's support.
152. *Rising* can be purchased as a CD/downloaded at wwwgilalai.com.
153. See page 457.
154. Hung Song (inward pointed undertones) can balance the endocrine system. This subject is described in my book *Heal the Pineal*.
155. Gerald Pollack, American professor in neurobiology, has found that our cells are built by EZ water – Exclusion Zone Water, which is also called structured water. This is further mentioned in my books: *Help* and *Heal the Pineal*.
156. Further information: *Illustreret Videnskab* nr.2/2008.
157. Elizabeth von Muggenthaler is a bioacoustician, a scientist that studies natural sound, in the air, underwater and seismically. She is president of Fauna Communications Research Institute.
158. Sources: "Naturligvis", Malene Wonsbek and "Nyt Aspekt", Annegrethe Ballegaard, 1995.
159. https://www.youtube.com/watch?v=o92nbZGEsQ4
160. Published March 27 in the journal *Scientific Reports*: https://www.nature.com/articles/s41598-018-23062-6 and also https://www.livescience.com/62128-interstitium-organ.html
161. Royal Raymond Rife invented the "Rife machine" which cured 16 out of 16 terminal cancer patients in a scientific research controlled by Medical Doctors. See *Help*.
162. See my books Heal the Pineal and Help, and Ted Talk link below.

Inspirational Film Links

Link for practice CD – The Note from Heaven:
https://en.gilalai.com/the-note-from-heaven/

"Water, The Great Mystery": Covering worldwide scientific
   research about water's amazing ability to remember:
   https://www.youtube.com/watch?v=_QEuwFOvJ9o0
Water Memory (Documentary of 2014 about Nobel Prize
   laureate Luc Montagnier):
   https://www.youtube.com/watch?v=R8VyUsVOic0&t=228s
   https://www.youtube.com/watch?v=_4HwM3rAOPU

The Fibonacci Sequence:
   https://www.youtube.com/watch?v=aB_KstBiou4

TEDx talk by Gerald Pollack about structured water:
   https://www.youtube.com/watch?v=i-T7tCMUDXU

John Stuart Reid, inventor of the Cymascope which makes
   sound visible/Cymatics:
https://vimeo.com/325628968

As It Is in Heaven, an Oscar-nominated film by the Swedish
   author and director, Kay Pollak:
https://www.youtube.com/

Bibliography

Bailey, Alice. Herkules' Arbejder (Esoterisk Center)

Becker, Annesofie (ed). At Skrive er en Kærlighedshandling (om H.C. Andersen) (Thorvaldsens Museum, 2005)

Ben-David, Githa. Lyd er Liv (Gilalai, 2011)

Ben-David, Githa. Syng dig Fri (UG, 2008)

Ben-David, Githa. Tonen fra himlen (Borgen, 2002)

Ben-David, Githa & Lars Muhl. Terapeuternes Mysterieskole (Gilalai, 2012)

Christensen, Dan Charly. Naturens Tanker, en biografi af H.C. Ørsted (Tusculanum)

Ehdin, Susanna. Det Selvhelbredende Menneske (Aschehoug, 2004)

Favrholdt, David. Filosoffen Niels Bohr (Informations Forlag, 2010)

Frankl, Victor E. Psykologi og Eksistens (Gyldendal)

Gass, Robert. Chanting: Discovering Spirit in Sound (Broadway Books, 1999)

Giversen, Søren. Thomas Evangelist (Gyldendal, 2005)

Jammer, Max. Einstein and Religion (Princeton University Press, 2002)

Johnson, Robert A. Owning Your Own Shadow (HarperOne)

Khan, Hazrat Inayat. The Mysticism of Music, Sound and Word (Banarsidass Pub.)

Khan, Hazrat Inayat. Sufi-Perler (Lemuel Books, 2011)

Levitin, Daniel. The World in Six Songs (Aurum Press)

Maman, Fabien. The Role of Music in the Twenty-First Century (Tama-do Press, 1997)

Muhl, Lars. Det Aramæiske Mysterium (Lemuel Books)

Muhl, Lars. Det Knuste Hjertes Visdom (Lemuel Books)

Myskja, Audun. Den Musiske Medisin (Norsk Forening for Musik Terapi, 2002)

Pollack, Gerald. The Fourth Phase of Water (Ebner & Sons 2013)

Ritskes, Rients and Merel Ritskes-Hoitinga. Endorfiner [Endorphins] (Bogan)

Sørensen, Emmanuel. Sunyata: En dansk mystikers liv og visdomsord (Ørnens Forlag)

www.illustreretvidenskab.dk

The Internet/Google

About the Author

Biography

Githa Ben-David was born in Juelsminde, Denmark, 23 November 1961, into an atheist family from a Protestant background. From 1985-1993 Githa went to India six times to study classical Khyal singing with Mangala Tiwari. She lived in Israel 1994-1998 working as a musician, therapist and composer. Today Githa Ben-David lives in Denmark.

Education

Trained in classical saxophone at the Royal Danish Music Conservatory.

Studied classical Khyal/Indian song in Varanasi, India, sponsored by the Danish Music Council and the Danish Royal Music Conservatory.

Educated as a healer in Mystical Therapy by Master José (from Spain) in Israel.

Educated as a regression therapist by André Corell in Copenhagen.

Musical Career

Performed with classical music, blues, oriental, jazz, experimental, African, Salsa bands and Indian inspired music, primarily in Denmark and in Israel (storytelling for kids with music). Today she performs alone or with Lars Muhl and her two sons. Songwriting and recording music is a fully integrated part of Githa Ben-David's career and life. Since a deaf person regained hearing from her singing, her main focus is Vocal Sound Therapy using "The Note from Heaven" as a fundament.

Current Work

Leader of Certified International Education in The Note from Heaven (Vocal Sound Therapy).

Runs Gilalai Institute of Energy and Consciousness (including Gilalai Publishing) with Lars Muhl.

Runs courses in Denmark and throughout Europe/ Worldwide.

Gives concerts and works as composer and author.

Internet Resources

www.thenotefromheaven.com

www.gilalai.com (courses, books, CDs, education, downloads)

https://online.gilalai.com (online courses and webinars)

www.cosmoporta.com (film page of Gilalai)

www.facebook.com/GithaBenDavid1

https://en.gilalai.com/subscribe-newsletter

Book Publications

Tonen fra himlen, Borgen 2002

Syng dig Fri, Universal Gratefulness 2008

Lyd er Liv, Gilalai 2011

Terapeuternes Mysterieskole (with Lars Muhl), Gilalai 2012

The Songs of Lars Muhl & Githa Ben-David, Gilalai 2015

Liluja (novel), Gilalai 2015

The Note from Heaven, Watkins 2016

Hjælp, Gilalai 2018

Heal the Pineal, Gilalai 2020

Help, Gilalai 2022

CD Releases

Tonen fra himlen – øve-CD i bog. Borgen 2002

The Note from Heaven, practice CD. Gilalai (download)

Rising. Ug-records 2005

Tryllesange – musisk indlæring af tabeller. Ug-Records 2007
To Heal the Space Between Us (with Lars Muhl). Gilalai 2011
Zeros (with Lars Muhl). Gilalai 2015
Sound in Silence (Danish version). Gilalai 2015
Sound in Silence (English version). Gilalai 2016
Hung Song (Danish version). Gilalai 2019 (download)
Hung Song (English version). Gilalai 2019 (download)

Books, CDs, downloads can be purchased at www.gilalai.com.
Find Practice Guidance for The Note from Heaven and Sa, Re,
Gha training in free downloads.

Practical Information

At www.thenotefromheaven.com you will find information
about The Open International Education in Vocal Sound
Healing; Sound Healers educated in the Note from Heaven and
a calendar of activities.

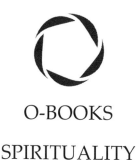

O-BOOKS

SPIRITUALITY

O is a symbol of the world, of oneness and unity; this eye represents knowledge and insight. We publish titles on general spirituality and living a spiritual life. We aim to inform and help you on your own journey in this life.

If you have enjoyed this book, why not tell other readers by posting a review on your preferred book site?

Recent bestsellers from O-Books are:

Heart of Tantric Sex
Diana Richardson
Revealing Eastern secrets of deep love and intimacy to Western couples.
Paperback: 978-1-90381-637-0 ebook: 978-1-84694-637-0

Crystal Prescriptions
The A-Z guide to over 1,200 symptoms and their healing crystals
Judy Hall
The first in the popular series of eight books, this handy little guide is packed as tight as a pill-bottle with crystal remedies for ailments.
Paperback: 978-1-90504-740-6 ebook: 978-1-84694-629-5

Take Me To Truth
Undoing the Ego
Nouk Sanchez, Tomas Vieira
The best-selling step-by-step book on shedding the Ego, using the teachings of *A Course In Miracles*.
Paperback: 978-1-84694-050-7 ebook: 978-1-84694-654-7

The 7 Myths about Love...Actually!
The Journey from your HEAD to the HEART of your SOUL
Mike George
Smashes all the myths about LOVE.
Paperback: 978-1-84694-288-4 ebook: 978-1-84694-682-0

The Holy Spirit's Interpretation of the New Testament
A Course in Understanding and Acceptance
Regina Dawn Akers
Following on from the strength of *A Course In Miracles*, NTI teaches us how to experience the love and oneness of God.
Paperback: 978-1-84694-085-9 ebook: 978-1-78099-083-5

The Message of A Course In Miracles
A translation of the Text in plain language
Elizabeth A. Cronkhite
A translation of *A Course in Miracles* into plain, everyday language for anyone seeking inner peace. The companion volume, *Practicing A Course In Miracles*, offers practical lessons and mentoring.
Paperback: 978-1-84694-319-5 ebook: 978-1-84694-642-4

Your Simple Path
Find Happiness in every step
Ian Tucker
A guide to helping us reconnect with what is really important in
our lives.
Paperback: 978-1-78279-349-6 ebook: 978-1-78279-348-9

365 Days of Wisdom
Daily Messages To Inspire You Through The Year
Dadi Janki
Daily messages which cool the mind, warm the heart and guide
you along your journey.
Paperback: 978-1-84694-863-3 ebook: 978-1-84694-864-0

Body of Wisdom
Women's Spiritual Power and How it Serves
Hilary Hart
Bringing together the dreams and experiences of women across
the world with today's most visionary spiritual teachers.
Paperback: 978-1-78099-696-7 ebook: 978-1-78099-695-0

Dying to Be Free
From Enforced Secrecy to Near Death to True Transformation
Hannah Robinson
After an unexpected accident and near-death experience, Hannah
Robinson found herself radically transforming her life, while a
remarkable new insight altered her relationship with her father, a
practising Catholic priest.
Paperback: 978-1-78535-254-6 ebook: 978-1-78535-255-3

Quantum Bliss

The Quantum Mechanics of Happiness, Abundance, and Health
George S. Mentz
Quantum Bliss is the breakthrough summary of success and
spirituality secrets that customers have been waiting for.
Paperback: 978-1-78535-203-4 ebook: 978-1-78535-204-1

The Upside Down Mountain

Mags MacKean
A must-read for anyone weary of chasing success and happiness
– one woman's inspirational journey swapping the uphill slog for
the downhill slope.
Paperback: 978-1-78535-171-6 ebook: 978-1-78535-172-3

Your Personal Tuning Fork

The Endocrine System
Deborah Bates
Discover your body's health secret, the endocrine system, and
'twang' your way to sustainable health!
Paperback: 978-1-84694-503-8 ebook: 978-1-78099-697-4

Readers of ebooks can buy or view any of these bestsellers by
clicking on the live link in the title. Most titles are published
in paperback and as an ebook. Paperbacks are available in
traditional bookshops. Both print and ebook formats are
available online.
Find more titles and sign up to our readers' newsletter at
http://www.johnhuntpublishing.com/mind-body-spirit
Follow us on Facebook at https://www.facebook.com/OBooks/
and Twitter at https://twitter.com/obooks

Printed and bound by CPI Group (UK) Ltd, Croydon, CR0 4YY

02/01/2025

01814444-0010

The concept of *The Ultimate Book on Vocal Sound Healing* is The Note from Heaven — a condition of bliss, where time disappears and the voice seems to sing you, rather than you sing the voice.

The experience of surrendering to The Note from Heaven is overwhelming and leads the singer into a state of Oneness, where present, past and future merge together and energetic patterns and traumas can be transformed and profound healings happen.

BOOK I

The Note from Heaven — How to sing yourself into contact with Oneness.

BOOK II

Regressive Cell-Singing — How to sing yourself free of traumas and change emotional programming.

BOOK III

Sound Healing — How to sound-scan a fellow being with your voice, plus a Q&A with members from the White Brotherhood.

"A very important contribution, indeed a gift, for people who want to exercise their innate power to experience wholeness."
Richard Moss, physician, author and spiritual teacher

Githa Ben-David is educated in the Royal Danish Academy of Music, has studied Indian singing, regression therapy, healing and is a recognized pioneer in Vocal Sound Therapy. She is a singer, composer, author and leader of International Education in Vocal Sound Therapy.

thenotefromheaven.com   **gilalai.com**   **cosmoporta.com**

MIND, BODY & SPIRIT
UK £28.99
US $37.95

Cover image © Adobe Stock
Cover design by Design Deluxe
www.o-books.com

US $37.95
ISBN 978-1-78904-862-9

9 781789 048629